AF449365

Macular Edema

Developments in Ophthalmology

Vol. 58

Series Editor

F. Bandello   Milan

Macular Edema

2nd, revised and extended edition

Volume Editor

Gabriel Coscas Créteil

Co-Editors

Anat Loewenstein Tel Aviv
José Cunha-Vaz Coimbra
Gisèle Soubrane Créteil, Paris

127 figures, 89 in color, and 9 tables, 2017

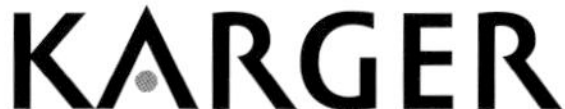

Basel · Freiburg · Paris · London · New York · Chennai · New Delhi ·
Bangkok · Beijing · Shanghai · Tokyo · Kuala Lumpur · Singapore · Sydney

Prof. Gabriel Coscas
Service Universitaire d'Ophtalmologie
Hôpital Intercommunal de Créteil
40, Avenue de Verdun
FR–94010 Créteil (France)

Library of Congress Cataloging-in-Publication Data

Names: Coscas, Gabriel, editor. | Loewenstein, Anat, editor. | Cunha-Vaz,
  José G., editor. | Soubrane, Gisèle, editor.
Title: Macular edema / volume editor, Gabriel Coscas ; co-editors, Anat Loewenstein,
  José Cunha-Vaz, Gisèle Soubrane.
Other titles: Developments in ophthalmology ; v. 58. 0250-3751
Description: 2nd, revised and extended edition. | Basel ; New York : Karger, 2017. |
  Series: Developments in ophthalmology, ISSN 0250-3751 ; vol. 58 |
  Includes bibliographical references and index.
Identifiers: LCCN 2017010160| ISBN 9783318060324 (hard cover : alk. paper) |
  ISBN 9783318060331 (e-ISBN)
Subjects: | MESH: Macular Edema
Classification: LCC RE661.M3 | NLM WW 270 | DDC 617.7/35--dc23
LC record available at https://lccn.loc.gov/2017010160

Bibliographic Indices. This publication is listed in bibliographic services, including Current Contents® and Index Medicus.

© Copyright 2017 by S. Karger AG, P.O. Box, CH–4009 Basel (Switzerland)
www.karger.com
Printed on acid-free and non-aging paper (ISO 9706)
ISSN 0250–3751
e-ISSN 1662–2790
ISBN 978–3–318–06032–4
e-ISBN 978–3–318–06033–1

Contents

List of Contributors

Isabelle Audo, Dr.
Institut de la Vision
17, rue Moreau
FR–75012 Paris (France)
Email isabelle.audo@inserm.fr

Francesco Bandello, Prof.
Department of Ophthalmology
University Vita-Salute
Scientific Institute San Raffaele
Via Olgettina 60
IT–20132 Milano (Italy)
E-Mail bandello.francesco@hsr.it

Maurizio Battaglia Parodi, Dr.
Department of Ophthalmology
University Vita-Salute
Scientific Institute San Raffaele
Via Olgettina 60
IT–20132 Milano (Italy)
E-Mail battagliaparodi.maurizio@hsr.it

Francine Behar-Cohen, Prof.
University of Lausanne
Avenue de France 15
CH–1004 Lausanne (Switzerland)
E-Mail francine.behar@gmail.com

Sébastien Bonnel, Dr.
Centre Hospitalier National d'Ophtalmologie (CHNO)
des Quinze-Vingts
28, rue de Charenton
FR–75012 Paris (France)
E-Mail sbonnel@15-20.fr

Carlo Cagini, Dr.
Section of Ophthalmology
Department of Biomedical and Surgical Sciences
S. Maria della Misericordia Hospital
University of Perugia
IT–06165 Perugia, Italy
E-Mail carlocagini@hotmail.com

Florence Coscas, Dr.
Service Universitaire d'Ophtalmologie
Hôpital Intercommunal de Créteil
40, Avenue de Verdun
FR–94010 Créteil (France)
E-Mail coscas.f@gmail.com

Gabriel Coscas, Prof.
Service Universitaire d'Ophtalmologie
Hôpital Intercommunal de Créteil
40, Avenue de Verdun
FR–94010 Créteil (France)
E-Mail gabriel.coscas@gmail.com

Catherine Creuzot-Garcher, Prof.
Service d'Ophtalmologie
Centre Hospitalier Universitaire Dijon
Boulevard Gaffarel
FR–21000 Dijon (France)
E-Mail catherine.creuzot-garcher@chu-dijon.fr

José Cunha-Vaz, Prof.
AIBILI
Azinhaga de Santa Comba
Celas
PT–3000-548 Coimbra (Portugal)
E-Mail cunhavaz@aibili.pt

Alejandra Daruich, Dr.
Department of Ophthalmology
University of Lausanne
Avenue de France 15
CH–1004 Lausanne (Switzerland)
E-Mail adaruich.matet@gmail.com

Marc D. de Smet, Prof.
MicroInvasive Ocular Surgery Center
Avenue du Léman 32
1003 Lausanne (Switzerland)
E-Mail mddesmet1@mac.com

Agnès Glacet-Bernard, Dr.
Service Universitaire d'Ophtalmologie
Hôpital Intercommunal de Créteil
40, Avenue de Verdun
FR–94010 Créteil (France)
E-Mail Agnes.Glacet@chicreteil.fr

Alessandro Invernizzi, Dr.
Eye Clinic
Department of Biomedical and
Clinical Science "Luigi Sacco"
Sacco Hospital
Via G.B. Grassi 74
IT–20157 Milan (Italy)
E-Mail alessandro.invernizzi@gmail.com

Jost B. Jonas, Prof.
Department of Ophthalmology
Faculty of Clinical Medicine Mannheim
University of Heidelberg
Theodor-Kutzer-Ufer 1–3
DE–68167 Mannheim (Germany)
E-Mail Jost.Jonas@umm.de

Baruch D. Kuppermann, Prof.
Gavin Herbert Eye Institute
University of California, Irvine
850 Health Sciences Rd.
Irvine, CA 92697 (USA)
E-Mail bdkupper@uci.edu

Paolo Lanzetta, Prof.
Department of Ophthalmology
University of Udine
Piazzale S. Maria della Misericordia
IT–33100 Udine (Italy)
E-Mail paolo.lanzetta@uniud.it

Anat Loewenstein, Prof.
Division of Ophthalmology
Tel Aviv Sourasky Medical Center
Sackler Faculty of Medicine
Tel Aviv University
6, Weizman St.
64239 Tel Aviv (Israel)
E-Mail anatl@tlvmc.gov.il

Marco Lupidi, Dr.
Department of Biomedical and Surgical Sciences
Section of Ophthalmology
University of Perugia
"S. Maria della Misericordia" Hospital
Loc. S.Andrea Delle Fratte
IT–06156 Perugia (Italy)
E-Mail dr.marco.lupidi@gmail.com

Pascale Massin, Prof.
Department of Ophthalmology
Lariboisiere Hospital
2, rue Ambroise-Paré
FR–75475 Paris Cedex 10 (France)
E-Mail p.massin@lrb.ap-hop-paris.fr

Alexandre Matet, Dr.
Department of Ophthalmology
University of Lausanne
Avenue de France 15
CH–1004 Lausanne (Switzerland)
E-Mail alexmatet@gmail.com

Francesca Menchini, Dr.
Department of Ophthalmology
University of Udine
Piazzale S. Maria della Misericordia
IT–33100 Udine (Italy)
E-Mail francescamenchini@gmail.com

Elad Moisseiev, Dr.
Division of Ophthalmology
Tel Aviv Sourasky Medical Center
Sackler Faculty of Medicine
Tel Aviv University
6, Weizman St.
64239 Tel Aviv (Israel)
Email elad_moi@netvision.net.il

Jordi Monés, Dr.
Institut de la Màcula i de la Retina
Centro Médico Teknon
Vilana 12
ES–08022 Barcelona (Spain)
E-Mail jmones@institutmacularetina.com

Sarah Mrejen, Dr.
Centre Hospitalier National d'Ophtalmologie (CHNO)
des Quinze-Vingts
28, rue de Charenton
FR–75012 Paris (France)
E-Mail smrejen@15-20.fr

Raja Narayanan, Dr.
Clinical Research
Suite 603C
L.V. Prasad Eye Institute
L.V. Prasad Marg
Banjara Hills
Hyderabad 500034 (India)
E-Mail narayanan@lvpei.org

Marco Pellegrini, Dr.
Eye Clinic
Department of Biomedical and
Clinical Science "Luigi Sacco"
Sacco Hospital
Via G.B. Grassi 74
IT–20157 Milan (Italy)
E-Mail mar.pellegrini@gmail.com

Chiara Preziosa, Dr.
Eye Clinic
Department of Biomedical and
Clinical Science "Luigi Sacco"
Sacco Hospital
Via G.B. Grassi 74
IT–20157 Milan (Italy)
E-Mail preziosachiara@gmail.com

José Sahel, Prof.
Vision Institute
Pierre et Marie Curie University
17, Rue Moreau
FR–75012 Paris (France)
E-Mail j.sahel@gmail.com

Gisèle Soubrane, Prof.
Hotel Dieu
University Paris V Centre
1, place du Parvis Notre Dame
FR–75004 Paris (France)
E-Mail soubraneg@gmail.com

Giovanni Staurenghi, Prof.
Eye Clinic
Department of Biomedical and
Clinical Science "Luigi Sacco"
Sacco Hospital
Via G.B. Grassi 74
IT–20157 Milan (Italy)
E-Mail giovanni.staurenghi@unimi.it

Daniele Veritti, Dr.
Department of Ophthalmology
University of Udine
Piazzale S. Maria della Misericordia
IT–33100 Udine (Italy)
E-Mail verittidaniele@gmail.com

Thomas J. Wolfensberger, Prof.
Jules Gonin Eye Hospital
Department of Ophthalmology
University of Lausanne
Avenue de France 15
CH–1000 Lausanne 7 (Switzerland)
E-Mail Thomas.Wolfensberger@fa2.ch

Dinah Zur, Dr.
Division of Ophthalmology
Tel Aviv Sourasky Medical Center
Sackler Faculty of Medicine
Tel Aviv University
6, Weizman St.
64239 Tel Aviv (Israel)
E-Mail dinahzur@gmail.com

Prefaces

Preface, 2nd, revised and extended edition

Cystoid macular edema is still one of the most important causes of vision decrease related to retinal vascular disease.

In recent years, many advances have been made related to the pathophysiology of macular edema (especially Müller cells). These have been made possible mainly due to remarkable modern imaging, particularly optical coherence tomography (OCT) techniques and new approaches, including "en face" OCT and OCT angiography.

Moreover, treatment approaches have been considerably improved with the use of anti-VEGF and anti-inflammatory drugs that allow flattening of the retina without lasers and their irreversible scars, as well as avoiding additional surgery, but including prolonged long-term follow-up and recurrent treatment.

Gabriel Coscas, 2017

Preface, 1st edition

Macular edema has for a long time been one of the most important issues in retinal pathologies, as damage to the macula has an immediate effect on central visual acuity and may substantially affect a patient's quality of life.

For more than 40 years, clinicians have attempted to identify macular edema in its initial state and to define its various etiologies. Diagnosing macular edema with certitude at an early stage has proven difficult despite the progress in contact lens biomicroscopy.

Fluorescein angiography has been critical for detecting macular edema and currently remains the 'gold standard' for the diagnosis, identifying the characteristic stellar pattern of cystoid macular edema. Fluorescein angiography also provides a qualitative assessment of vascular leakage, which is essential for identifying treatable lesions. However, it is only since the use of laser photocoagulation that it became possible to offer an effective modality of treatment for macular edema, despite the destructive localized laser scars.

During the last decade, the clinical diagnosis of macular edema and its treatment have been greatly improved due to multiple and remarkable advances of modern imaging technologies, which allow recognition of the main etiologies of this complication. By correlating results from fluorescein angiography, optical coherence tomography, and especially spectral domain optical coherence tomography, fluid accumulation within and under the sensory retina can be confirmed and located. This fluid accumulation, frequently associated with subretinal fluid and serous retinal detachment, may not otherwise be clinically detected.

Moreover, spectral domain optical coherence tomography can characterize the presence and integrity of the external limiting membrane and the photoreceptor inner and outer segments, which is useful information for prognosis as well as a guide for treatment. The diagnosis of macular edema and its clinical forms is now based primarily on the correlation of these imaging techniques.

One of the most important innovations in the field of macular edema has been the advent of intravitreal drug delivery approaches for the treatment of posterior segment pathologies. These emerging modalities treat posterior eye disease or restore the permeability of the blood-retinal barrier by delivering drug compounds either systemically, locally, or intravitreally with anti-inflammatory or anti-vascular endothelial growth factor drugs.

Multicenter controlled clinical trials testing these new compounds as well as biologic delivery systems and treatment strategies have already been completed or are currently under way. From this research, the care of macular edema will soon be more efficient and effective due to increased target specificity, noninvasive drug administration routes, and sustained-release compounds that will allow sufficient levels of therapeutic efficacy for longer durations.

Macular Edema: A Practical Approach describes the different patterns and etiologies of macular edema and the importance of preserving the photoreceptors at the early stage in order to retain central visual acuity. The book was designed to bring together the most recent data and evidence-based medicine while also including the multiple areas still unknown and debated.

Macular Edema: A Practical Approach presents the pathophysiological basis of macular edema and the different approaches of drug delivery to the posterior segment. Recommendations for treatment procedures or different therapies have been carefully analyzed and considered prior to inclusion.

The authors bring their personal experience and full teaching acumen to each chapter, culminating in a single book that brings to the forefront the importance of macular edema.

Macular Edema: A Practical Approach provides the ophthalmologist with a synthesis of knowledge to diagnose, determines the etiology, and offers viable treatment options for the benefit of all our patients.

Gabriel Coscas, 2010

Chapter 1

Coscas G (ed): Macular Edema. 2nd, revised and extended edition.
Dev Ophthalmol. Basel, Karger, 2017, vol 58, pp 1–10 (DOI: 10.1159/000455264)

Macular Edema: Definition and Basic Concepts

Gabriel Coscas[a] · José Cunha-Vaz[b] · Gisèle Soubrane[a]

[a]Service Universitaire d'Ophtalmologie, Hôpital Intercommunal de Créteil, Créteil, France; [b]AIBILI, Coimbra, Portugal

Abstract

Macular edema is the result of an accumulation of fluid in the retinal layers around the fovea. It contributes to vision loss by altering the functional cell relationship in the retina and promoting an inflammatory reparative response. Macular edema may be intracellular or extracellular. Intracellular accumulation of fluid, also called cytotoxic edema, is an alteration of the cellular ionic distribution. Extracellular accumulation of fluid, which is more frequent and clinically more relevant, is directly associated with an alteration of the blood-retinal barrier (BRB). The following parameters are relevant for clinical evaluation of macular edema: extent of the macular edema (i.e., the area that shows increased retinal thickness); distribution of the edema in the macular area (i.e., focal versus diffuse macular edema); central foveal involvement (central area 500 µm); fluorescein leakage (evidence of alteration of the BRB or 'open barrier') and intraretinal cysts; signs of ischemia (broken perifoveolar capillary arcade and/or areas of capillary closure); presence or absence of vitreous traction; increase in retinal thickness and cysts in the retina (inner or outer), and chronicity of the edema (i.e., time elapsed since initial diagnosis and response to therapy). It is essential to establish associations and correlations of all the different images obtained, regardless of whether the same or different modalities are used.

Macular edema is the result of an accumulation of fluid in the retinal layers around the fovea. It contributes to vision loss by altering the functional cell relationship in the retina and promoting an inflammatory reparative response.

Macular edema is a *nonspecific sign of ocular disease* and not a specific entity. It should be viewed as a special and clinically relevant type of macular response to an altered retinal environment. In most cases, it is associated with an alteration of the blood-retinal barrier (BRB).

Macular edema may occur in a wide variety of ocular situations including uveitis, trauma, intraocular surgery, vascular retinopathies, vitreoretinal adhesions, hereditary dystrophies, diabetes, and age-related macular degeneration.

The *histopathological picture* of this condition is an accumulation of fluid in the outer plexiform (Henle's) and inner nuclear and plexiform layers of the retina (fig. 1). The increase in water content of the retinal tissue characterizing macular edema may be *intracellular* or *extracellular*. Intracellular accumulation of fluid, also called cytotoxic edema, is an alteration of the cellular ionic distribution. Extracellular accu-

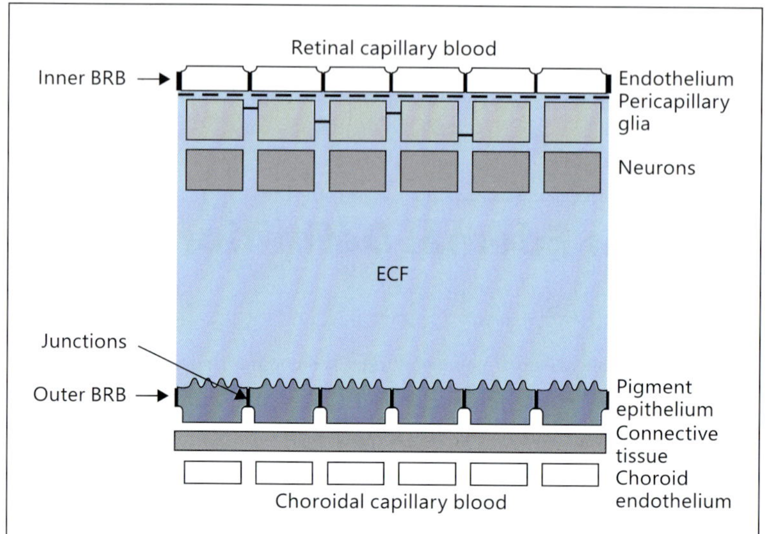

Fig. 1. Schematic presentation of the inner and outer BRBs and their relative location. ECF = Extracellular fluid.

mulation of fluid, which is more frequent and clinically more relevant, is directly associated with an alteration of the BRB.

Intracellular Edema

Intracellular edema in the retina may occur when there is an intact BRB and the retinal cells are swollen due to an alteration of the cellular ionic distribution, resulting in excessive accumulation of sodium ions (Na^+) inside the cells.

This is known as cytotoxic edema. It may be the immediate result of ischemia, trauma, or toxic cell damage.

Extracellular Edema

Extracellular edema is directly associated with an open BRB (i.e., it is caused by a breakdown of the inner or outer BRB). The increase in tissue volume is due to an increase in the retinal extracellular space.

Breakdown of the BRB is identified by *fluorescein leakage*, which can be detected in a clinical environment by fluorescein angiography (FA) or vitreous fluorometry measurements. Starling's law[a], which governs the movements of fluids, applies in this type of edema (Cunha-Vaz and Travassos, 1984)[1].

---

[a] Starling's law: In extracellular edema, the 'force' driving water across the capillary wall is the result of a hydrostatic pressure difference (ΔP) and an effective osmotic pressure difference ($\Delta \pi$). The equation regulating fluid movements across the BRB is: driving force $= L_p[(P_{plasma} - P_{tissue}) - \sigma(\pi_{plasma} - \pi_{tissue})]$, where L_p is the membrane permeability of the BRB; σ is an osmotic reflection coefficient; P_{plasma} is blood pressure, and P_{tissue} is the retinal tissue osmotic pressure. An increase in ΔP, contributing to retinal edema, may be due to an increase in P_{plasma} and/or a decrease in P_{tissue}. An increase in P_{plasma} due to increased systemic blood pressure contributes to retinal edema formation only after loss of autoregulation of retinal blood flow and alteration of the characteristics of the BRB. A decrease in P_{tissue} is an important component that has previously not been given sufficient attention. Any loss in the cohesiveness of the retinal tissue due to pathologies, such as cyst formation, vitreous traction, or pulling at the inner limiting membrane, will lead to a decrease in P_{tissue}. A decrease in P_{tissue} (i.e., increased retinal tissue compliance) may lead to fluid accumulation, edema formation, and an increase in retinal thickness. A decrease in $\Delta \pi$ contributing to retinal edema may occur due to increased protein accumulation in the retina after breakdown of the BRB. Extravasation of proteins will draw more water into the retina. This is the main factor provoking a decrease in $\Delta \pi$, as a reduction in plasma osmolarity high enough to contribute to edema formation is an extremely rare event.

After a breakdown of the BRB, the progression of retinal edema depends directly on the hydrostatic pressure difference (ΔP) and osmotic pressure difference ($\Delta \pi$) gradients. In these conditions, tissue compliance becomes more important, directly influencing the rate of edema progression. Thus, in the presence of retinal edema, it is essential to recognize whether the edema has arisen due to an intact or open BRB.

BRB breakdown leading to macular edema may be mediated by locally released cytokines, and it induces an inflammatory reparative response creating the conditions for further release of cytokines and growth factors. The BRB cells, retinal endothelial cells, and retinal pigment epithelium (RPE) cells are both the target and producer of eicosanoids, growth factors, and cytokines.

Macular edema is one of the most serious consequences of inflammation in the retinal tissue. Inflammatory cells can alter the permeability of the tight junctions that maintain the inner and outer BRB. Cell migration may occur primarily through splitting of the junctional complexes or through the formation of channels or pores across the junctional complexes.

Clinical Evaluation of Macular Edema

The clinical evaluation of macular edema has been difficult to characterize, but evaluation has become more precise with the help of modern imaging such as FA and optical coherence tomography (OCT).

The following parameters are relevant for clinical evaluation of macular edema: extent of the macular edema (i.e., the area that shows increased retinal thickness); distribution of the edema in the macular area (i.e., focal versus diffuse macular edema); central fovea involvement (central area 500 µm); fluorescein leakage (evidence of alteration of BRB or 'open barrier') and intraretinal cysts; signs of ischemia (broken perifoveolar capillary arcade and/or areas of capillary closure); presence or absence of vitreous traction; increase in retinal thickness and cysts in the retina (inner or outer), and chronicity of the edema (i.e., time elapsed since first diagnosis and response to therapy).

Direct and Indirect Ophthalmoscopy
Direct and indirect ophthalmoscopy may show only an alteration of the foveal reflexes. Slit lamp biomicroscopy and stereoscopic fundus photography have played an important role in demonstrating changes in retinal volume in the macular area, but they are dependent on the observer's experience, and the results do not offer a reproducible measurement of the volume change (Gonzalez et al., 1995)[2].

The Early Treatment Diabetic Retinopathy Study specified the following characteristics as indicating clinically significant macular edema: (1) thickening of the retina (as seen by slit lamp biomicroscopy or stereoscopic fundus photography) at or within 500 µm of the center of the macula; (2) hard exudates at or within 500 µm of the center of the macula associated with thickening of the adjacent retina (but not residual hard exudates remaining after disappearance of retinal thickening), and (3) a zone or zones of retinal thickening 1 disk in area or larger in size, any part of which is within 1 disk diameter of the center of the macula. This definition of macular edema specifically takes into consideration the involvement of the center of the macula and its relationship to visual loss.

Fluorescein Angiography
FA documents if there is fluorescein leakage, which in turn determines whether a barrier is classified as open or intact. Clinical use of FA has contributed significantly to the present understanding of retinal disease, and it is considered the 'gold standard'.

The dye used in FA is sodium fluorescein, a small molecule that diffuses freely through the

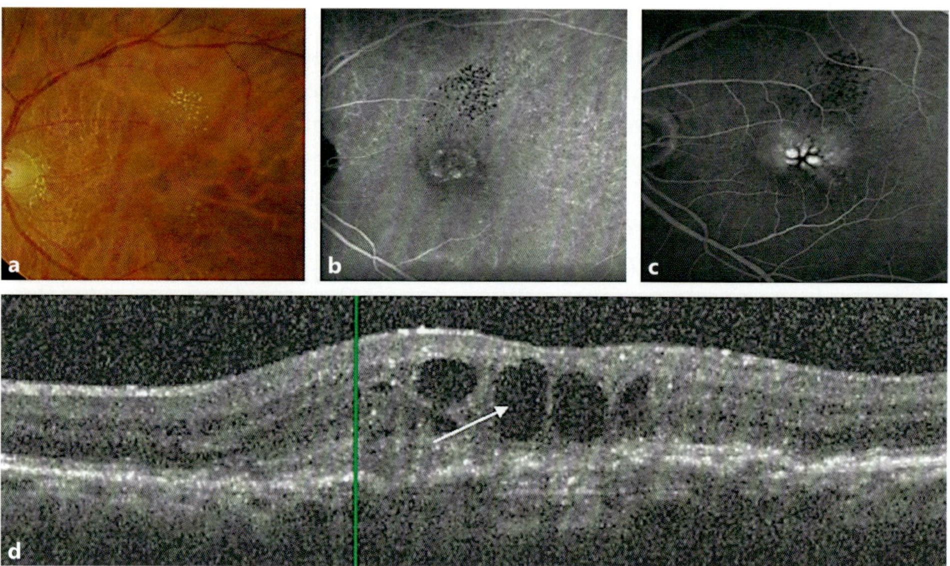

Fig. 2. Cystoid macular edema. **a** Color photo. **b, c** FA (early and late stage); capillary dilation and leakage; fluorescein dye pools in cystoid spaces located in the outer plexiform layer (Henle's layer) and arranged radially from the fovea. **d** Spectral domain OCT (Spectralis): typical image of cystoid spaces. OCT imaging allows precise analysis of large cystoid spaces, and their location, the extent of an area of increased thickness, and the extent of the involvement of the central macula are essential in determining the presence of macular edema. Moreover, the analysis of the outer retinal layers could give valuable prognostic indications.

choriocapillaris and Bruch's membrane but does not diffuse through the tight junctions of the retinal endothelial cells and the RPE, which are the inner and outer BRBs. Understanding these barriers is the key to understanding and interpreting a fluorescein angiogram (Cunha-Vaz and Travassos, 1984)[1].

FA also fundamentally contributes to our understanding of vascular retinopathy. FA will help for the identification of areas of capillary leakage and/or capillary closure or capillary dropout. Capillary closure and fluorescein leakage were first clinically identified with FA, and they are accepted as the determinant alterations occurring in the diabetic retina, retinal vein occlusion, and other retinal vasculopathies identifying the progression of retinopathy (Kohner and Henkind,1970; Coscas and Dhermy, 1978)[3, 4].

Intravenous injection of sodium fluorescein is generally safe and easy to perform. It is routinely used in ophthalmological clinics despite severe anaphylactic reactions that may occur on rare occasions (1 in 200,000) (Yannuzzi et al., 1986)[5].

The noncystoid form of macular edema is characterized by diffuse abnormal permeability of the retinal capillary bed with diffuse leakage and intraretinal fluid accumulation that has not accumulated in cystoid spaces but may still do so in the later course of the disease. It is displayed as a diffusely outlined and ill-delimited area of hyperfluorescence.

In cystoid macular edema, early capillary dilation and leakage can be detected. In the late phase of the angiogram, fluorescein pools in cystoid spaces located in the outer plexiform layer (Henle's layer) displayed as the classic petaloid stain-

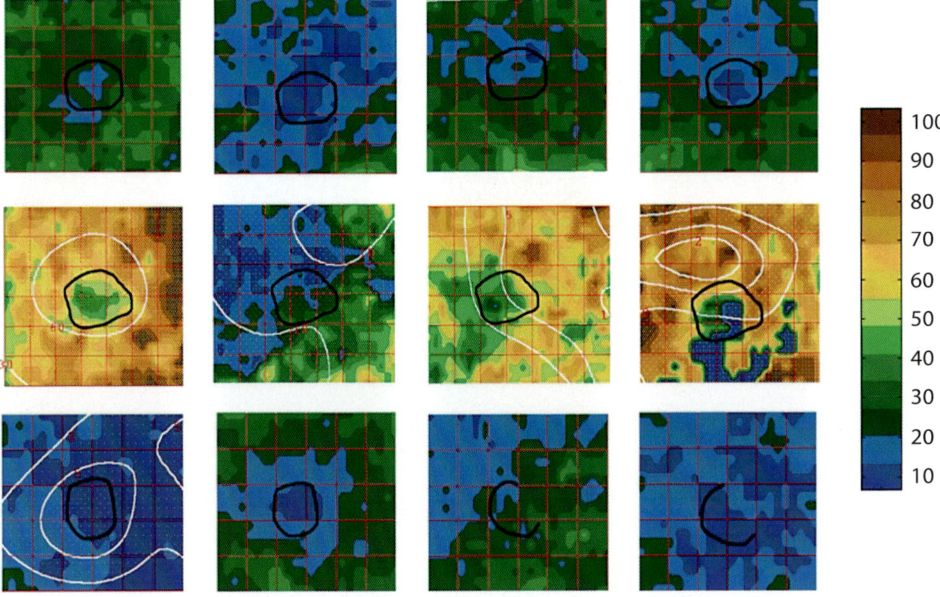

Fig. 3. Multimodal images from 3 patients (rows 1, 2, and 3) from visits 0, 12, 24, and 36 months showing the foveal avascular zone contour, retinal leakage analyzer results, and retinal thickness analyzer results. The retinal leakage analyzer color-coded maps of the BRB permeability indexes are shown. Retinal thickness analyzer views show white dot density maps of the percentage increases in retinal thickness. Patterns a, b, and c are shown on rows 1, 2, and 3, respectively.

ing pattern (Guyer et al., 1999)[6]. These cystoid spaces are usually arranged radially from the fovea (fig. 2). In long-standing cystoid macular edema, the cystoid spaces enlarge and may merge, representing irreversible damage of the retina.

The extent of dye leakage alone does not completely correlate with functional damage and visual acuity. Duration of the edema and associated changes (RPE photoreceptor and neuroglial damage) must also be taken into account.

Fundus imaging using *indocyanine green dye*, particularly with the scanning laser, may provide additional direct signs for macular edema but also for the precise analysis of RPE alterations and for the detection and delimitation of cystoid spaces progressively filled with the dye. Analogous to the Rosetta Stone, the key to interpretation is correlation of the data acquired from the different imaging systems.

Optical Coherence Tomography
OCT provides images of retinal structures that could not previously be obtained by any other noninvasive, noncontact, transpupillary diagnostic method. OCT allows assessment and detection of subretinal and intraretinal fluid related to changes in the inner and outer BRBs and abnormal exudation from the retinal capillary bed.

OCT provides anteroposterior images by measuring the echo time and intensity of reflected or backscattered light from intraretinal microstructures. These anteroposterior 2-dimensional or B-scan images (analogous to those of ultrasound) were demonstrated for the first time in 1991 by Huang et al. (1991)[7] and in the human retina in 1993 by Fercher et al. (1993)[8] and Swanson et al. (1993)[9]. These optical scans are based on the principle of low-coherence light interferometry (Puliafito et al., 1995; Schuman et al., 2004)[10, 11].

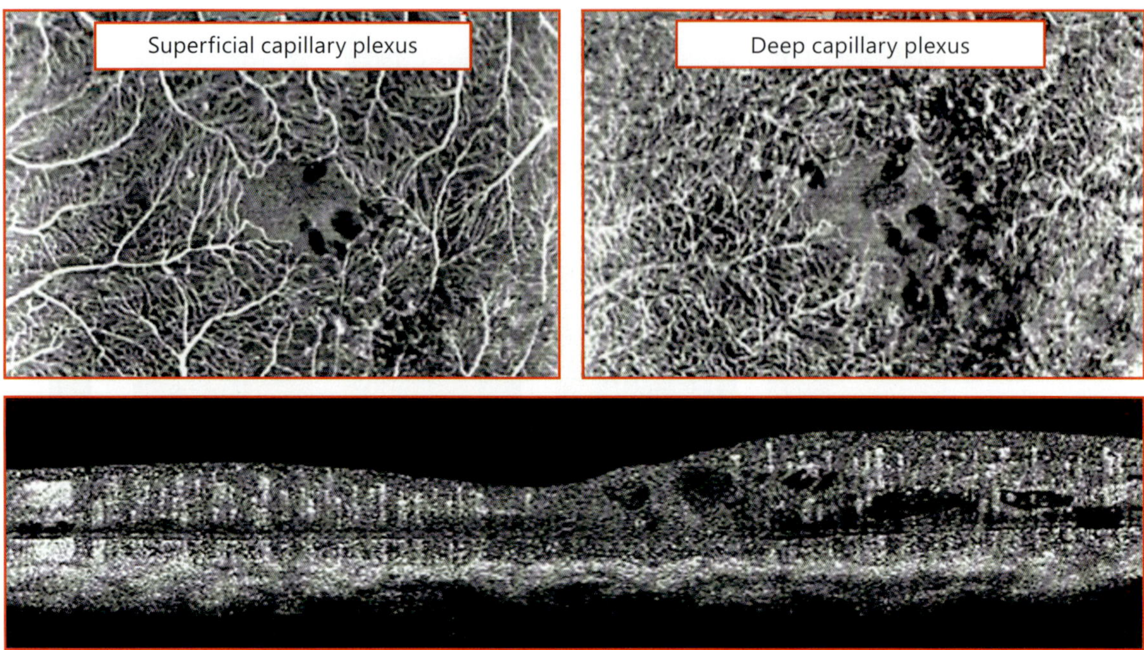

Fig. 4. Comprehensive assessment of a DME patient on OCT angiography. The imaging approach includes a C-scan at the ganglion cell layer (**a**), a C-scan at the inner nuclear layer (**b**), and a corresponding B-scan (**c**). **a** C-scan section taken at the level of the ganglion cell layer *(superficial capillary plexus),* The enlargement of the foveal avascular zone is associated with focal capillary dilations and small areas of capillary nonperfusion. The presence of large, roundish, hypointense lesions (dark black*)* are due to cystoid spaces in the perifoveal area. Smaller cystoid lesions are also visible in the extrafoveal area. **b** C-scan at the inner nuclear layer *(deep capillary plexus)*. A diffuse reduction of the vascularity is visible coupled with an enlargement of the foveal avascular zone, focal capillary dilations, and areas of capillary nonperfusion. Numerous hypointense (dark black) lesions *(cystoid spaces)* are appreciable in macular area. **c** Corresponding B-scan passing through the foveal depression. The hyperintense structures that are visible at the level of the inner retinal layers are referred to transverse sections of retinal capillaries. It is difficult to visualize the eventual vascular abnormalities with the cross-sectional OCT (B-scan), but it is highly useful to evaluate the morphofunctional correlation with the corresponding structural B-scan (Coscas et al., 2016)[19].

Schematically, in time domain OCT, the light beam emitted by a super luminescent diode is split into two beams by a beam splitter: an incident beam enters the ocular media and is reflected by the various layers of the fundus, while the other beam is reflected by a reference mirror. Displacement of the mirror placed on the path of the reference light beam allows analysis of structures situated at various depths during each light echo acquisition, forming an A-scan. The time necessary for this scanning and for the acquisition of these sections is the essential determinant of the quality of the signal, hence the name time domain OCT.

Spectral domain OCT, a method based on the famous Fourier transform mathematical equation (1807), eliminates the need for a moving mirror in the path of the reference beam, which allows for much more rapid image acquisition and provides excellent resolution (axial resolution of <10 μm). This property enables spectral domain OCT systems to capture a large number of high-resolution images: 50 times faster than standard time domain OCT and 100 times faster than the

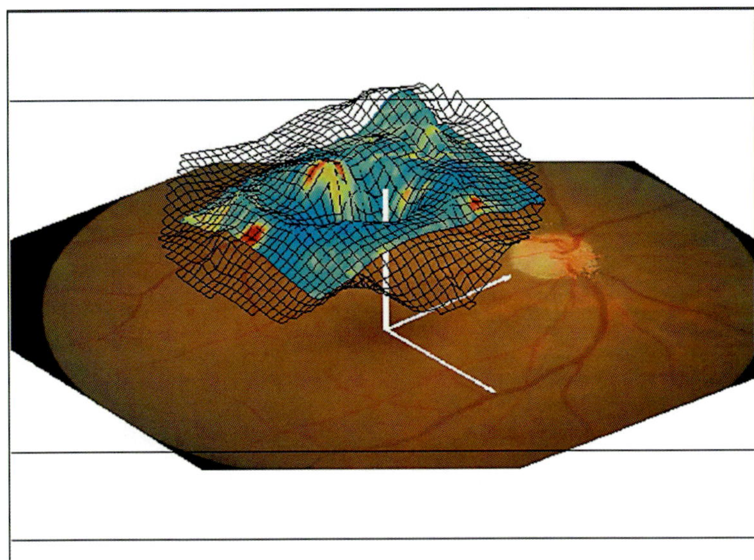

Fig. 5. The same information presented in figure 2 is now shown 3-dimensionally. The differences in the information presented are significant. Although the shape of the thickness is now clear, it occurs at the expense of having fewer details on the leakage itself and the location of both the thickness and leakage within the macular area.

first ultrahigh-resolution OCT. As the examination can be performed simultaneously in various planes, real high-speed 3-dimensional reconstructions can be obtained with hundreds of images per second.

Rapid scanning allows an increased number and density of scans of the retina to be obtained in a very short time, with a marked reduction of artifacts related to patient movements (eye and respiratory movements) during the examination. The use of image processing systems based on *real-time averaging* reduces the signal-to-noise ratio and increases image definition and image quality.

OCT has rapidly become a noninvasive optical imaging modality for medical diagnosis in ophthalmology, allowing in vivo visualization of the internal microstructures of the retina on these sections and evaluation of variations of *retinal thickness*. Images are obtained in 2 or 3 dimensions and represent variations of these reflections (and backscatter) of light either in a plane of section or in a volume of tissue. This anteroposterior dimension of OCT provides a spectacular complement to angiographic data.

OCT scans can visualize exudative reactions with fluid accumulation (intraretinal and/or subretinal). Comparative quantitative evaluation of these images during the course of the disease is particularly useful. OCT may allow discovery at a stage often difficult to assess by other imaging methods, considerably enhancing the ability to diagnose and follow macular edema.

After the introduction of new spectral domain OCT instruments, studies were published comparing retinal thickness measurements. These studies demonstrated that retinal thickness measurements are dependent on the segmentation of the inner and outer retinal borders. The new spectral domain OCT systems image the outer retinal layers as 3 hyperreflective bands: the external limiting membrane, the junction (or interface) of the photoreceptor outer and inner segments, and the RPE.

The *outer layers of the retina* can now be analyzed due to these recent technological progresses allowing high-definition, high-speed volume imaging. This allows analysis of structural changes particularly affecting photoreceptors and the IS/

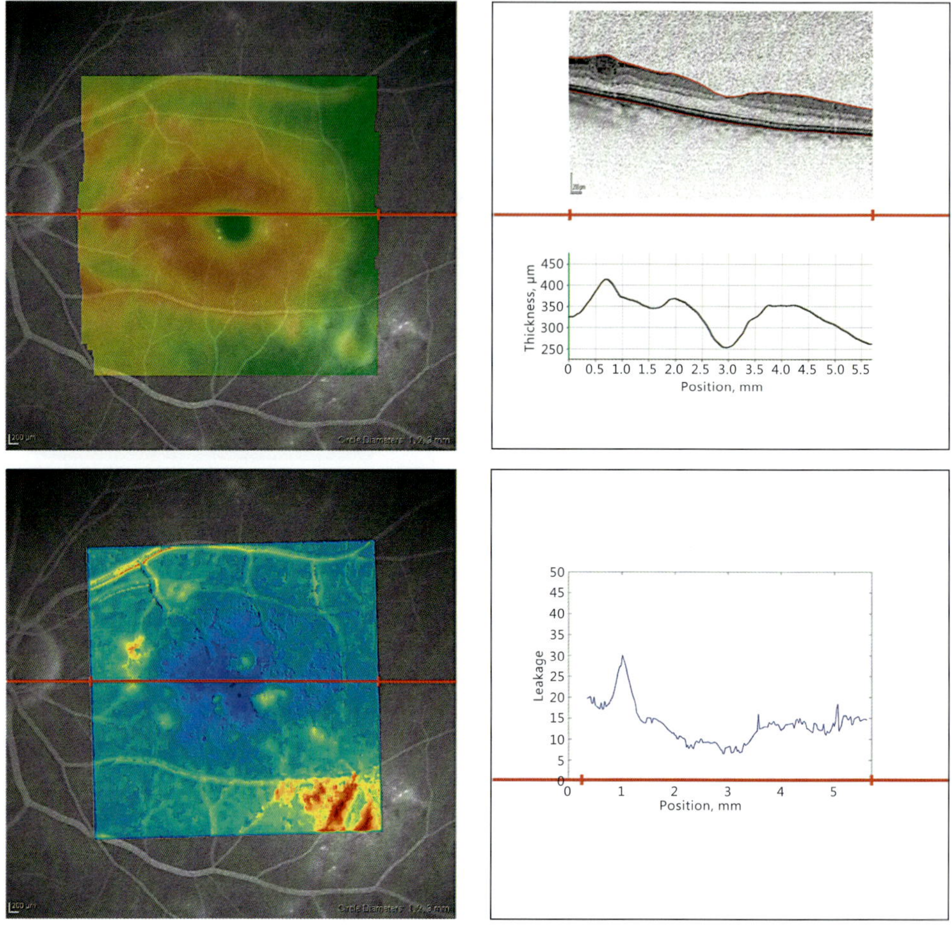

Fig. 6. This new approach on the representation of a multimodal imaging system integrates the fundus reference (left column), the color-coded thickness, and leakage maps (left column, top and bottom rows, respectively). A selected location (marked as a red horizontal line on the left column images) allows choosing the location where details are to be shown on the right. On the top right image, the detailed structure of the retina and the respective thickness profile is shown. On the bottom right image, the plotted profile of the leakage information for the same location is shown, allowing correlation of the structure, thickness, and leakage at the local level.

OS interface, thereby providing functional information on these tissues. The possibility of integrated structural imaging and functional imaging will play an increasingly important role in clinical applications (Coscas, 2009)[12].

Real-time images of the microscopic retinal tissues have been termed 'optical biopsy' and closely reflect histological sections of the macula and fovea.

Increasingly, they resemble a real anatomical representation, especially with the development of ultrahigh-resolution techniques and the upcoming combination with adaptive optics (Soubrane, 2009)[13].

In macular edema, the process begins with diffuse swelling of the outer retinal layers, advancing to the typical image of cystoid spaces. Later, the large cystoid spaces can extend from the RPE to the internal limiting membrane and even rupture, causing macular holes. Hence, OCT is becoming a very efficient tool for following the distribution, evolution, and location of macular edema. The extent of an area of increased thickness and the involvement of the central macula are essential to describe a clinical case of macular edema and predict visual loss. The presence of cysts and vitreous traction are particularly well documented using OCT. The analysis of the outer retinal layers may provide valuable prognostic indications (fig. 2).

OCT angiography (OCTA) is a transformative approach for imaging ocular vessels based on flow rather than simple reflectance intensity. It is therefore a functional extension of OCT that can be used to visualize microvascularization by detecting motion contrast from flowing blood. The resultant image looks like an angiogram but is derived only from signals intrinsically generated from tissue, without the need for contrast agent injection (Coscas et al., 2016)[14].

A key advantage of OCT angiography over traditional FA is that it provides depth-resolved functional information of blood flow in vessels. In comparison, FA provides only a bidimensional image that simplifies all of the perfused layers of the retinal and choroidal blood vessels.

Finally, OCT-Leakage is a new method of analysis of OCT data which uses a novel algorithm to identify the location of the sites of lower optical reflectivity performing automated analysis and mapping of the retinal extracellular space, i.e., extracellular fluid (Cunha-Vaz et al., 2016)[15]. OCT-Leakage permits the identification, location, and mapping of areas of fluid accumulation, and allows their correlation with sites of BRB breakdown and changes in retinal thickness.

Location and quantification of retinal edema by OCT-Leakage is expected to complement OCT angiography.

To *establish a correlation between different images*, either from the same or from different modalities, it is essential to associate and to correlate them all. Multimodal macula mapping, for example, uses a variety of diagnostic tools and techniques to obtain additional information (fig. 3–6) (Lobo et al., 2004; Bernardes et al., 2002; Cunha-Vaz, 2006)[16–18].

Spectral domain OCT facilitates correlations with clinical data, angiographies, and functional investigations.

These imaging techniques are essential to guide the indications for current treatment and to assess the response to treatment.

References

1 Cunha-Vaz JG, Travassos A: Breakdown of the blood-retinal barriers and cystoid macular edema. Surv Ophthalmol 1984; 28:485–492.

2 Gonzalez ME, Gonzalez C, Stern MP, Arredondo B, Martinez S; Mexico City Diabetes Study Retinopathy Group: Concordance in diagnosis of diabetic retinopathy by fundus photography between retina specialists and a standardized reading center. Arch Med Res 1995; 26:127–131.

3 Kohner EM, Henkind P: Correlation of fluorescein angiogram and retinal digest in diabetic retinopathy. Am J Ophthalmol 1970;69:403–414.

4 Coscas G, DhermyP: Occlusions veineuses rétiniennes. Rapport Société Française d'Ophtalmologie. Paris, Masson, 1978.

5 Yannuzzi LA, Rohrer KJ, Tinder LJ, et al: Fluorescein angiography complications survey. Ophthalmology 1986;93,611–617.

6 Guyer D, Yannuzzi LA, Chang S, Shields JA, Green WR: Retina-Vitreous-Macula, ed 1. Philadelphia, Saunders, 1999.

7 Huang D, Swanson E, Lin C, et al: Optical coherence tomography. Science 1991;254:1178–1181.

8 Fercher AF, Hitzenberger CK, Drexler W, et al: In vivo optical coherence tomography. Am J Ophthalmol 1993;116:113–114.

9 Swanson EA, Izatt JA, Hee MR, et al: In vivo retinal imaging by optical coherence tomography. Opt Lett 1993;18:1864–1866.

10 Puliafito CA, Hee MR, Lin CP, et al: Imaging of macular diseases with optical coherence tomography. Ophthalmology 1995;102:217–229.

11 Schuman JS, Puliafito CA, Fujimoto JG: Optical Coherence Tomography of Ocular Diseases, ed 2. Thorofare, SLACK Inc., 2004.

12 Coscas G: Optical Coherence Tomography in Age-Related Macular Degeneration, ed 2. Berlin, Springer, 2009.

13 Soubrane G: Personal communication, unpublished data. 2009.

14 Coscas G, Lupidi M, Coscas F: Optical Coherence Tomography Angiography in Healthy Subjects in OCT Angiography in Retinal and Macular Diseases. Dev Ophthalmol 2016;56:37–44.

15 Cunha-Vaz J, Santos T, Ribeiro L, Alves D, Marques I, Goldberg M: OCT-Leakage. A new method to identify and locate abnormal fluid accumulation in diabetic retinal edema. Invest Ophthalmol Vis Sci 2016;57:6776–6783.

16 Lobo CL, Bernardes RC, Figueira JP, de Abreu JR, Cunha-Vaz JG: Three-year follow-up study of blood-retinal barrier and retinal thickness alterations in patients with type 2 diabetes mellitus and mild non proliferative diabetic retinopathy. Arch Ophthalmol 2004;122:211–217.

17 Bernardes R, Lobo C, Cunha-Vaz JG: Multimodal macula mapping: a new approach to study diseases of the macula. Surv Ophthalmol 2002;47:580–589.

18 Cunha-Vaz JG: Clinical characterization of diabetic macular edema. Int Ophthalmol 2006;1:99–100.

19 Coscas G, Lupidi M, Coscas F: Atlas of Oct-Angiography in Diabetic Maculopathy. Paris, L'Européenne d'Edition, 2016, p 150.

Prof. Gabriel Coscas
Service Universitaire d'Ophtalmologie
Hôpital Intercommunal de Créteil
40, Avenue de Verdun
FR–94010 Créteil (France)
E-Mail gabriel.coscas@gmail.com

Coscas G (ed): Macular Edema. 2nd, revised and extended edition.
Dev Ophthalmol. Basel, Karger, 2017, vol 58, pp 11–20 (DOI: 10.1159/000455265)

Mechanisms of Retinal Fluid Accumulation and Blood-Retinal Barrier Breakdown

José Cunha-Vaz

AIBILI – Association for Innovation and Biomedical Research on Light and Image, Azinhaga de Santa Comba, Celas, Coimbra, Portugal

Abstract

Macular edema is the swelling of the central portion of the human retina and it is associated with increased retinal thickness. It can be simply defined as an excess of fluid within the retinal tissue. It must be realized that the normal retina possesses a functional extracellular space. With regard to the extracellular volume of the retina, there have been few physiologic studies, but there are reported values of 24.8% for the cerebrum and 23.6% for the cerebellum. It is accepted that the retinal extracellular space is similar to the brain. It is generally agreed that the proximate cause of macular edema and retinal fluid accumulation is a breakdown of the blood-retinal barrier (BRB). When there is a breakdown of the BRB, retinal edema can be interpreted in terms of basic principles of capillary filtration (Starling's law). Therefore, the main factors influencing retinal edema formation are BRB permeability, capillary hydrostatic pressure, tissue hydrostatic pressure, tissue osmotic pressure, and plasma osmotic pressure. Active transport by the retinal pigment epithelium is necessary to remove water that percolates through the retina from intraocular pressure and is also as a safety mechanism against fluid accumulation in disease. Clinical evaluation of the BRB and retinal edema can be performed noninvasively by using an OCT-based method designated OCT-Leakage, which is capable of identifying and quantifying sites of alteration of the BRB, and by mapping sites of low optical reflectivity, i.e., changes in the retinal extracellular fluid.

© 2017 S. Karger AG, Basel

Macular edema is the swelling of the central portion of the human retina and is, therefore, associated with increased retinal thickness. It can be simply defined as an excess of fluid within the retinal tissue (Henkind et al., 1980)[1].

In order to understand the mechanisms of retinal edema it is necessary to consider data from many sources including anatomy, physiology, pathology, and clinical ophthalmology, as well as information obtained when dealing with the parallel situation in the brain.

Like in the brain, free leakage of fluid and protein from the retinal blood vessels is prevented by the blood-retinal barrier (BRB), which in the retina is located at the retinal vessels and retinal pigment epithelium (RPE). Thus, the interstitial spaces of the retina are normally relatively dry. There may a slow percolation of water into the retina from intraocular pressure, but without solutes it is not retained and active transport across the RPE removes this water as fast as it gets through (Marmor, 1999)[2].

It must be realized that a normal retina possess a functional extracellular space. Smelser and Ishikawa (1965)[3] injected thorotrast particles into the vitreous humor of cats and were able to detect its presence within 6 h throughout the retinal extracellular space, between the internal and external limiting membranes. They concluded that the intercellular space in the retina is available for diffusion of even particulate matter and that such clefts are important for retinal nutrition and could potentially play a role in pathological processes.

With regard to the extracellular volume of the retina, there have been few physiologic studies although there have been numerous studies conducted in brain tissue of various species. In a major review of the subject, Cheek and Holt (1978)[4] concluded that the distribution of chloride gave the most accurate assessment of the brain extracellular space. They reported values of 24.8% in the cerebrum and 23.6% in the cerebellum of adult rhesus monkeys. It is, therefore, accepted that the retinal extracellular space, like in the brain, is a system of interconnected pathways of varying dimensions and present throughout the retinal tissue.

There is, in the retina, a situation of restricted permeability between the blood and retina, which is called the BRB and is comparable to the blood-brain barrier (Cunha-Vaz et al., 1975)[5].

The BRB is located at two levels, retinal vessels and chorioretinal interface, the former designated as the inner BRB and the latter as the outer BRB. The main structures involved are the endothelial cells of the retinal vessels for the inner BRB and the RPE for the outer BRB. Both of these membranes function as 'epithelial-like' structures because they have zonulae occludentes, i.e., tight junctions of the 'non-leaky' type.

It is generally agreed that the most frequent proximate cause of macular edema associated with any systemic or ocular disease or drug is a breakdown of the inner BRB. Although the contents of the vascular lumina can reach the extravascular space by transcellular mechanisms directly through the endothelial cell cytoplasm, most data available indicate that the most frequent pathologic mechanism is the breakdown of the interendothelial junctional complexes (Cunha-Vaz and Shakib, 1967)[6]. The accumulation of fluid in edema may be extracellular, intracellular, or a combination of both. In the retina, we may follow the classification proposed by Klatzo (1967)[7] for brain edema.

Cytotoxic edemas are those in which the primary lesion is initiated in the cells, neurons, or glia. Intracellular swelling of the retina may occur primarily in certain intoxications and in hypoxic/ischemic damage, where breakdown of the BRB is a secondary event (Parikh et al., 2016)[8]. Vasogenic edemas, by far the most frequent, are those in which the primary defect is in the BRB, leading to abnormal accumulation of extracellular fluid. In this situation a secondary cellular response may occur in an effort to deal with the excess fluid in the extracellular space. Müller cells and aquaporin 4 channels may indeed be involved in the reabsorption of the abnormal fluid entering the retina due to alterations of the BRB.

Understanding Retinal Edema Based on Starling's Law for Capillary Filtration

When there is a breakdown of the BRB in vasogenic edema, it is possible to interpret retinal edema in terms of basic principles of capillary filtration. In 1896, Starling suggested originally that edema occurs in a tissue when the rate of capillary filtration exceeds the rate of fluid removal from the perivascular interstitium. Lymphatics remove fluid from peripheral tissues, but fluid from retinal capillaries must percolate through the retina to reach the vitreous or return into the circulation.

We proposed in 1984 how Starling's law could be applied to the retina (Cunha-Vaz and Travassos, 1984)[9]. The 'force' driving water across the capillary wall is the result of a hydrostatic pressure difference ΔP and an effective osmotic pressure difference $\sigma \Delta \pi$. This equation is, therefore:

$$(\text{flow}) = Lp \, [P^{plasma} - P^{tissue} - \sigma(\pi^{plasma} - \pi^{tissue})]$$

where Lp is the hydraulic conductivity or 'membrane permeability' and σ is an osmotic reflection coefficient.

Retinal capillaries are different from most other peripheral capillaries, being almost impermeable to proteins, electrolytes, and water-soluble nonelectrolytes. The capillaries are lined by continuous endothelial cells with tight junctions, across which each of these solutes exerts a full effective osmotic pressure.

At a first approximation, protein osmotic pressure equals zero in the retinal tissue because protein is negligible in the vitreous and retinal extracellular space. Normally, capillary hydrostatic and protein osmotic pressures dominate the force term in the equation. π^{plasma} is 25 mm Hg higher than π^{tissue} because of protein osmotic pressure. P^{plasma} can be estimated by assuming that arteriolar resistance reduces carotid artery pressure from 65 mm Hg by about 50%. If P^{plasma} = 30 mm Hg, the driving force for filtration is less than 5 mm Hg, depending on the value of P^{tissue}.

Edema develops when fluid accumulates within the retina so as to increase retinal volume. The rate of fluid accumulation depends on a fundamental factor, retinal compliance, and is more rapid in a compliant tissue than in tissue that resists deformation when P^{tissue} rises.

Breakdown of the Blood-Retinal Barrier and Macular Edema

The main factors influencing retinal edema formation are:

1 *BRB permeability.* An increase in BRB permeability is induced by direct damage to the retinal vessel wall and/or to the choroid-RPE complex. Another mechanism is loss of autoregulation of blood flow. Increased permeability is reflected in the equation above as an increase in hydraulic conductivity and a fall in σ, both effects of increasing BRB filtration.

2 *Capillary hydrostatic pressure.* An increase in systemic blood pressure does not normally produce retinal edema because autoregulation of blood flow prevents capillary hypertension, dilatation, and breakdown of the barrier. However, edema often develops when autoregulation is overcome. Disease and loss of autoregulation leads to abnormal BRB permeability, allowing a full direct effect of systemic blood pressure on fluid accumulation in the retina (fig. 1).

3 *Tissue hydrostatic pressure.* This term counterbalances the capillary pressure and is altered in a situation of edema. In this situation there is more fluid between the cells, less tissue, and increased tissue compliance. Increased tissue compliance allows easier fluid accumulation to occur in situations of increased extracellular space (fig. 2) and when there is vitreoretinal traction (fig. 3). A normal low retinal compliance in the closed eye could prevent measurable retinal edema in response to small increases in BRB filtration. The concept of retinal compliance may have particular importance and should be well understood. Low compliance of a tissue represents its resistance to deformation and accumulation of fluid within its limits. The retina has closely interwoven cellular processes, many junctions between the glial cells, and reduced extracellular space. The Müller cells form a relatively rigid framework that holds together the remaining retinal tissue. It is this skeleton that must yield as a result of tissue damage or breakdown of the BRB, resulting in edema and thickening of the retina. In a situation of breakdown of the BRB, the

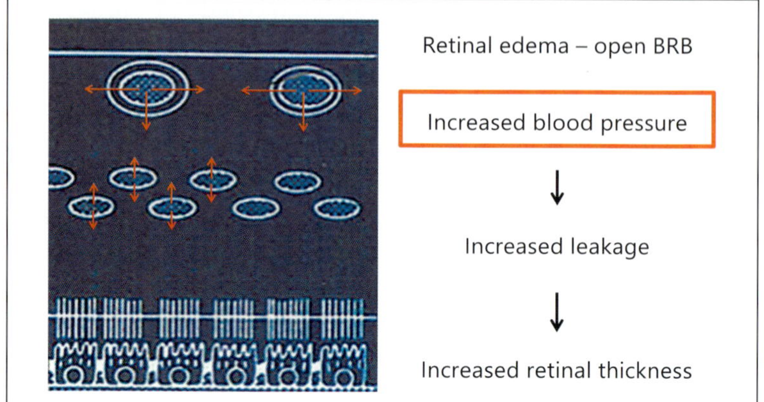

Fig. 1. Schematic drawing of the retina indication how increased blood pressure may play a role in retinal edema when there is an alteration of the inner BRB.

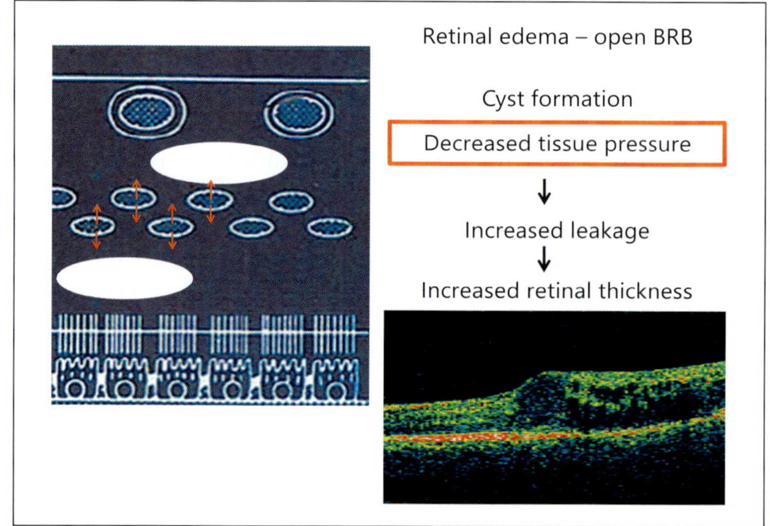

Fig. 2. Schematic drawing of the retina in a situation of retinal edema where decreased tissue pressure and increased compliance play a major role in the abnormal fluid accumulation.

accumulation of fluid in the retina increases its compliance, creating conditions for lower tissue resistance and further accumulation of fluid.

4 *Tissue osmotic pressure.* Assuming that protein in the vitreous equals that in the retinal extracellular space, protein osmotic pressure in the retina is close to zero. Barrier opening allows proteins to enter the retina, contributing to edema formation. Tissue osmotic pressure may also increase as a result of an increase in nonproteic solutes such as tissue lactate or products of cell cytolysis. This elevation of tissue osmotic pressure is a major contributor to increased capillary filtration and abnormal accumulation of fluid in the retina (fig. 4).

5 *Plasma osmotic pressure.* In the brain, for edema to develop it is necessary to have a rapid reduction of 35 mOsmols in plasma osmolarity. The threshold for edema formation in the retina may reflect the low compliance of the retinal tissue within the closed eye.

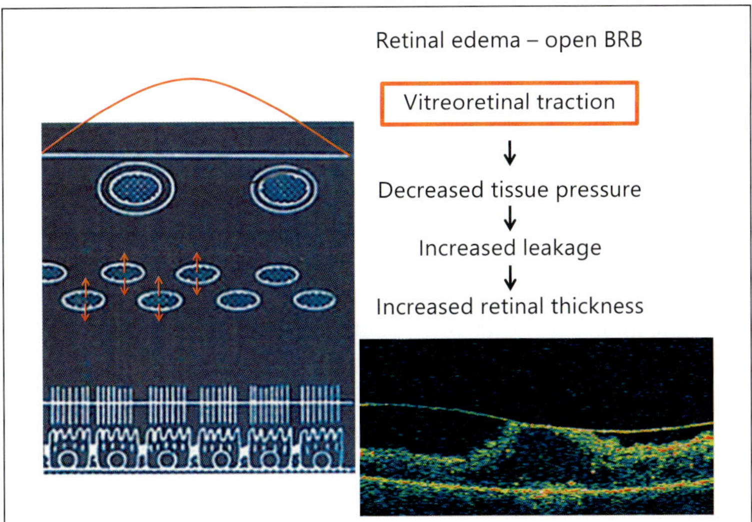

Fig. 3. Schematic drawing of the retina in a situation of retinal edema where vitreoretinal traction contributes to decreased tissue pressure and abnormal collection of fluid in the retina.

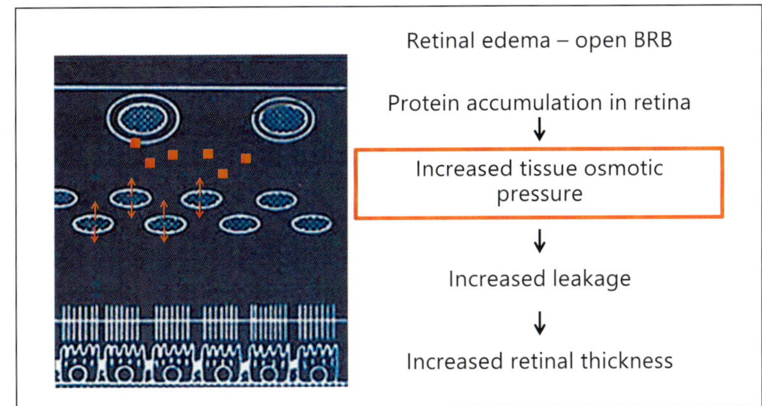

Fig. 4. Schematic drawing of the retina in a situation of retinal edema indication how abnormal protein accumulation may contribute to increased tissue osmotic pressure and fluid accumulation.

In summary, retinal edema can develop when the rate of capillary filtration exceeds the rate of fluid transport out of the retina. Accumulation of edema fluid depends mainly on tissue compliance and changes in tissue osmotic pressure.

Anatomic Considerations and Protein Movement

Although the tight junctions of the retinal endothelial cells and the RPE are the main barriers protecting and modulating the microenvironment of the retinal cells, other structural features of the retina function as relative barriers to water and protein movement and are relevant to the formation of edema.

The retinal extracellular space as a whole limits the free flow of water to the degree at which water leaves the eye across the RPE (Fatt and Shantinath, 1971)[10]. The normal RPE is capable of pumping a lot more water per minute than what actually leaves the eye under normal conditions (Marmor, 1998)[11] because water cannot exit through the retina any faster. The internal limiting membrane consists only of matrix material and condensed vitreous collagen, and is probably not a significant impediment to water or solute movement (Hogan et al., 1971)[12]. The intercellular pathway from the vitreous to subretinal space is convoluted and ends with a band of zonulae adherentes that form the external limiting membrane (ELM). The zonulae adherentes of the ELM are not as tight as the zonulae occludentes of the inner and outer BRB, but they limit particularly the movement of large molecules, i.e., larger than albumin. The rate of albumin movement across the retina is substantial, accounting for 4–5% of the concentration difference across the retina per hour (Takeuchi et al., 1995)[13].

These observations have relevant implications for retinal edema. Large molecules do not diffuse freely and are blocked partially by the ELM. Thus, protein that is released within the retina will tend to remain for a period of time and will tend to back up behind the ELM. To the extent that protein is retained, water will also be retained osmotically and contribute to the maintenance of retinal edema.

Absorptive Forces

In a normal eye, both passive and active forces work to move water across the retina and out of the subretinal space. First, intraocular pressure is continuously pushing water into the retina. Second, choroidal osmotic pressure draws water towards the choroid. The two forces are strong enough to keep the retina in place and the subretinal space dry without the intervention of active RPE transport (Marmor, 1999)[2].

Active transport across the RPE is needed mainly because of the requirement for a protein-free neural environment which dictates that the BRB on the RPE side is necessary for the RPE tight junctions to impede the passive absorption of fluid. Active transport is necessary to remove water that percolates through the retina from intraocular pressure and perhaps also as a safety mechanism against fluid accumulation in disease.

Therefore, it is likely, that almost any retinal disorder which involves metabolic dysfunction or choroidal vascular insufficiency will alter RPE transport to some degree. A diffuse diminution of RPE transport may explain why subretinal fluid accumulates and persists in a disease such as central serous chorioretinopathy, where there is only a small focal source of fluid entry (Marmor, 1997)[14].

Role of Proteins and Osmotic Pressure in Driving Retinal Edema

It is important to ask how extracellular fluid can accumulate in a thin tissue such as the retina with no barriers against water escaping into the vitreous. One of the answers must be the abnormal presence of proteins. In diseases with a breakdown of the BRB, albumin and other proteins will be forced by blood pressure and diffusion gradients into the extracellular space of the retina. At the internal limiting membrane, the protein will leave the retina freely but at the ELM, protein will tend to back up, creating a localized increase in oncotic pressure, bind water, and create conditions for retinal edema. Accumulation of fluid will be greater near the sites of leakage (layers where the retinal vessels are located) and at sites of protein build-up (ELM). The active transport located at the RPE, on the other hand, is able to transport water counteracting the protein effect.

Studies using methods to analyze retinal thickness have shown a relatively poor correlation, in some situations, between fluorescein leakage and retinal thickness. Some sites of fluorescein leakage lead to little fluid accumulation and thickness, whereas other sites of alteration of the BRB evidenced by fluorescein leakage are associated with situations of great and prolonged fluid accumulation. The degree of alteration of the BRB allowing less or more protein leakage into the retina may be the relevant factor.

Clinical Evaluation of the Blood-Retinal Barrier

Fluorescein angiography (FA) permits a dynamic evaluation of extracellular fluid changes resulting from retinal circulatory disturbances. FA was the first method to demonstrate in a clinical setting the sites of fluorescein leakage, indicating the location of the alteration of the BRB. Its reproducibility depends, however, on the variable quality of the angiography.

With the development of vitreous fluorometry, a method that was developed to quantify fluorescein leakage, a large number of clinical and experimental studies demonstrated the major role played by alterations of the BRB as a posterior segment disease (Strauss, 2005)[15]. More recently, confocal retinal leakage mapping was introduced to identify the sites of BRB breakdown. However, all of these methods require an intravenous injection of fluorescein, which can cause nausea, vomiting, and (rarely) anaphylaxis (Yannuzzi et al., 1986)[16].

An OCT-based method has been recently described by our group, designated OCT-Leakage, which is capable of noninvasively identifying and quantifying sites of alteration of the BRB by mapping sites of lower-than-normal optical reflectivity, thus reflecting the changes in retinal extracellular fluid. Extracellular fluid distribution in the retina is represented on OCT by the distribution of sites of lower-than-normal optical reflectivity. Increases or decreases in extracellular fluid distribution of a given area of the retina can, therefore, be measured by the ratio of sites of low optical reflectivity (LOR) identified in the area under evaluation (fig. 5, 6).

OCT-Leakage, using a proprietary algorithm to identify the sites of lower-than-normal optical reflectivity, reliably locates and quantifies increases in extracellular space in retinal disease showing that changes in the retinal extracellular space correlate well with the occurrence and degree of retinal edema (Cunha-Vaz et al., 2016)[17].

A coregistration procedure allows the mapping of fluorescein leakage locations identified in the FA image onto the OCT data, so that locations of OCT LOR and leakage can be compared (fig. 1, 2). There is good correspondence between the location of increased LOR area ratios and sites of fluorescein leakage in FA. The changes in extracellular space, represented by the LOR area ratio, corresponded well with the main sites of leakage on FA (fig. 2). Similar correlations were found for all eyes with nonproliferative diabetic retinopathy and other retinal diseases examined by FA and the OCT-Leakage method.

It is to be noted that the LOR ratios identify the main sites of leakage and also the areas of late leakage shown in FA. Furthermore, in OCT-Leakage the areas of abnormal fluid accumulation can be identified in specific retinal layers, demonstrating different involvement in different eyes of the different retinal layers. Note that similar degrees of fluorescein leakage are associated with different degrees of extracellular fluid accumulation, supporting the view that the amount of extracellular fluid and its spread to the different retinal layers will be a better indicator of the severity of the BRB breakdown.

Conclusions

Retinal edema develops not only because there is protein and fluid entering the extracellular space, but probably because the retinal stroma and the ELM limit the clearance of large osmotically active molecules. These molecules bind water osmotically and cause edema.

Most diseases causing macular edema involve a degree of damage to both the inner and outer BRB. OCT-Leakage is expected to help identify fluid movement in the retina and contribute to a better understanding of retinal edema.

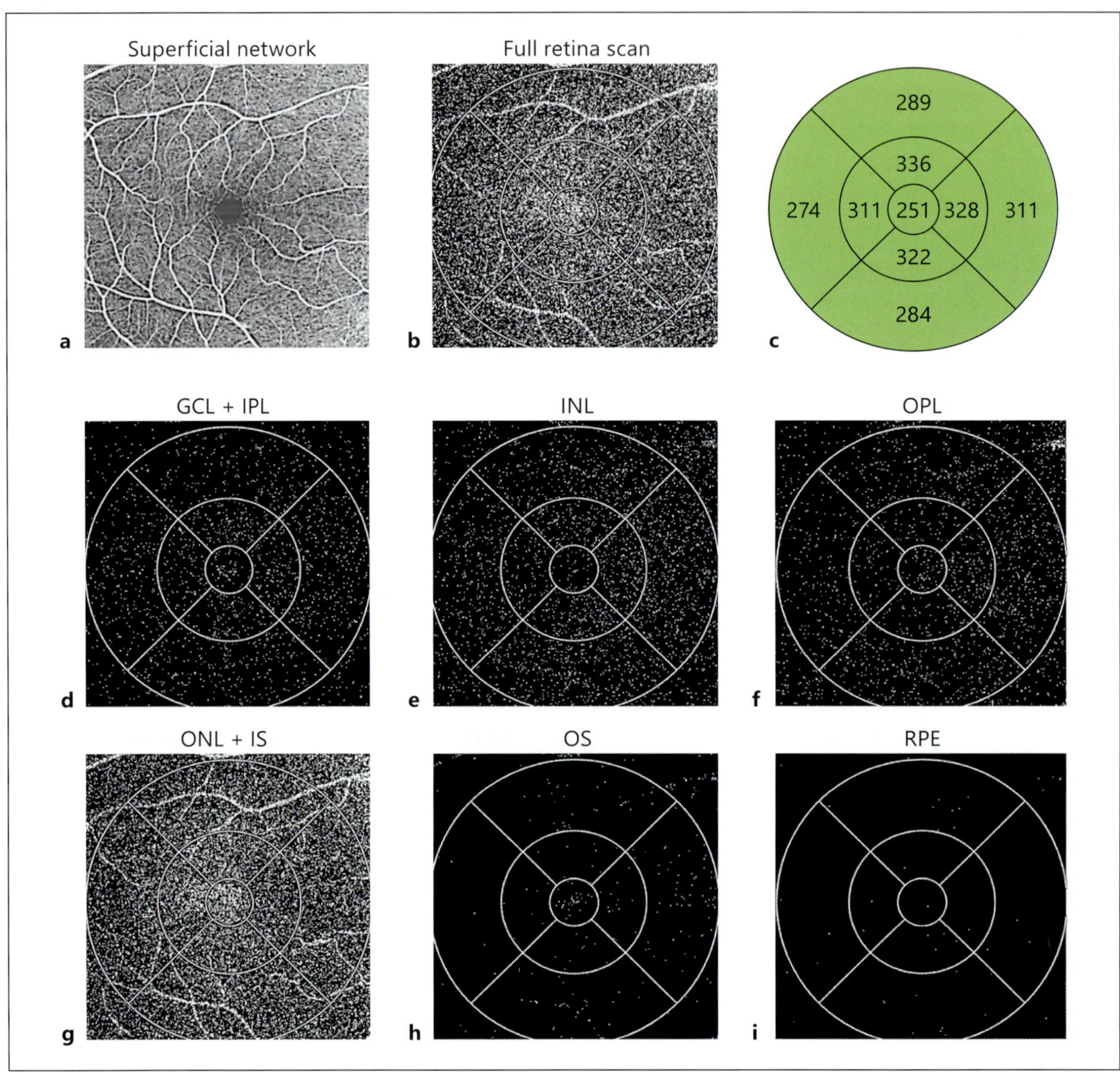

Fig. 5. OCT-Leakage maps for the right eye of a healthy subject for the full retina scan and for each of the segmented retinal layers. **a** Superficial vascular network acquired by the AngioPlex system. **b** Full retina scan LOR map. **c** ETDRS grid of the retinal thickness obtained by the Cirrus 5000. **d–i** LOR maps layer by layer for the GCL+IPL, INL, OPL, ONL+IS, OS, and RPE, respectively. Locations of LOR are identified in white. The ETDRS grid is centered at the fovea. GCL = Ganglion cell layer; IPL = inner plexiform layer; INL = inner nuclear layer; OPL = outer plexiform layer; ONL = outer nuclear layer; IS = inner segment; OS = outer segment.

Finally, any therapeutic strategy for retinal edema needs to address the BRB breakdown in order to impede fluid and protein leakage into the retina, and take into consideration the structural changes in the retina associated with spe- cific involvement of the different retinal layers that condition protein and water movement out of the retina and the fluid absorptive transport of water at the RPE.

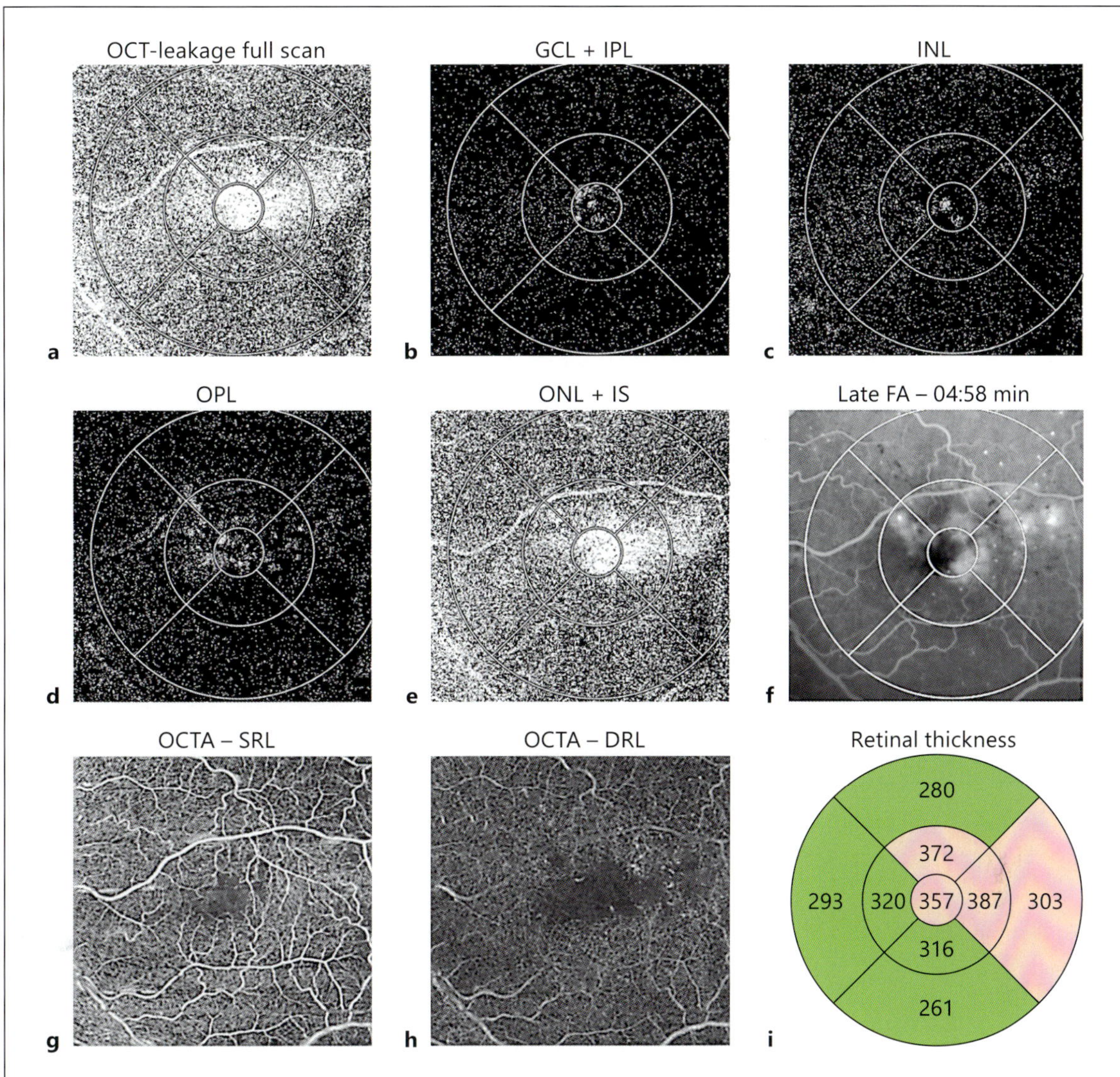

Fig. 6. Eye with diabetic macular edema and evidence of localized leakage on FA, corresponding well with the increase in extracellular space detected in the OCT-Leakage maps of the full retina scan and different retinal layers (GCL+IPL, INL, OPL and ONL+IS) and vascular abnormalities of the deep retinal vascular layer. **a–e** OCT-Leakage maps of the different retinal layers showing different levels of involvement but corresponding to fluorescein leakage detected in the FA. **f** FA showing the localization of the fluorescein leakage. **g** OCTA superficial retinal vascular layer. **h** OCTA deep retinal layer showing microaneurysms and other vascular changes in the same location of the increased extracellular space (OCT-Leakage maps) and fluorescein leakage (FA). **i** OCT thickness map showing the zone of increased retinal thickness. GCL = Ganglion cell layer; IPL = inner plexiform layer; INL = inner nuclear layer; OPL = outer plexiform layer; ONL = outer nuclear layer; IS = inner segment; OCTA = optical coherence tomography angiography; SRL = superficial retinal vascular layer; DRL = deep retinal layer.

References

1 Henkind P, Bellhorn R, Schall B: Retinal edema: postulated mechanism(s); in Cunha-Vaz J (ed): The Blood-Retinal Barriers. Boston, Springer US, 1980, pp 251–268.

2 Marmor MF: Mechanisms of fluid accumulation in retinal edema. Doc Ophthalmol 1999;97:239–249.

3 Smelser GK, Ishikawa T PY: Electron Microscopic Studies of Intra-retinal Spaces: Diffusion of Particulate Materials; in JW R (ed): The Structure of the Eye. Stuttgart, Schattauer, 1965, p 109.

4 Cheek DB, Holt AB: A review: extracellular volume in the brain – the relevance of the chloride space. Pediatr Res 1978; 12:635–645.

5 Cunha-Vaz J, Faria de Abreu JR, Campos AJ: Early breakdown of the blood-retinal barrier in diabetes. Br J Ophthalmol 1975;59:649–656.

6 Cunha-Vaz JG, Shakib M: Ultrastructural mechanisms of breakdown of the blood-retina barrier. J Pathol Bacteriol 1967;93:645–652.

7 Klatzo I: Presidental address. Neuropathological aspects of brain edema. J Neuropathol Exp Neurol 1967;26:1–14.

8 Parikh VS, Modi YS, Au A, Ehlers JP, Srivastava SK, Schachat AP, Singh RP: Nonleaking cystoid macular edema as a presentation of hydroxychloroquine retinal toxicity. Ophthalmology 2016; 123:664–666.

9 Cunha-Vaz JG, Travassos A: Breakdown of the blood-retinal barriers and cystoid macular edema. Surv Ophthalmol 1984; 28(suppl):485–492.

10 Fatt I, Shantinath K: Flow conductivity of retina and its role in retinal adhesion. Exp Eye Res 1971;12:218–226.

11 Marmor MF: Control of subretinal fluid and mechanisms of serous detachment; in Marmor MF, Wolfensberger TJ (eds): The Retinal Pigment Epithelium: Current Aspects of Function and Disease. New York, Oxford University Press, 1998, pp 420–438.

12 Hogan M, Alvarado J, Weddell J: Histology of the Human Eye. Philadelphia, WB Saunders, 1971, pp 488–490.

13 Takeuchi A, Kricorian G, Marmor MF: Albumin movement out of the subretinal space after experimental retinal detachment. Invest Ophthalmol Vis Sci 1995;36:1298–1305.

14 Marmor M: On the cause of serous detachments and acute central serous chorioretinopathy. Br J Ophthalmol 1997; 81:812–813.

15 Strauss O: The retinal pigment epithelium in visual function. Physiol Rev 2005;85:845–881.

16 Yannuzzi LA, Rohrer KT, Tindel LJ, Sobel RS, Costanza MA, Shields W, Zang E: Fluorescein angiography complication survey. Ophthalmology 1986;93: 611–617.

17 Cunha-Vaz J, Santos T, Ribeiro L, Alves D, Marques I, Goldberg M: OCT-Leakage. A new method to identify and locate abnormal fluid accumulation in diabetic retinal edema. Invest Ophthalmol Vis Sci 2016;57:6776–6783.

José Cunha-Vaz
AIBILI – Association for Innovation and Biomedical Research on Light and Image
Azinhaga de Santa Comba, Celas
PT–3000-548 Coimbra (Portugal)
E-Mail cunhavaz@aibili.pt

Chapter 3

Coscas G (ed): Macular Edema. 2nd, revised and extended edition.
Dev Ophthalmol. Basel, Karger, 2017, vol 58, pp 21–26 (DOI: 10.1159/000455266)

Intracellular Edema

Raja Narayanan[a] · Baruch D. Kuppermann[b]

[a] Smt Kanuri Santhamma Vitreoretina Center, L.V. Prasad Eye Institute, Hyderabad, India; [b] Gavin Herbert Eye Institute, University of California, Irvine, Irvine, CA, USA

Abstract

The macula is predisposed to edema in various retinal conditions, even when the insult is remote from the macula. The various factors that may predispose the macula to edema include high metabolic activity, radial arrangement of the Henle's layer, lack of inner layers at the fovea, and lack of blood supply at the fovea. The edema is most pronounced in the outer plexiform layer (Henle's layer). Alteration in the blood-retinal barrier and ischemia cause disturbances in vascular permeability as well as with the function of Müller cells. K+ ions and aquaporin-4 play an important role in maintaining the dryness of the macula in physiological conditions. Intracellular edema of Müller cells contributes significantly to macular edema. Steroids and anti-VEGF agents reduce intracellular edema, apart from extracellular edema. Therapeutic targets for improving Müller cell function could play a key role in the development of new molecules.

© 2017 S. Karger AG, Basel

Macular edema is the accumulation of fluid in the outer plexiform layer (Henle's layer) and the inner nuclear layer at the macula (fig. 1), along with intracellular edema of Müller cells. Macular edema is the final common pathway for the decrease in vision in many conditions, such as age-related macular degeneration, diabetic retinopathy, reti-nal vein occlusion, and uveitis. Damage to the blood-retinal barrier formed by intercellular junctions results in macular edema.

The macula is predisposed to edema even though the insult may not be directly at the macula, such as in anterior uveitis, peripheral vasculitis, or vein occlusion. The various factors that may predispose the macula to edema include high metabolic activity, radial arrangement of the Henle's layer, lack of inner layers at the fovea, and lack of blood supply at the fovea. Cystoid macular edema (CME) is typically seen as radially oriented cysts, centered on the fovea, and is best appreciated clinically by slit-lamp biomicroscopy. The central fluid is more prominent in Henle's layer. A petaloid appearance due to leakage from the retinal vessels as seen during fluorescein angiography is a classic feature of CME. This chapter deals with the intracellular mechanisms of CME.

Pathogenesis of Cystoid Macular Edema

Macular edema occurs due to leakage of proteins through capillaries, either due to damage to endothelial cells or following an ischemic event (Marmor, 1999; Bringmann et al., 2004; Coscas et al., 2010; Finkelstein, 1992; Scholl et al., 2010)[1–5].

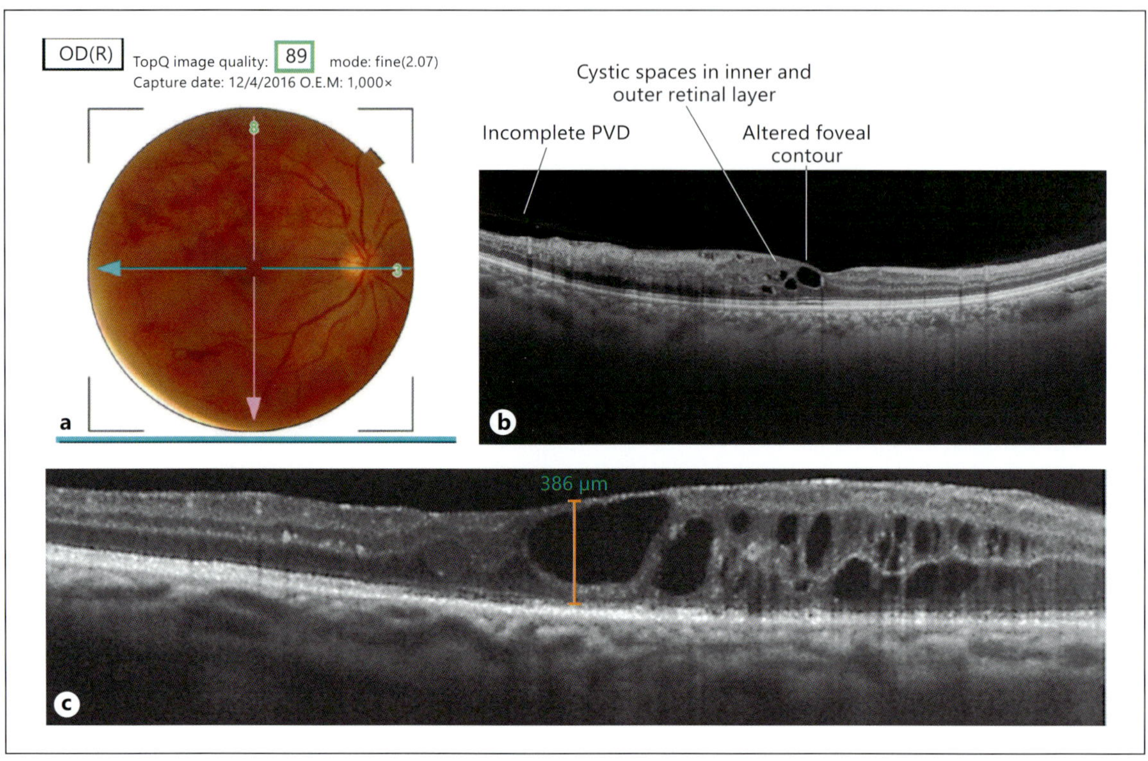

Fig. 1. a Hemorrhages in the superotemporal quadrant suggestive of a branch retinal vein occlusion. **b** Horizontal optical coherence tomography scan showing cystoid spaces in the inner and outer retinal layers. **c** Long-standing chronic edema secondary to diabetic retinopathy. It is difficult to distinguish intracellular and extracellular edema with the current imaging technology. PVD = Posterior vitreous detachment.

Under physiologic conditions, various factors such as osmotic forces, hydrostatic forces, capillary permeability, and tissue compliance prevent accumulation of fluid in the macula. The rate of capillary filtration equals the rate of fluid removal from the extracellular retinal tissue. Therefore, the interstitial spaces of the retina can be kept dry in physiological conditions. Active transport of fluid across the retinal pigment epithelium is efficient at removing subretinal fluid, but the flow resistance of the retina limits removal of intraretinal edema by the retinal pigment epithelium.

The two most common vascular diseases that cause macular edema are diabetic retinopathy and retinal vein occlusion. The mechanisms by which high glucose levels directly lead to diabetic reti-nopathy are not well known. Activation of protein kinase C, accumulation of polyols through the aldose reductase pathway, increased formation of advanced glycation end products, and overproduction of free radicals may occur due to hyperglycemia (Tang and Kern, 2011)[6]. These metabolic changes increase proinflammatory cytokines, chemokines, and other inflammatory mediators that stimulate an influx of leukocytes and alter vascular permeability (Tang and Kern, 2011)[6]. Elevated levels of interleukin 6 (IL-6), IL-8, tumor necrosis factor-α, vascular endothelial growth factor (VEGF), interferon-induced protein-10, intercellular adhesion molecule 1, and monocyte chemoattractant protein-1 (MCP-1) have been demonstrated in eyes with diabetic retinopathy (Tang

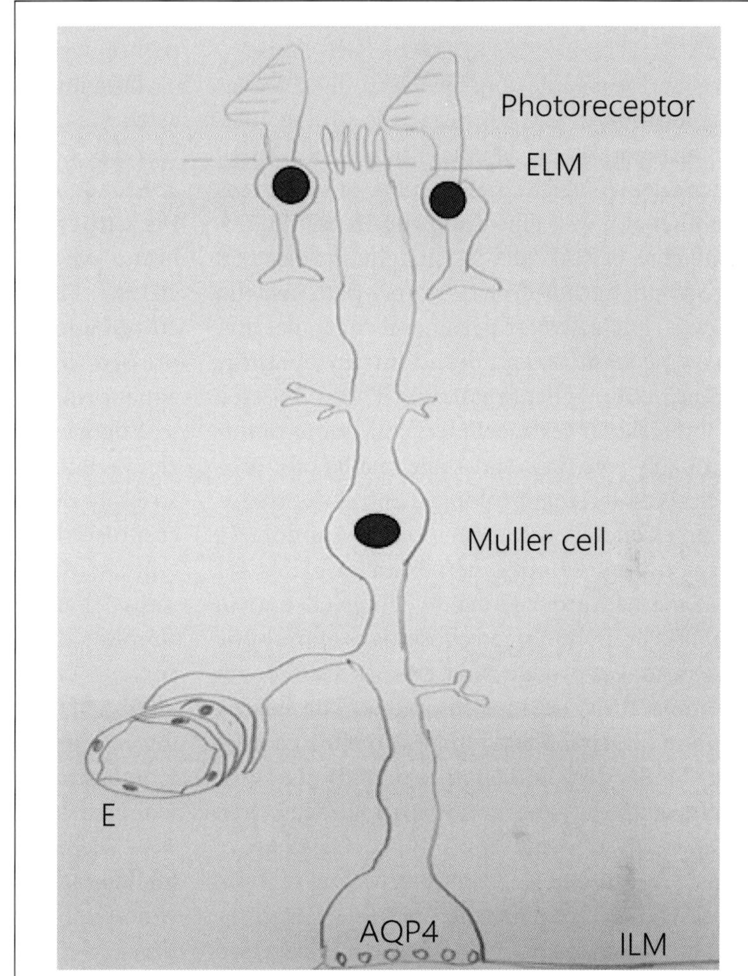

Fig. 2. Pericytes and endothelial cells (E) constitute the blood-retinal barrier that is covered by multiple processes of the Müller cells. These processes over the pericytes have aquaporin-4 (AQP4) channels (not shown). Müller cells traverse the entire retina and are the major determinant of retinal fluid movement. The footplates of the Müller cells form the internal limiting membrane (ILM) of the retina. At the inner border of the Müller cell, there is a high concentration of aquaporin-4 channels (vesicles). ELM = External limiting membrane.

and Kern, 2011)[6]. A number of inflammatory cytokines and growth factors may be elevated in RVO patients, including IL-1α, IL-6, IL-8, monocyte chemoattractant protein-1, platelet-derived growth factor AA, and VEGF relative to control eyes (Lee et al., 2012; Noma et al., 2005)[7, 8].

Ischemia and Hypoxia

Hypoxia plays a central role in the development of macular edema. In neuronal cells, there is excessive water production due to a high rate of ATP synthesis. The uptake of metabolic substrates such as glucose is related to an influx of water into cells. Under physiological conditions, fluid is absorbed by Müller cells and is released into the blood or the vitreous. The release of fluid from the Müller cells into the retina occurs through their perivascular end-feet facing the vitreous. Aquaporin-4 channels play a significant role in mediating these water fluxes (fig. 2). In postischemic cerebral edema, the swelling of glial cell end-feet around blood vessels is enhanced by an altered expression of the aquaporin 4 water channels in cell membranes (Pannicke et al., 2004)[9].

Location of Edema

There has been some controversy about the anatomic location of CME in regard to Müller cells. The histopathologic studies published about CME have involved a small number of specimens (Yanoff et al, 1984; Fine and Brucker, 1981)[10, 11]. Yanoff et al. (1984)[10] described light and electron microscopic findings reviewed in 2 patients who had eyes enucleated for peripheral choroidal malignant melanomas, and found intracytoplasmic swelling of the Müller (glial) cells. They suggested that intercellular (extracellular) collections of fluid probably were late end-stage results of a process that results from prolonged and excessive intracellular edema, cell death, and disruption. In the patient whose optic nerve was available for study, marked intracellular swelling (edema) of the glial cells in the lamina choroidalis of the optic nerve head was present, and was associated with compression of the adjacent axons. The nearby temporal, parapapillary retina also showed edema of Müller cells and compression of the nerve fibers, suggesting a more widespread process than was clinically evident. Fine and Brucker (1981)[11] described light and electron microscopy of 3 patients. The electron microscopic findings common to all 3 eyes were widespread swelling and necrosis of Müller cell cytoplasm. There was no enlargement of intercellular spaces. The retinal vascular changes were probably the cause of CME. Gass et al. (1985)[12] suggested the edema to be extracellular, although there were very few cases in his series. The size of the cystoid spaces seems to be much more than the diameter of a Müller cell. It seems unlikely that all the fluid accumulation in macular edema is intracellular.

Hydrodynamics of Macula

While the body of literature on the pathophysiology of cerebral edema is extensive, research on macular edema is quite limited. Understanding cerebral edema may provide insights into the pathophysiology of macular edema.

Distribution of water in the brain is done by astrocytes, with their end-feet surrounding the blood vessels. These cells have densely packed arrays of aquaporin-4, occupying a large surface of the astrocyte in apposition to the basement membrane of the vessels (Nagelhus and Ottersen, 2013)[13]. The aquaporins are a family of more than 10 homologous water-transporting proteins expressed in many mammalian cells. At least five aquaporins are expressed in the eye.

Edema of retinal cells occurs when their K^+ channels are blocked. During ischemia, glial cells strongly downregulate their K^+ conductance. In contrast, the expression of the aquaporin-4 protein is only slightly altered after ischemia of the retina (Pannicke et al., 2004)[9]. There may be a coupling of transmembranous water fluxes to K^+ currents in glial cells. Ischemia causes a downregulation of the K^+ conductance of glial cells, resulting in osmotically driven water fluxes from the blood into the glial cells through aquaporins. Retinal glial cells progressively lose K^+ conductivity with increasing age. This fact may explain the higher incidence of macular edema under ischemic/hypoxic conditions in the elderly population.

Macular edema is a complication of various retinal diseases, resulting in the degeneration of photoreceptors and the death of neuronal cells. In the development of macular edema, it is believed that a swelling of Müller cells occurs before the formation of extracellular edema. The amount of edema would be affected by the amount of fluid produced, tissue conductance and architecture, osmotic pressures, and fluid absorption (Nagashima et al., 1990; Marmarou et al., 1980; Hatashita and Hoff; 1988)[14–16].

Fluid entry into and out of the macula may occur at four sites: the subretinal space, retinal border with the vitreous, and the superficial and deep vascular plexus. If the external limiting membrane is intact, exudation from below the retina would cause serous detachment of the retina. The inner and deep plexiform layers hinder movement of fluid and molecules within the retina. Therefore, the retinal tissue forms a complex series of potential sources of fluid and natural barriers to fluid passage.

Müller Cells

The control of fluid movement into and out of the retina from the vitreous and the retinal blood vessels shares many similarities, largely because both involve Müller cells, the central glial cells of the retina. Müller cells are one of the most important cells in homeostasis of fluid and ions in the retinal interstitial areas (Newman, 1993)[17]. Müller cells can buffer changes in intracellular K^+ concentration chiefly through Kir2.1 and Kir4.1 channels (Newman, 1993; Nagelhus et at., 2004)[17, 18]. After a light-evoked potassium increase within the retina, there is a substantial transfer of potassium from the retina to the vitreous humor by potassium current flow through Müller cells (Karwoski et al., 1989)[19]. Along with the potassium ions, water is induced to move through aquaporin-4 channels. The spatial buffering by Müller cells pumping K^+ into the vitreous or blood vessels is called potassium siphoning (Verkman, 2003)[20]. For each K^+ ion transported, approximately 140 water molecules are also transferred. The aquaporin channels are densely packed at the Müller cell footplate and on the Müller cell processes surrounding the retinal vessels in the superficial and deep vascular plexus (fig. 2). The packing density is high at these sites and the aquaporin-4 molecules form 2-dimensional crystalline supramolecular assemblies that are also called orthogonal arrays of particles (Newman, 1994)[21]. The retina is one of the mostly highly metabolic tissues in the body, and in addition to producing metabolic water it also generates CO_2, which is cleared with the help of Müller cells. As a consequence, Müller cells have huge amounts of active carbonic anhydrase (Newman, 1994; Ochrietor et al., 2005)[21, 22]. There is a cellular compartmentalization of the two isoforms of carbonic anhydrase in Müller cells, one cytoplasmic and the other on the plasma membrane.

Breakdown of the blood-ocular barrier can allow excessive water, electrolytes, and potentially larger macromolecules from the serum into the extravascular space. Fluid entry into the retinal parenchyma could occur by Müller cell trafficking or by paracellular movement around the Müller cell processes. Ischemia and inflammation can cause alteration in the density and pattern of aquaporin and Kir4.1 channels (Reichenbach et al., 2007)[23].

Pharmacological reactivation of the retinal water clearance by Müller cells may represent an approach to the development of new drugs for macular edema. Corticosteroids, which are clinically used to resolve edema, prevent osmotic swelling of Müller cells as they induce the release of endogenous adenosine and subsequent A1 receptor activation, which results in the opening of ion channels. Apparently, steroids resolve edema by both inhibition of vascular leakage and stimulation of retinal fluid clearance by Müller cells (Reichenbach et al., 2007)[23].

Multiple cytokines and chemokines are involved in the pathogenesis of diabetic macular edema, with multiple cellular involvements affecting the neurovascular unit. Corticosteroids are unique in that they are the one class of agents that acts upon most of the multiple processes in the pathophysiology of macular edema. For example, corticosteroids are capable of inhibiting prostaglandin and leukotriene synthesis as well as interfering with intercellular adhesion molecule-1, IL-6, VEGF-A, and stromal cell derived factor-1 pathways. Corticosteroids also have been shown to decrease paracellular permeability and increase tight junction integrity both by directly restoring tight junctional proteins to their proper location at the cell border and by increasing the gene expression of those proteins. VEGF is 50,000 times more potent than histamine as a vasopermeability factor. Anti-VEGF agents act by reducing the vasopermeability effect of VEGF (Das et al., 2015)[24]. While most drugs for macular edema act by reducing vasopermeability, improving the activity of Müller cells to reduce intracellular edema, as well as pumping out extracellular edema, should be the target of new molecules for the treatment of macular edema.

In conclusion, intracellular edema is a significant component in eyes with macular edema. Müller cells play a key role in the hydrodynamics of macula, and Müller cell dysfunction in different pathologies of the macula results in alteration of fluid equilibrium. Therapeutic targets for improving Müller cell function could play a key role in the treatment of macular edema in the future.

References

1 Marmor MF: Mechanisms of fluid accumulation in retinal edema. Doc Ophthalmol 1999;97:239–249.

2 Bringmann A, Reichenbach A, Wiedemann P: Pathomechanisms of cystoid macular edema. Ophthalmic Res 2004; 36:241–249.

3 Coscas G, Cunha-Vaz J, Soubrane G: Macular edema: definition and basic concepts. Dev Ophthalmol 2010;47:1–9.

4 Finkelstein D: Ischemic macular edema. Recognition and favorable natural history in branch vein occlusion. Arch Ophthalmol 1992;110:1427–1434.

5 Scholl S, Kirchhof J, Augustin AJ: Pathophysiology of macular edema. Ophthalmologica 2010;224(suppl 1):8–15.

6 Tang J, Kern TS: Inflammation in diabetic retinopathy. Prog Retin Eye Res 2011;30:343–358.

7 Lee WJ, Kang MH, Seong M, Cho HY: Comparison of aqueous concentrations of angiogenic and inflammatory cytokines in diabetic macular oedema and macular oedema due to branch retinal vein occlusion. Br J Ophthalmol 2012; 96:1426–1430.

8 Noma H, Funatsu H, Yamasaki M, Tsukamoto H, Mimura T, Sone T, et al: Pathogenesis of macular edema with branch retinal vein occlusion and intraocular levels of vascular endothelial growth factor and interleukin-6. Am J Ophthalmol 2005;140:256–261.

9 Pannicke T, Iandiev I, Uckermann O, Biedermann B, Kutzera F, Wiedemann P, et al: A potassium channel-linked mechanism of glial cell swelling in the postischemic retina. Mol Cell Neurosci 2004;26:493–502.

10 Yanoff M, Fine BS, Brucker AJ, Eagle RC Jr: Pathology of human cystoid macular edema. Surv Ophthalmol 1984;28(suppl):505–511.

11 Fine BS, Brucker AJ: Macular edema and cystoid macular edema. Am J Ophthalmol 1981;92:466–481.

12 Gass JD, Anderson DR, Davis EB: A clinical, fluorescein angiographic, and electron microscopic correlation of cystoid macular edema. Am J Ophthalmol 1985; 100:82–86.

13 Nagelhus EA, Ottersen OP: Physiological roles of aquaporin-4 in brain. Physiol Rev 2013;93:1543–1562.

14 Nagashima T, Horwitz B, Rapoport SI: A mathematical model for vasogenic brain edema. Adv Neurol 1990;52:317–326.

15 Marmarou A, Takagi H, Shulman K: Biomechanics of brain edema and effects on local cerebral blood flow. Adv Neurol 1980;28:345–358.

16 Hatashita S, Hoff JT: Biomechanics of brain edema in acute cerebral ischemia in cats. Stroke 1988;19:91–97.

17 Newman EA: Inward-rectifying potassium channels in retinal glial (Müller) cells. J Neurosci 1993;13:3333–3345.

18 Nagelhus EA, Mathiisen TM, Ottersen OP: Aquaporin-4 in the central nervous system: cellular and subcellular distribution and coexpression with KIR4.1. Neuroscience 2004;129:905–913.

19 Karwoski CJ, Lu HK, Newman EA: Spatial buffering of light-evoked potassium increases by retinal Müller (glial) cells. Science 1989;244:578–580.

20 Verkman AS: Role of aquaporin water channels in eye function. Exp Eye Res 2003;76:137–143.

21 Newman EA: A physiological measure of carbonic anhydrase in Müller cells. Glia 1994;11:291–299.

22 Ochrietor JD, Clamp MF, Moroz TP, Grubb JH, Shah GN, Waheed A, et al: Carbonic anhydrase XIV identified as the membrane CA in mouse retina: strong expression in Müller cells and the RPE. Exp Eye Res 2005;81:492–500.

23 Reichenbach A, Wurm A, Pannicke T, Iandiev I, Wiedemann P, Bringmann A: Müller cells as players in retinal degeneration and edema. Graefes Arch Clin Exp Ophthalmol 2007;245:627–636.

24 Das A, McGuire PG, Rangasamy S: Diabetic macular edema: pathophysiology and novel therapeutic targets. Ophthalmology 2015;122:1375–1394.

Baruch D. Kuppermann
Gavin Herbert Eye Institute
University of California, Irvine
850 Health Sciences Rd.
Irvine, CA 92697 (USA)
E-Mail bdkupper@uci.edu

Chapter 4

Coscas G (ed): Macular Edema. 2nd, revised and extended edition.
Dev Ophthalmol. Basel, Karger, 2017, vol 58, pp 27–38 (DOI: 10.1159/000455267)

Central Serous Chorioretinopathy

Alejandra Daruich[a] · Alexandre Matet[a] · Francine Behar-Cohen[b–e]

[a]Department of Ophthalmology, University of Lausanne, Jules-Gonin Eye Hospital, Fondation Asile des Aveugles, and [b]University of Lausanne, Lausanne, Switzerland; [c]Teams 1 and 17, Centre de Recherche des Cordeliers, UMR 1138, Sorbonne Universités, UPMC Université Paris 06, [d]Centre de Recherche des Cordeliers, INSERM, UMR 1138, and [e]Centre de Recherche des Cordeliers, UMR 1138, Université Paris Descartes, Sorbonne Paris Cité, Paris, France

Abstract

Central serous is an atypical form of macular edema with mostly accumulation of fluid under the retina. It contitutes a pure phenotype of retinal pigment epithelium barrier breakdown. Another particularity is the good visual preservation despite important fluid volume increase in the macula.   © 2017 S. Karger AG, Basel

Definition and Epidemiology

Central serous chorioretinopathy (CSCR or CSC) is a chorioretinal disease affecting predominantly middle-aged men and characterized by serous retinal detachments (SRD) frequently involving the macular area and associated with focal pigment epithelial detachments (PED). CSCR is often unilateral, but variable contralateral involvement has been detected in up to 40% of cases (Gäckle et al., 1998)[1]. A population-based study reported an annual incidence of 9.9 per 100,000 for men and 1.7 for women, confirming the male predilection (Kitzmann et al., 2008)[2]. The mean age at disease onset has been estimated between 39 and 51 years (Kitzmann et al., 2008; Spaide et al., 1996; Tsai et al., 2013)[2–4].

Clinical Presentation

The term 'CSCR' covers two distinct entities classically defined as acute and chronic. This distinction is ambiguous because it relies either on the duration of SRD (4–6 months), or on the presence of severe retinal pigment epithelium (RPE) alterations. The term 'nonresolving' or 'persistent' CSCR may be more appropriate to describe cases with long-lasting SRD, and thus avoid confusion with the chronic form characterized by a diffuse pigment epitheliopathy (Loo et al., 2002)[5].

Acute CSCR

In acute CSCR (fig. 1), patients report symptoms related to the detachment of the macula: blurred vision, relative central scotoma, variable meta-

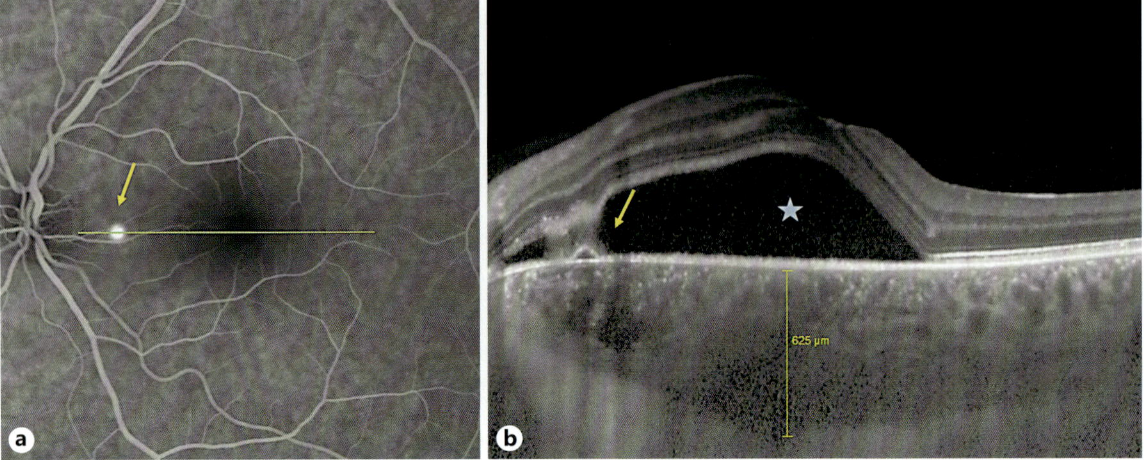

Fig. 1. Acute CSCR. Thirty-five-year-old man who reported blurred vision in his left eye for 4 days. Midphase fluorescein angiogram (**a**) revealed a single leaking point (yellow arrow). **b** SD-OCT identified a pigment epithelium detachment (yellow arrow) at the level of the leaking point, confirmed the presence of a subretinal detachment involving the fovea (blue star), and revealed an increased choroidal thickness (625 μm).

morphopsia, dyschromatopsia, hypermetropization, micropsia, and reduced contrast sensitivity (Wang et al., 2008)[6]. In addition to SRD visible on fundus examination, spectral domain optical coherence tomography (SD-OCT) may show limited RPE alterations, such as small PEDs. A leakage site through the RPE is frequently identified on fluorescein angiography (FA). The SRD usually resolves within 3–4 months, without sequelae (Baran et al., 2005)[7].

Recurrent CSCR is defined as a new episode of acute CSCR following a previous resolved episode. Recurrences are estimated to occur in 15–50% of cases (Daruich et al., 2015)[8]. The evolution to recurrent or persistent CSCR has been identified as a risk factor of visual acuity worse than 20/40 (Loo et al., 2002)[5].

Chronic CSCR

The chronic form was initially named 'diffuse retinal epitheliopathy' (Yannuzzi et al., 1992)[9]. It presents with widespread tracks of RPE atrophy associated with decreased fundus autofluorescence (FAF) (fig. 2) (Imamura et al., 2011; Teke et al., 2014)[10, 11]. Symptoms are permanent with moderate-to-severe visual acuity loss and decreased light sensitivity depending on the extent of photoreceptor damage (Ooto et al., 2010; Piccolino et al., 2005)[12, 13]. SD-OCT shows variable chronic SRD, multifocal RPE atrophy, and irregular RPE detachments. Intraretinal cystoid cavities can also be observed (Iida et al., 2003; Piccolino et al., 2008)[14, 15], more frequently with disease duration longer than 5 years (fig. 2) (Piccolino et al., 2008)[16].

Choroidal neovascularization (CNV) may complicate CSCR, either as the natural course of the disease (prevalence: 2–9%) or as a complication of focal treatments (Spaide et al., 1996; Loo et al., 2002)[3, 5].

Diagnosis: Multimodal Imaging of Central Serous Chorioretinopathy

SD-OCT is instrumental for the diagnosis and follow-up of CSCR. FA identifies the origin of leakage. FAF noninvasively detects RPE altera-

Daruich · Matet · Behar-Cohen

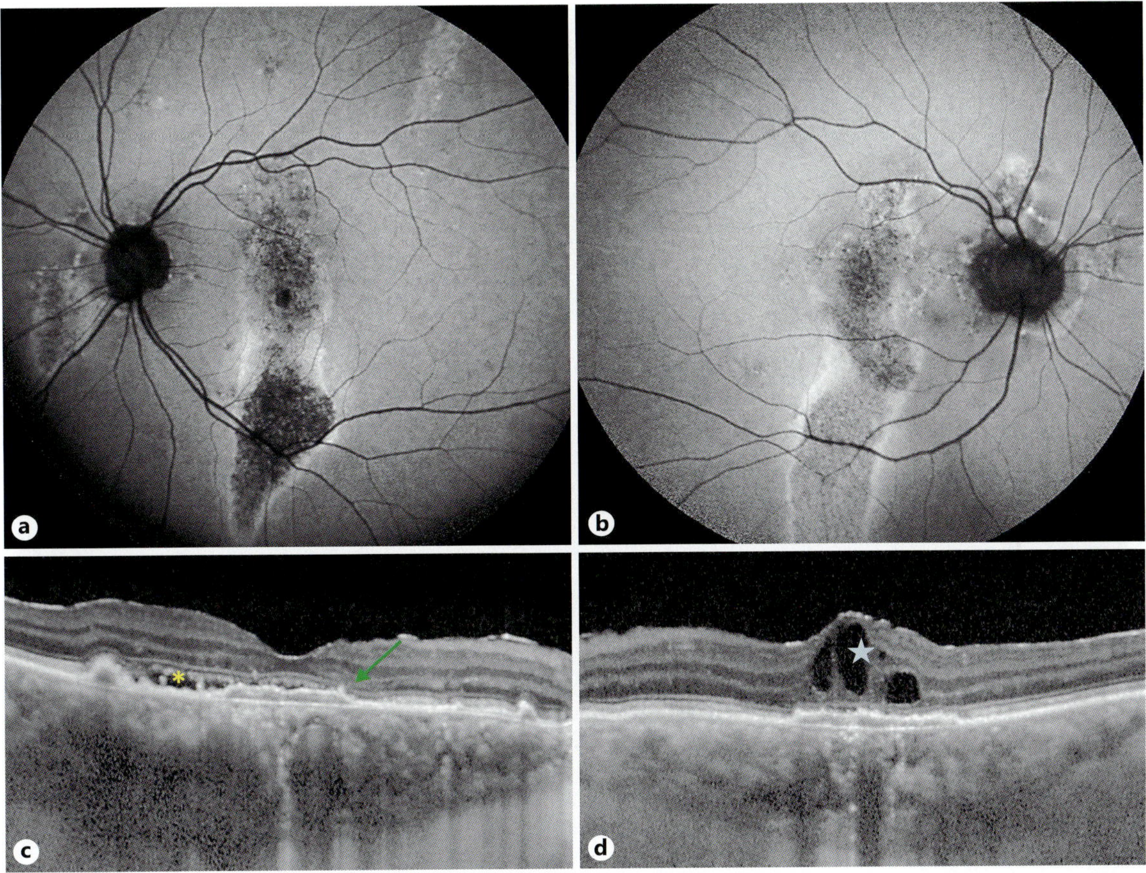

Fig. 2. Chronic CSCR. **a, b** FAF in a 70-year-old man showing bilateral oblong descending hypoautofluorescent tracks, a pathognomonic feature of a severe chronic CSCR with diffuse atrophy of the RPE. **c, d** SD-OCT revealed a small subretinal detachment (asterisk), a shallow PED (arrows) and the presence of intraretinal cysts (star).

tions. Recurrent, nonresolving, and chronic CSCR should benefit from multimodal imaging with SD-OCT, FAF, FA, and indocyanine green (ICG) angiography to guide treatment, follow extension, and detect neovascular components.

Spectral Domain Optical Coherence Tomography
Retinal Findings
In acute CSCR, retinal layers are preserved despite the presence of subretinal fluid. Elongation of photoreceptor outer segments above the SRD is frequent (fig. 3a) (Matsumoto et al., 2008)[17]. In-

traretinal cysts and loss of photoreceptor outer segments are seen in very long-standing cases. Hyperreflective dots (fig. 3a) can be observed in the subretinal space (Kon et al., 2008; Maruko et al., 2011; Spaide and Klancnik, 2005)[18–20] and within the neuroretina (Kon et al., 2008; Ahlers et al., 2009; Yalcinbayir et al., 2014)[18, 21, 22]. Variable alterations of RPE, as PEDs, areas of RPE atrophy, or hypertrophy, may be observed in all CSCR subtypes (fig. 1, 2) (Piccolino et al., 2008; Yalcinbayir et al., 2014; Lim and Wong, 2008; Yang et al., 2013)[15, 22–24].

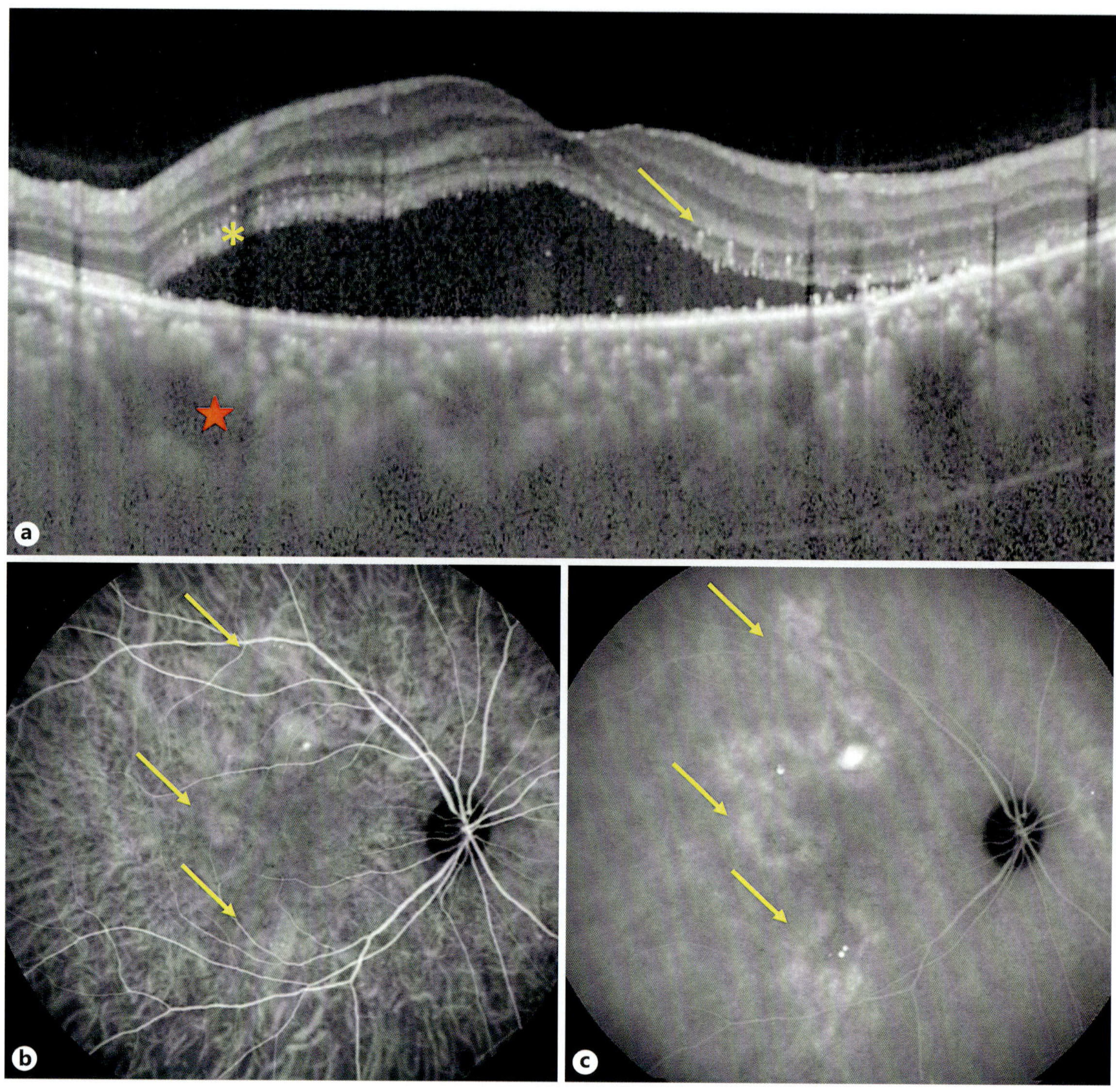

Fig. 3. Imaging of the choroid in CSCR. Forty-year-old woman presenting a first episode of CSCR. **a** SD-OCT identified a subretinal detachment associated with elongation of photoreceptor outer segments (asterisk). The enhanced-depth imaging acquisition mode visualized enlarged choroidal vessels (star) and the classical aspect of pachychoroid. Hyper-reflective dots were visible in the neuroretina (arrow). ICG angiography showed multifocal hyperfluorescence areas with blurred contours during midphase, indicating choroidal vascular hyperpermeability (arrows) (**b**) that evolved into persistent hyperfluorescence, or peripheral extension forming hyperfluorescent rings at the late phase (arrows) (**c**).

Choroidal Findings
Increased choroidal thickness (>395 μm) (Lehmann et al., 2015)[25] is often observed in affected (Yang et al., 2013; Imamura et al., 2009; Jiraratanasopa et al., 2012; Kim et al., 2011; Kuroda et al., 2013)[24, 26–29] and contralateral eyes of CSCR patients (Goktas, 2014; Maruko et al., 2011; Yang et al., 2013)[30–32]. Choroidal thickening (pachychoroid) can result from focal or diffuse dilatation of large choroidal vessels (fig. 1b, 3a). These dilated vessels are commonly localized within areas of increased choroidal vascular permeability on ICG angiography (Yang et al., 2013; Jiraratanasopa et al., 2012; Kuroda et al., 2013; Maruko et al., 2011; Razavi et al., 2014)[24, 27, 29, 31, 33].

Fundus Autofluorescence
FAF imaging reflects RPE status. In chronic CSCR, FAF is pathognomonic with oblong descending hypofluorescent tracks, originating from the optic disc or the macula, and described as 'gravitational tracks' (fig. 2a, b).

Fluorescein Angiography
By identifying single (fig. 1a) or multiple leakage points, FA confirms the diagnosis and guides laser treatment (for extrafoveal leakages) (Yannuzzi et al., 2000)[34]. In acute cases, leakage sites (Burumcek et al., 1997)[35] present as a pinpoint of increasing fluorescence along the sequence, with a possible 'ink-blot' (progressive circular expansion), or 'smokestack' aspect (ascending expansion). In the mid- and late phases, a circular hyperfluorescence appears within the SRD. PED are characterized by early fluorescein pooling with hyperfluorescence persisting in late phases.

In chronic forms, diffuse RPE defects provoke multifocal leakage points visible in the mid- and late phases as patchy, granular hyperfluorescence (Yannuzzi et al., 1984)[36].

Indocyanine Green Angiography
ICG angiography has become the gold standard to analyze the choroidal vasculature. It helps differentiate other CSCR from differential diagnoses and identifies CNV when complicating CSCR (Spaide et al., 1996; Yannuzzi, 2011)[3, 37].

The choroidal modifications observed by ICG angiography in CSCR eyes are:
- Early phase: delayed filling of arteries and coriocapillaris (Prünte, 1995)[38], hypofluorescent areas corresponding to decreased choriocapillaris filling (persisting in the mid- and late phases) (Kitaya et al., 2003)[39]
- Midphase: dilation of large choroidal veins, geographic areas of hyperfluorescence with blurred contours described as choroidal vascular hyperpermeability, one of the hallmarks of CSCR (fig. 3b) (Piccolino and Borgia, 1994; Spaide et al., 1996)[40, 41]
- Late phase: midphase hyperfluorescent areas evolve into persistent hyperfluorescence, wash-out, or a peripheral extension forming hyperfluorescent rings (fig. 3c) (Tsujikawa et al., 2010)[42]

Pathogenesis

Risk Factors
Corticosteroids
The systemic or local administration of corticosteroids [inhalation (Haimovici et al., 1997; Kleinberger et al., 2011)[43, 44], epidural (Iida et al., 2001; Kao, 1998; Pizzimenti and Daniel, 2005)[45–47] or intra-articular injections (Hurvitz et al., 2009; Kassam et al., 2011; Mondal et al., 2005)[48–50], topical dermal (Ezra et al., 2011; Fernandez et al., 2004; Karadimas and Bouzas, 2004; Romero et al., 2005)[51–54], and periocular injections (Baumal et al., 2004)[55]] has been associated with the triggering, prolongation, aggravation, and recurrences of CSCR (Khairallah et al., 2012)[56].

Endocrine Changes
The risk of CSCR is higher during pregnancy (Haimovici et al., 2004)[57] and may resolve spontaneously after delivery (Chumbley and Frank,

1974; Errera et al., 2013; Schultz et al., 2005)[58–60]. CSCR develops in up to 5% of patients with endogenous Cushing syndrome (Bouzas et al., 1993; Carvalho-Recchia et al., 2002)[61, 62]. Morning serum cortisol levels (Garg et al., 1997; Zakir et al., 2009)[63, 64] and 24-hour urine cortisol levels (Garg et al., 1997; Kapetanios et al., 1998)[63, 65] are higher in acute CSCR patients than in healthy subjects.

Psychopathology
An association was suggested between CSCR and 'type A' personality, characterized by a competitive drive, a sense of urgency, and an aggressive and hostile temperament (Yannuzzi, 1986)[66]. Antipsychotropic medication use and psychological stress were described as independent risk factors for CSCR (Tittl et al., 1999)[67]. Depression has been associated with an increased risk of recurrence (Fok et al., 2011)[68].

Genetic Predisposition
Several sporadic familial cases of CSCR have been reported (Amalric et al., 1971; Haik et al., 1968; Lin et al., 2000; Oosterhuis, 1996; Park et al., 1998; Wyman, 1963)[69–74]. Additional evidence comes from the observation of fundus atrophic lesions or pachychoroid suggestive of CSCR in relatives of CSCR patients (Lehmann et al., 2015; Weenink et al., 2001)[25, 75]. Genetic studies based on single nucleotide polymorphisms have been performed on CSCR subjects. An association between 5 common complement factor H polymorphisms (Miki et al., 2014)[76] and 4 common cadherin-5 single nucleotide polymorphisms have been identified (Schubert et al., 2014)[77].

Cardiovascular Diseases and Hypertension
Patients with hypertension have higher risk of developing CSCR (Tittl et al., 1999; Eom et al., 2012)[67, 78]. Men with CSCR have a significantly higher rate of coronary heart disease (Chen et al., 2014)[79]. CSCR is also an independent risk factor for ischemic stroke (Tsai et al., 2012)[80] and organic and psychogenic erectile dysfunction (Tsai et al., 2013)[81].

Sympathetic-Parasympathetic Activity and Reactivity
Based on cardiac monitoring, patients with CSCR have shown significantly decreased parasympathetic activity and increased sympathetic activity (Tewari et al., 2006)[82].

Gastroesophageal Disorders
A higher risk of gastroesophageal reflux and more frequent use of antiacid or antireflux medications were found in CSCR patients (Mansuetta et al., 2004)[83]. Additional studies reported that CSCR patients have a high prevalence of *Helicobacter pylori* infection (Ahnoux-Zabsonre et al., 2004; Cotticelli et al., 2006; Giusti, 2001; Mateo-Montoya and Mauget-Faÿsse, 2002; Roshani et al., 2014)[84–89].

Drug-Induced CSCR
CSCR episodes have been associated with the use of phosphodiesterase-5 inhibitors (sildenafil, tadalafil, vardenafil) (Aliferis et al., 2012; Fraunfelder and Fraunfelder, 2008)[90, 91]. Up to 65% of patients under oral MEK inhibitors (binimetinib) for metastatic cancer develop transient bilateral SRD and moderately blurred vision suggestive of CSCR (McCannel et al., 2014; Urner-Bloch et al., 2014)[92, 93].

Sleep Disturbance
The role of obstructive sleep apnea in CSCR remains controversial (Eom et al., 2012; Kloos et al., 2008; Brodie et al., 2015)[78, 94, 95].

Mechanism of CSCR
Choroidopathy and Epitheliopathy
The major mechanistic steps involved in CSCR pathogenesis are choroidal vascular hyperpermeability and congestion (choroidopathy), damage of the overlying RPE (epitheliopathy), and abnormal movement of plasma proteins and water through the RPE into the subretinal space (SRD).

Molecular Hypothesis: Involvement of the Aldosterone/Mineralocorticoid Receptor Pathway in CSCR

Recent evidence from clinical and animal studies supports the hypothesis that inappropriate activation of the mineralocorticoid receptor (MR) pathway involvement leads to choroidal vasodilatation in CSCR. Indeed, MR activation in the choroidal endothelial cells, either by its natural ligand, aldosterone, or by glucocorticoids that have a high affinity for MR, induces upregulation of the vasodilator potassium channel KCa2.3 (calcium-dependent channel) and smooth muscle cell relaxation in the choroidal vasculature (fig. 4) (Daruich et al., 2015; Zhao et al., 2012; Zhao et al., 2010; Bousquet et al., 2013)[8, 96–98].

Treatments

Since acute CSCR is a self-limited disease (Yannuzzi, 2010)[99], observation is the recommended first-line attitude.

For persistent CSCR, there is no consensus about the optimal treatment and timing. Classically, treatment is justified in case of persistent macular SRD for more than 4 months, a new episode with history of multiple recurrences, reduced visual acuity, history of CSCR in the fellow eye with poor visual outcome, and professional need of rapid recovery (Nicholson et al., 2013)[100].

Eviction of Risk Factors

Interruption of glucocorticoid treatment appears beneficial to facilitate the resolution of CSCR episodes (Polak et al., 1995; Sharma et al., 2004; Wakakura et al., 1997; Williamson and Nuki, 1970)[101–104]. Improvement after management of obstructive sleep apnea has also been reported (Jain et al., 2010)[105]. Psychological support associated or not with pharmacotherapy should also be discussed when a clear psychopathology is identified.

Laser Photocoagulation

Laser photocoagulation has been attempted to 'seal' the RPE leakage site when located outside the macular area. Besides the direct thermal effect on the RPE, it is thought to increase fluid movements out of the subretinal space into the choroid (Robertson and Ilstrup, 1983)[106] or to allow the expansion of surrounding RPE cells after destruction of altered RPE cells (Lim et al., 2011)[107].

Laser photocoagulation accelerates the resolution of SRD without an impact on the final visual acuity (Burumcek et al., 1997; Robertson and Ilstrup, 1983; Leaver and Williams, 1979; Gilbert et al., 1984; Brancato et al., 1987)[35, 106, 108–110] or on the rate of recurrences. The few reported adverse effects include paracentral scotoma and iatrogenic CNV (Gilbert et al., 1984; Ficker et al., 1988; Verma et al., 2004)[109, 111, 112].

Verteporfin Photodynamic Therapy

Verteporfin photodynamic therapy provokes short-term choriocapillaris hypoperfusion and long-term choroidal vascular remodeling, thus reducing choroidal congestion, vascular hyperpermeability and extravascular leakage (Chan et al., 2003; Schlötzer-Schrehardt et al., 2002)[113, 114]. Complete resolution of subretinal fluid has been obtained in 80–90% of eyes after 12 months. Possible long-term complications of photodynamic therapy include choriocapillaris nonperfusion, secondary CNV (Reibaldi et al., 2010)[115], and RPE atrophy (Lim et al., 2014)[116]. Reduction of verteporfin dosage and laser fluence/dose have been attempted to reduce these adverse effects while preserving the benefits of treatment.

Oral MR Antagonists: Spironolactone and Eplerenone

Both drugs have been evaluated for the treatment of nonresolving CSCR and have led to a significant improvement of foveal SRF and visual acuity (Bousquet et al., 2013; Bousquet et al., 2015; Herold et al., 2014; Singh et al., 2015)[98, 117–119]. Possible side effects of spironolactone include

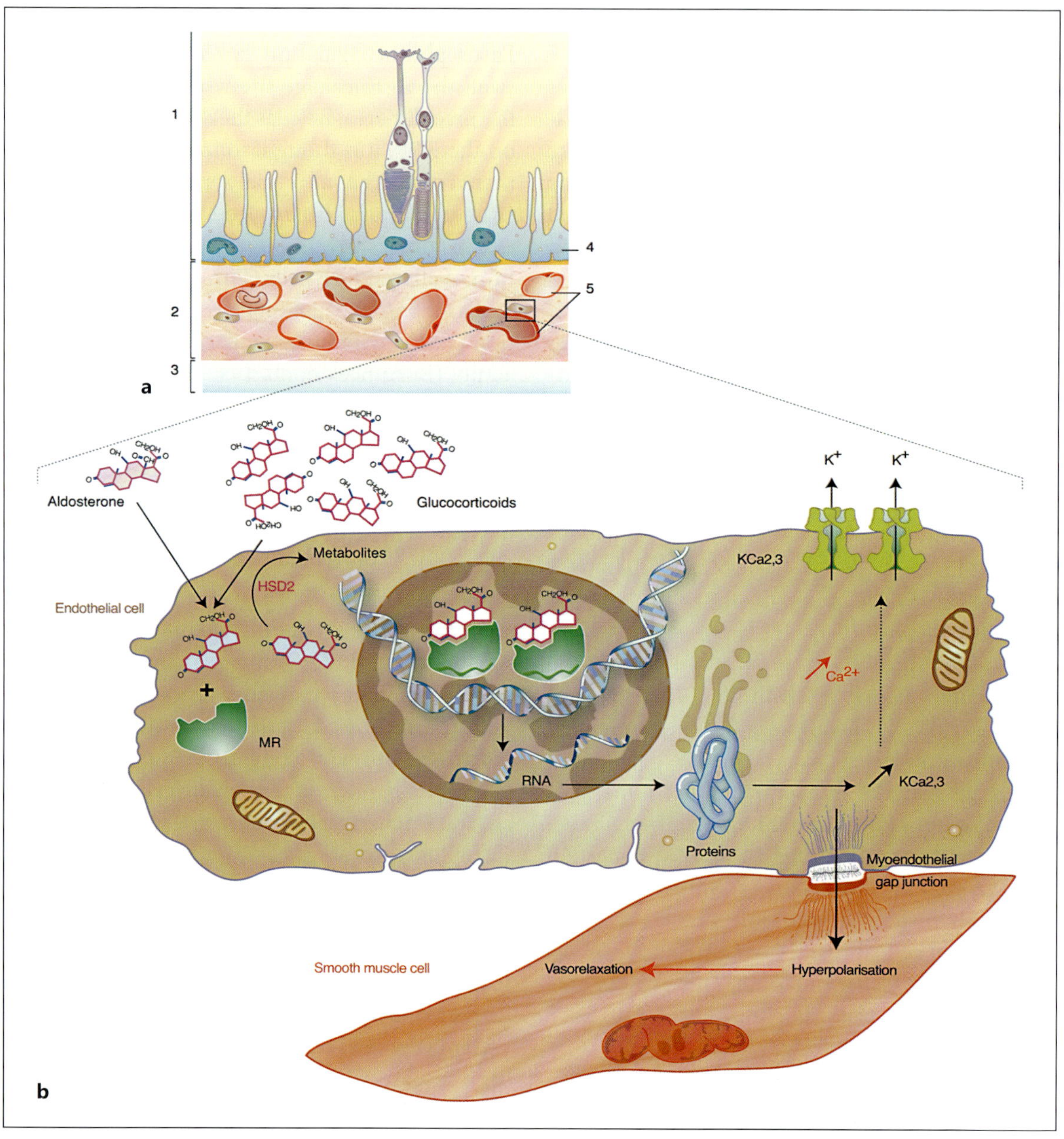

Fig. 4. Suggested mechanism leading to choroidal vascular dilatation by overactivation of the MR pathway in the choroidal vascular endothelial cells. Aldosterone and glucocorticoids bind to the MR. Permanent activation of the MR by glucocorticoids is prevented by the metabolizing enzyme 11-β-hydroxysteroid dehydrogenase type 2 (HSD2), which degrades the glucocorticoids into subproducts with a weaker affinity for the MR. However, the MR pathway can be activated by an excess of glucocorticoids or overexpression of the MR. MR activation increases the calcium-dependent, endothelial vasodilatory potassium channel KCa2.3. As a result, this leads to the hyperpolarization of endothelial cells and the underlying smooth muscle cells (via electric coupling through myoendothelial gap junctions), finally inducing choroidal vasodilation. K^+ = Potassium; Ca^{2+} = calcium. Adapted from Daruich (2015)[8].

hyperkalemia, gynecomastia, erectile dysfunction, decrease in libido, and menstrual irregularities (Funder, 2013)[120]. Eplerenone has been designed to reduce these side effects.

Anti-VEGF Agents
A few case series indicate a beneficial effect of intravitreal anti-VEGFs (Chan et al., 2007; Konstantinidis et al., 2010; Broadhead and Chang, 2015)[121–123] on CNV complicating CSCR.

Central Serous Chorioretinopathy-Related Entities and Differential Diagnosis

Several entities may present with retinal or choroidal changes mimicking CSCR. Clinical history and multimodal imaging are crucial to distinguish them from CSCR:
- Type 1 CNV complicating age-related macular degeneration
- Polypoidal choroidal vasculopathy
- Cavitary optic disc anomalies: optic disc pit and optic disc coloboma
- Circumscribed choroidal hemangioma
- Dome-shaped macula with subretinal fluid
- 'Pachychoroid neovasculopathy'

Conclusion

CSCR is a chorioretinal disease with a wide presentation spectrum and different prognoses. Pathogenesis of CSCR is not fully understood but recent findings have suggested an overactivation of the MR pathway that opens new therapeutic perspectives in addition to laser/photodynamic therapy treatments. Despite the high prevalence of CSCR, the best treatment option and the ideal timing of intervention still need to be specified.

References

1 Gäckle HC, Lang GE, Freissler KA, Lang GK: Central serous chorioretinopathy. Clinical, fluorescein angiography and demographic aspects (in German). Ophthalmologe 1998;95:529–533.

2 Kitzmann AS, Pulido JS, Diehl NN, et al: The incidence of central serous chorioretinopathy in Olmsted County, Minnesota, 1980–2002. Ophthalmology 2008; 115:169–173.

3 Spaide RF, Campeas L, Haas A, et al: Central serous chorioretinopathy in younger and older adults. Ophthalmology 1996;103:2070–2079; discussion 2079–2080.

4 Tsai D-C, Chen S-J, Huang C-C, et al: Epidemiology of idiopathic central serous chorioretinopathy in Taiwan, 2001–2006: a population-based study. PLoS One 2013;8:e66858.

5 Loo RH, Scott IU, Flynn HW, et al: Factors associated with reduced visual acuity during long-term follow-up of patients with idiopathic central serous chorioretinopathy. Retina 2002;22:19–24.

6 Wang M, Munch IC, Hasler PW, et al: Central serous chorioretinopathy. Acta Ophthalmol 2008;86:126–145.

7 Baran NV, Gürlü VP, Esgin H: Long-term macular function in eyes with central serous chorioretinopathy. Clin Exp Ophthalmol 2005;33:369–372.

8 Daruich A, Matet A, Dirani A, et al: Central serous chorioretinopathy: recent findings and new physiopathology hypothesis. Prog Retin Eye Res 2015;48: 82–118.

9 Yannuzzi LA, Slakter JS, Kaufman SR, Gupta K: Laser treatment of diffuse retinal pigment epitheliopathy. Eur J Ophthalmol 1992;2:103–114.

10 Imamura Y, Fujiwara T, Spaide RF: Fundus autofluorescence and visual acuity in central serous chorioretinopathy. Ophthalmology 2011;118:700–705.

11 Teke MY, Elgin U, Nalcacioglu-Yuksekkaya P, et al: Comparison of autofluorescence and optical coherence tomography findings in acute and chronic central serous chorioretinopathy. Int J Ophthalmol 2014;7:350–354.

12 Ooto S, Tsujikawa A, Mori S, et al: Thickness of photoreceptor layers in polypoidal choroidal vasculopathy and central serous chorioretinopathy. Graefes Arch Clin Exp Ophthalmol 2010;248: 1077–1086.

13 Piccolino FC, de la Longrais RR, Ravera G, et al: The foveal photoreceptor layer and visual acuity loss in central serous chorioretinopathy. Am J Ophthalmol 2005;139:87–99.

14 Iida T, Yannuzzi LA, Spaide RF, et al: Cystoid macular degeneration in chronic central serous chorioretinopathy. Retina 2003;23:1–7; quiz 137–138.

15 Piccolino FC, De La Longrais RR, Manea M, Cicinelli S: Posterior cystoid retinal degeneration in central serous chorioretinopathy. Retina 2008;28:1008–1012.

16 Piccolino FC, De La Longrais RR, Manea M, et al: Risk factors for posterior cystoid retinal degeneration in central serous chorioretinopathy. Retina 2008;28: 1146–1150.

17 Matsumoto H, Kishi S, Otani T, Sato T: Elongation of photoreceptor outer segment in central serous chorioretinopathy. Am J Ophthalmol 2008;145:162–168.

18 Kon Y, Iida T, Maruko I, Saito M: The optical coherence tomography-ophthalmoscope for examination of central serous chorioretinopathy with precipitates. Retina 2008;28:864–869.

19 Maruko I, Iida T, Ojima A, Sekiryu T: Subretinal dot-like precipitates and yellow material in central serous chorioretinopathy. Retina 2011;31:759–765.

20 Spaide RF, Klancnik JM: Fundus autofluorescence and central serous chorioretinopathy. Ophthalmology 2005;112:825–833.

21 Ahlers C, Geitzenauer W, Stock G, et al: Alterations of intraretinal layers in acute central serous chorioretinopathy. Acta Ophthalmol 2009;87:511–516.

22 Yalcinbayir O, Gelisken O, Akova-Budak B, et al: Correlation of spectral domain optical coherence tomography findings and visual acuity in central serous chorioretinopathy. Retina 2014;34:705–712.

23 Lim Z, Wong D: Retinal pigment epithelial rip associated with idiopathic central serous chorioretinopathy. Eye (Lond) 2008;22:471–473.

24 Yang L, Jonas JB, Wei W: Optical coherence tomography-assisted enhanced depth imaging of central serous chorioretinopathy. Invest Ophthalmol Vis Sci 2013;54:4659–4665.

25 Lehmann M, Bousquet E, Beydoun T, Behar-Cohen F: Pachychoroid: an inherited condition? Retina 2015;35:10–16.

26 Imamura Y, Fujiwara T, Margolis R, Spaide RF: Enhanced depth imaging optical coherence tomography of the choroid in central serous chorioretinopathy. Retina 2009;29:1469–1473.

27 Jirarattanasopa P, Ooto S, Tsujikawa A, et al: Assessment of macular choroidal thickness by optical coherence tomography and angiographic changes in central serous chorioretinopathy. Ophthalmology 2012;119:1666–1678.

28 Kim YT, Kang SW, Bai KH: Choroidal thickness in both eyes of patients with unilaterally active central serous chorioretinopathy. Eye (Lond) 2011;25:1635–1640.

29 Kuroda S, Ikuno Y, Yasuno Y, et al: Choroidal thickness in central serous chorioretinopathy. Retina 2013;33:302–308.

30 Goktas A: Correlation of subretinal fluid volume with choroidal thickness and macular volume in acute central serous chorioretinopathy. Eye (Lond) 2014;28:1431–1436.

31 Maruko I, Iida T, Sugano Y, et al: Subfoveal choroidal thickness in fellow eyes of patients with central serous chorioretinopathy. Retina 2011;31:1603–1608.

32 Yang L, Jonas JB, Wei W: Choroidal vessel diameter in central serous chorioretinopathy. Acta Ophthalmol 2013; 91:e358–e362.

33 Razavi S, Souied EH, Cavallero E, et al: Assessment of choroidal topographic changes by swept source optical coherence tomography after photodynamic therapy for central serous chorioretinopathy. Am J Ophthalmol 2014;157:852–860.

34 Yannuzzi LA, Freund KB, Goldbaum M, et al: Polypoidal choroidal vasculopathy masquerading as central serous chorioretinopathy. Ophthalmology 2000;107:767–777.

35 Burumcek E, Mudun A, Karacorlu S, Arslan MO: Laser photocoagulation for persistent central serous retinopathy: results of long-term follow-up. Ophthalmology 1997;104:616–622.

36 Yannuzzi LA, Shakin JL, Fisher YL, Altomonte MA: Peripheral retinal detachments and retinal pigment epithelial atrophic tracts secondary to central serous pigment epitheliopathy. Ophthalmology 1984;91:1554–1572.

37 Yannuzzi LA: Indocyanine green angiography: a perspective on use in the clinical setting. Am J Ophthalmol 2011; 151:745–751.e1.

38 Prünte C: Indocyanine green angiographic findings in central serous chorioretinopathy. Int Ophthalmol 1995;19:77–82.

39 Kitaya N, Nagaoka T, Hikichi T, et al: Features of abnormal choroidal circulation in central serous chorioretinopathy. Br J Ophthalmol 2003;87:709–712.

40 Piccolino FC, Borgia L: Central serous chorioretinopathy and indocyanine green angiography. Retina 1994;14:231–242.

41 Spaide RF, Hall L, Haas A, et al: Indocyanine green videoangiography of older patients with central serous chorioretinopathy. Retina 1996;16:203–213.

42 Tsujikawa A, Ojima Y, Yamashiro K, et al: Punctate hyperfluorescent spots associated with central serous chorioretinopathy as seen on indocyanine green angiography. Retina 2010;30:801–809.

43 Haimovici R, Gragoudas ES, Duker JS, et al: Central serous chorioretinopathy associated with inhaled or intranasal corticosteroids. Ophthalmology 1997;104:1653–1660.

44 Kleinberger AJ, Patel C, Lieberman RM, Malkin BD: Bilateral central serous chorioretinopathy caused by intranasal corticosteroids: a case report and review of the literature. Laryngoscope 2011;121:2034–2037.

45 Iida T, Spaide RF, Negrao SG, et al: Central serous chorioretinopathy after epidural corticosteroid injection. Am J Ophthalmol 2001;132:423–425.

46 Kao LY: Bilateral serous retinal detachment resembling central serous chorioretinopathy following epidural steroid injection. Retina 1998;18:479–481.

47 Pizzimenti JJ, Daniel KP: Central serous chorioretinopathy after epidural steroid injection. Pharmacotherapy 2005;25:1141–1146.

48 Hurvitz AP, Hodapp KL, Jadgchew J, et al: Central serous chorioretinopathy resulting in altered vision and color perception after glenohumeral corticosteroid injection. Orthopedics 2009;32:pii: orthosupersite.com/view. asp?rID=41926.

49 Kassam AA, White W, Ling RH, Kitson JB: Loss of visual acuity due to central serous retinopathy after steroid injection into the shoulder bursa. J Shoulder Elbow Surg 2011;20:e5–e6.

50 Mondal LK, Sarkar K, Datta H, Chatterjee PR: Acute bilateral central serous chorioretinopathy following intra-articular injection of corticosteroid. Indian J Ophthalmol 2005;53:132–134.

51 Ezra N, Taban M, Behroozan D: Central serous chorioretinopathy associated with topical corticosteroids in a patient with psoriasis. J Drugs Dermatol 2011; 10:918–921.

52 Fernandez CF, Mendoza AJ, Arevalo JF: Central serous chorioretinopathy associated with topical dermal corticosteroids. Retina 2004;24:471–474.

53 Karadimas P, Bouzas EA: Glucocorticoid use represents a risk factor for central serous chorioretinopathy: a prospective, case-control study. Graefes Arch Clin Exp Ophthalmol 2004;242:800–802.

54 Romero P, Martinez I, Salvat M: Diffuse retinal pigment epitheliopathy and corticoid ointment topical treatment in a patient with psoriasis (in French). J Fr Ophtalmol 2005;28:1101–1104.

55 Baumal CR, Martidis A, Truong SN: Central serous chorioretinopathy associated with periocular corticosteroid injection treatment for HLA-B27-associated iritis. Arch Ophthalmol 2004;122: 926–928.

56 Khairallah M, Kahloun R, Tugal-Tutkun I: Central serous chorioretinopathy, corticosteroids, and uveitis. Ocul Immunol Inflamm 2012;20:76–85.

57 Haimovici R, Koh S, Gagnon DR, et al: Risk factors for central serous chorioretinopathy: a case-control study. Ophthalmology 2004;111:244–249.

58 Chumbley LC, Frank RN: Central serous retinopathy and pregnancy. Am J Ophthalmol 1974;77:158–160.

59 Errera M-H, Kohly RP, da Cruz L: Pregnancy-associated retinal diseases and their management. Surv Ophthalmol 2013;58:127–142.

60 Schultz KL, Birnbaum AD, Goldstein DA: Ocular disease in pregnancy. Curr Opin Ophthalmol 2005;16:308–314.

61 Bouzas EA, Scott MH, Mastorakos G, et al: Central serous chorioretinopathy in endogenous hypercortisolism. Arch Ophthalmol 1993;111:1229–1233.

62 Carvalho-Recchia CA, Yannuzzi LA, Negrão S, et al: Corticosteroids and central serous chorioretinopathy. Ophthalmology 2002;109:1834–1837.

63 Garg SP, Dada T, Talwar D, Biswas NR: Endogenous cortisol profile in patients with central serous chorioretinopathy. Br J Ophthalmol 1997;81:962–964.

64 Zakir SM, Shukla M, Simi ZU, et al: Serum cortisol and testosterone levels in idiopathic central serous chorioretinopathy. Indian J Ophthalmol 2009;57:419–422.

65 Kapetanios AD, Donati G, Bouzas E, et al: Serous central chorioretinopathy and endogenous hypercortisolemia (in German). Klin Monbl Augenheilkd 1998; 212:343–344.

66 Yannuzzi LA: Type A behavior and central serous chorioretinopathy. Trans Am Ophthalmol Soc 1986;84:799–845.

67 Tittl MK, Spaide RF, Wong D, et al: Systemic findings associated with central serous chorioretinopathy. Am J Ophthalmol 1999;128:63–68.

68 Fok ACT, Chan PPM, Lam DSC, Lai TYY: Risk factors for recurrence of serous macular detachment in untreated patients with central serous chorioretinopathy. Ophthalmic Res 2011;46:160–163.

69 Amalric P, Gourinat P, Rebière P: Is central serous choroiditis sometimes hereditary? (in French). Bull Soc Ophtalmol Fr 1971;71:163–168.

70 Haik GM, Perez LF, Murtagh JJ: Central serous retinopathy. Consecutive development in daughter and mother. Am J Ophthalmol 1968;65:612–615.

71 Lin E, Arrigg PG, Kim RY: Familial central serous choroidopathy. Graefes Arch Clin Exp Ophthalmol 2000;238:930–931.

72 Oosterhuis JA: Familial central serous retinopathy. Graefes Arch Clin Exp Ophthalmol 1996;234:337–341.

73 Park DW, Schatz H, Gaffney MM, et al: Central serous chorioretinopathy in two families. Eur J Ophthalmol 1998;8:42–47.

74 Wyman GJ: Central serous retinopathy in twins. Am J Ophthalmol 1963;55: 1265.

75 Weenink AC, Borsje RA, Oosterhuis JA: Familial chronic central serous chorioretinopathy. Ophthalmologica 2001;215: 183–187.

76 Miki A, Kondo N, Yanagisawa S, et al: Common Variants in the Complement Factor H Gene Confer Genetic Susceptibility to Central Serous Chorioretinopathy. Ophthalmology 2014;121:1067–1072.

77 Schubert C, Pryds A, Zeng S, et al: Cadherin 5 is regulated by corticosteroids and associated with central serous chorioretinopathy. Hum Mutat 2014;35: 859–867.

78 Eom Y, Oh J, Kim SW, Huh K: Systemic factors associated with central serous chorioretinopathy in Koreans. Korean J Ophthalmol 2012;26:260–264.

79 Chen S-N, Chen Y-C, Lian I: Increased risk of coronary heart disease in male patients with central serous chorioretinopathy: results of a population-based cohort study. Br J Ophthalmol 2014;98: 110–114.

80 Tsai D-C, Huang C-C, Chen S-J, et al: Central serous chorioretinopathy and risk of ischaemic stroke: a population-based cohort study. Br J Ophthalmol 2012;96:1484–1488.

81 Tsai D-C, Huang C-C, Chen S-J, et al: Increased risk of erectile dysfunction among males with central serous chorioretinopathy – a retrospective cohort study. Acta Ophthalmol 2013;91:666–671.

82 Tewari HK, Gadia R, Kumar D, et al: Sympathetic-parasympathetic activity and reactivity in central serous chorioretinopathy: a case-control study. Invest Ophthalmol Vis Sci 2006;47:3474–3478.

83 Mansuetta CC, Mason JO 3rd, Swanner J, et al: An association between central serous chorioretinopathy and gastroesophageal reflux disease. Am J Ophthalmol 2004;137:1096–1100.

84 Ahnoux-Zabsonre A, Quaranta M, Mauget-Faÿsse M: Prevalence of *Helicobacter pylori* in central serous chorioretinopathy and diffuse retinal epitheliopathy: a complementary study (in French). J Fr Ophtalmol 2004;27:1129–1133.

85 Cotticelli L, Borrelli M, D'Alessio AC, et al: Central serous chorioretinopathy and *Helicobacter pylori*. Eur J Ophthalmol 2006;16:274–278.

86 Giusti C: Central serous chorioretinopathy: a new extragastric manifestation of *Helicobacter pylori*?: Analysis of a clinical case (in Italian). Clin Ter 2001;152: 393–397.

87 Mateo-Montoya A, Mauget-Faÿse M: *Helicobacter pylori* as a risk factor for central serous chorioretinopathy: literature review. World J Gastrointest Pathophysiol 2014;5:355–358.

88 Mauget-Faÿsse M, Kodjikian L, Quaranta M, et al: *Helicobacter pylori* in central serous chorioretinopathy and diffuse retinal epitheliopathy. Results of the first prospective pilot study (in French). J Fr Ophtalmol 2002;25:1021–1025.

89 Roshani M, Davoodi NA, Seyyedmajidi MR, et al: Association of *Helicobacter pylori* with central serous chorioretinopathy in Iranian patients. Gastroenterol Hepatol Bed Bench 2014;7:63–67.

90 Aliferis K, Petropoulos IK, Farpour B, et al: Should central serous chorioretinopathy be added to the list of ocular side effects of phosphodiesterase 5 inhibitors? Ophthalmologica 2012;227:85–89.

91 Fraunfelder FW, Fraunfelder FT: Central serous chorioretinopathy associated with sildenafil. Retina 2008;28:606–609.

92 McCannel TA, Chmielowski B, Finn RS, et al: Bilateral subfoveal neurosensory retinal detachment associated with MEK inhibitor use for metastatic cancer. JAMA Ophthalmol 2014;132:1005–1009.

93 Urner-Bloch U, Urner M, Stieger P, et al: Transient MEK inhibitor-associated retinopathy in metastatic melanoma. Ann Oncol 2014;25:1437–1441.

94 Kloos P, Laube I, Thoelen A: Obstructive sleep apnea in patients with central serous chorioretinopathy. Graefes Arch Clin Exp Ophthalmol 2008;246:1225–1228.

95 Brodie FL, Charlson ES, Aleman TS, et al: Obstructive sleep apnea and central serous chorioretinopathy. Retina 2015;35:238–243.

96 Zhao M, Célérier I, Bousquet E, et al: Mineralocorticoid receptor is involved in rat and human ocular chorioretinopathy. J Clin Invest 2012;122:2672–2679.

97 Zhao M, Valamanesh F, Celerier I, et al: The neuroretina is a novel mineralocorticoid target: aldosterone up-regulates ion and water channels in Müller glial cells. FASEB J 2010;24:3405–3415.

98 Bousquet E, Beydoun T, Zhao M, et al: Mineralocorticoid receptor antagonism in the treatment of chronic central serous chorioretinopathy: a pilot study. Retina 2013;33:2096–2102.

99 Yannuzzi LA: Central serous chorioretinopathy: a personal perspective. Am J Ophthalmol 2010;149:361–363.

100 Nicholson B, Noble J, Forooghian F, Meyerle C: Central serous chorioretinopathy: update on pathophysiology and treatment. Surv Ophthalmol 2013;58:103–126.

101 Polak BC, Baarsma GS, Snyers B: Diffuse retinal pigment epitheliopathy complicating systemic corticosteroid treatment. Br J Ophthalmol 1995;79:922–925.

102 Sharma T, Shah N, Rao M, et al: Visual outcome after discontinuation of corticosteroids in atypical severe central serous chorioretinopathy. Ophthalmology 2004;111:1708–1714.

103 Wakakura M, Song E, Ishikawa S: Corticosteroid-induced central serous chorioretinopathy. Jpn J Ophthalmol 1997;41:180–185.

104 Williamson J, Nuki G: Macular lesions during systemic therapy with depot tetracosactrin. Br J Ophthalmol 1970;54:405–409.

105 Jain AK, Kaines A, Schwartz S: Bilateral central serous chorioretinopathy resolving rapidly with treatment for obstructive sleep apnea. Graefes Arch Clin Exp Ophthalmol 2010;248:1037–1039.

106 Robertson DM, Ilstrup D: Direct, indirect, and sham laser photocoagulation in the management of central serous chorioretinopathy. Am J Ophthalmol 1983;95:457–466.

107 Lim JW, Kang SW, Kim Y-T, et al: Comparative study of patients with central serous chorioretinopathy undergoing focal laser photocoagulation or photodynamic therapy. Br J Ophthalmol 2011;95:514–517.

108 Leaver P, Williams C: Argon laser photocoagulation in the treatment of central serous retinopathy. Br J Ophthalmol 1979;63:674–677.

109 Gilbert CM, Owens SL, Smith PD, Fine SL: Long-term follow-up of central serous chorioretinopathy. Br J Ophthalmol 1984;68:815–820.

110 Brancato R, Scialdone A, Pece A, et al: Eight-year follow-up of central serous chorioretinopathy with and without laser treatment. Graefes Arch Clin Exp Ophthalmol 1987;225:166–168.

111 Ficker L, Vafidis G, While A, Leaver P: Long-term follow-up of a prospective trial of argon laser photocoagulation in the treatment of central serous retinopathy. Br J Ophthalmol 1988;72:829–834.

112 Verma L, Sinha R, Venkatesh P, Tewari HK: Comparative evaluation of diode laser versus argon laser photocoagulation in patients with central serous retinopathy: a pilot, randomized controlled trial [ISRCTN84128484]. BMC Ophthalmol 2004;4:15.

113 Chan WM, Lam DSC, Lai TYY, et al: Choroidal vascular remodelling in central serous chorioretinopathy after indocyanine green guided photodynamic therapy with verteporfin: a novel treatment at the primary disease level. Br J Ophthalmol 2003;87:1453–1458.

114 Schlötzer-Schrehardt U, Viestenz A, Naumann GO, et al: Dose-related structural effects of photodynamic therapy on choroidal and retinal structures of human eyes. Graefes Arch Clin Exp Ophthalmol 2002;240:748–757.

115 Reibaldi M, Cardascia N, Longo A, et al: Standard-fluence versus low-fluence photodynamic therapy in chronic central serous chorioretinopathy: a nonrandomized clinical trial. Am J Ophthalmol 2010;149:307–315.e2.

116 Lim JI, Glassman AR, Aiello LP, et al: Collaborative retrospective macula society study of photodynamic therapy for chronic central serous chorioretinopathy. Ophthalmology 2014;121:1073–1078.

117 Bousquet E, Beydoun T, Rothschild PR, et al: Spironolactone for nonresolving central serous chorioretinopathy: a randomized controlled crossover study. Retina 2015;35:2505–2515.

118 Herold TR, Prause K, Wolf A, et al: Spironolactone in the treatment of central serous chorioretinopathy – a case series. Graefes Arch Clin Exp Ophthalmol 2014;252:1985–1991.

119 Singh RP, Sears JE, Bedi R, et al: Oral eplerenone for the management of chronic central serous chorioretinopathy. Int J Ophthalmol 2015;8:310–314.

120 Funder JW: Mineralocorticoid receptor antagonists: emerging roles in cardiovascular medicine. Integr Blood Press Control 2013;6:129–138.

121 Chan W-M, Lai TYY, Liu DTL, Lam DSC: Intravitreal bevacizumab (avastin) for choroidal neovascularization secondary to central serous chorioretinopathy, secondary to punctate inner choroidopathy, or of idiopathic origin. Am J Ophthalmol 2007;143:977–983.

122 Konstantinidis L, Mantel I, Zografos L, Ambresin A: Intravitreal ranibizumab in the treatment of choroidal neovascularization associated with idiopathic central serous chorioretinopathy. Eur J Ophthalmol 2010;20:955–958.

123 Broadhead GK, Chang A: Intravitreal aflibercept for choroidal neovascularisation complicating chronic central serous chorioretinopathy. Graefes Arch Clin Exp Ophthalmol 2015;253:1217–1225.

Prof. Francine Behar-Cohen
University of Lausanne
Avenue de France 15
CH–1004 Lausanne (Switzerland)
E-Mail francine.behar@gmail.com

Chapter 5

Coscas G (ed): Macular Edema. 2nd, revised and extended edition.
Dev Ophthalmol. Basel, Karger, 2017, vol 58, pp 39–62 (DOI: 10.1159/000455268)

Diagnosis and Detection

Giovanni Staurenghi · Marco Pellegrini · Alessandro Invernizzi · Chiara Preziosa

Eye Clinic, Department of Biomedical and Clinical Science "Luigi Sacco", Sacco Hospital, University of Milan, Milan, Italy

Abstract

The aim of the chapter is to provide a practical but exhaustive guide in detecting macular edema and to describe its features according to the retinal condition that causes it. The most useful imaging techniques (biomicroscopy, retinography, optical coherence tomography, and fluorescein/indocyanine-green angiography will be analyzed in order to identify the best diagnostic algorithm in each pathology. There is a table at the end of the chapter which summarizes the important points of the chapter. © 2017 S. Karger AG, Basel

Broadly defined, macular edema is an abnormal thickening of the macula associated with the accumulation of excess fluid in the extracellular space of the neurosensory retina. Intracellular edema involving Müller cells has also been observed histopathologically. The term 'cystoid macular edema' (CME) is applied when there is evidence by biomicroscopy, fluorescein angiography (FA), and/or optical coherence tomography (OCT) of fluid accumulation into multiple cyst-like spaces within the macula. Although the classical pathology of CME consists of large cystoid spaces in the outer plexiform layer of Henle, such fluid-filled spaces can be seen in various layers of the retina depending in part on the underlying etiology (Johnson, 2009)[1].

The standard clinical method for determining macular edema is the subjective assessment of the presence or absence of macular thickening by slit lamp fundus stereo biomicroscopy. The traditional methods of evaluating macular thickening, including slit lamp biomicroscopy and fundus photography, are useful for visualizing signs correlated with retinal thickness such as hard and soft exudates, hemorrhages, and microaneurysms, but traditional evaluating methods are relatively insensitive to small changes in retinal thickness and are unable to detect specific anatomic details especially at the vitreomacular interface.

Observation of the fundus is obtained with the combined use of a slit lamp and a Goldmann contact lens or a 90- or 70-dpt noncontact lens. This is a complex psychomotor process that is highly dependent on the observer's skill and experience, the level of patient cooperation, the degree of pupillary dilation, the amount of media opacity, and the pattern and extent of retinal edema.

In diabetic retinopathy, macular edema is considered to be clinically significant if the following apply: (1) presence of any retinal thickening within 500 µm of the foveal center, (2) lipid exudates within 500 µm of the foveal center with adjacent thickening, and (3) an area of thickening >1

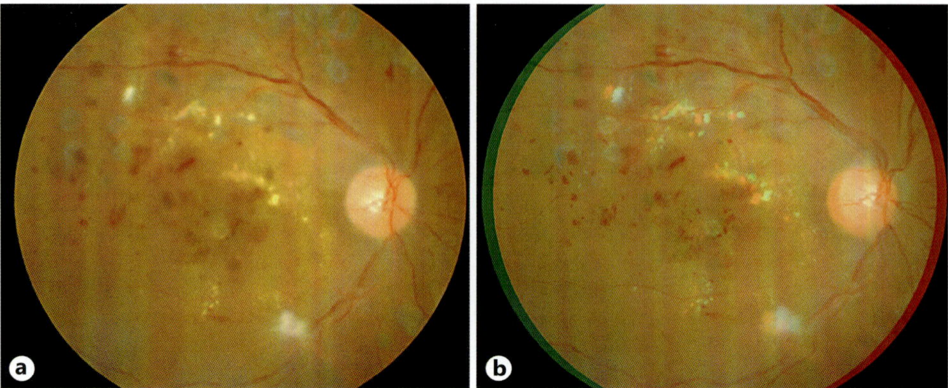

Fig. 1. Color pictures showing diabetic retinopathy. Macular edema and retinal thickness are better seen in a stereo image (wear red/cyan 3-dimensional goggles to visualize the stereo effect). **a** Single-frame image. **b** Stereo anaglyph image.

Macular Photocoagulation Study disk area (1 disk area = 1.767 mm^2) within 1 disk diameter (1.5 mm) of the foveal center (Early Treatment Diabetic Retinopathy Study Research Group, 1985)[2].

Fundus photography is used mainly for follow-up. This type of fundus photography is commonly used for clinical trials and used less in clinical practice. Stereo images, rather than a single image, are necessary to identify macular edema and retinal thickening (fig. 1).

Variations in the amount of stereopsis present in paired stereo photographs or in the threshold for thickening adopted by the observer may further complicate the accurate and reproducible detection of areas of edema. The lack of sensitivity of the clinical examination for detection of mild edema has been demonstrated for eyes with a foveal center thickness between 201 and 300 μm (200 defined as the upper limit of normal). Only 14% of eyes were noted to have foveal edema by contact lens biomicroscopy. The term 'subclinical foveal edema' describes such cases (Brown et al., 2004)[3]. Although the system proposed by Brown et al. is useful for the identification of foveal edema, it is not likely to identify cases of nonfoveal clinically significant macular edema – that is, if there was retinal thickening or hard exudates as-

sociated with adjacent retinal thickening observed within 500 ± 50 μm of the center of the foveal avascular zone or a zone or zones of retinal thickening 1 disk area or larger, any part of which was within 1 disk diameter of the center of the macula (Sadda et al., 2006)[4].

OCT is the criterion standard in the identification of CME. OCT is a noninvasive imaging modality that can determine the presence of CME by visualizing the fluid-filled spaces in the retina. The amount of CME can be monitored over time by quantifying the area of cystoid spaces on a cross-sectional image through the macula.

Studies have reported OCT to be comparable to FA in the evaluation of CME, especially with the newer high-resolution OCT scanners. The benefit of OCT is that it can quantify the thickness of the retina and allow quantitative measurements of macular edema over time. This noninvasive method is especially useful in monitoring the response to treatment. Newer OCT software has increased imaging resolution, which has led to the identification of specific patterns of CME (fig. 2).

While OCT provides an objective evaluation of macular edema and is displacing conventional subjective methods, the older evaluation tech-

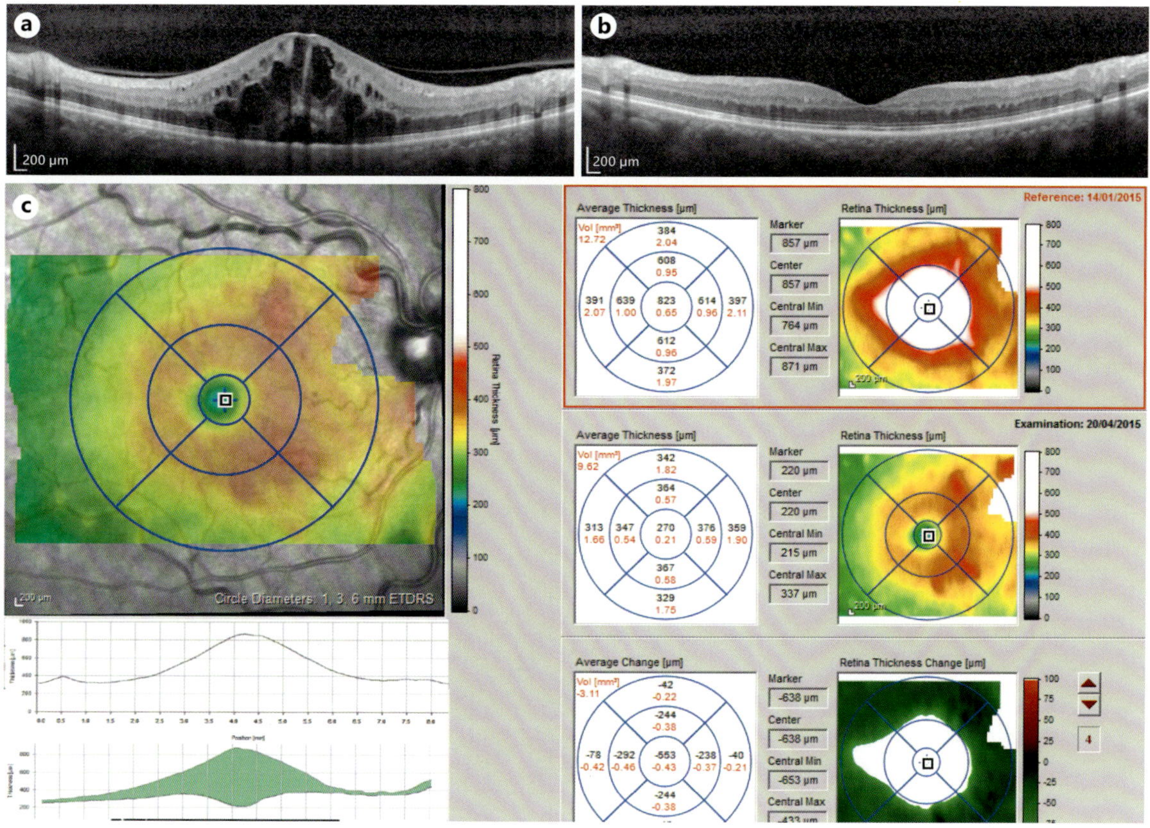

Fig. 2. OCT images of central vein occlusion with CME before (**a**) and after (**b**) treatment. The thickness map and differential thickness map (**c**) show resolution of the edema.

Table 1. Excitation and barrier wavelength for acquiring autofluorescence with different instruments

	Heidelberg HRA	Topcon	Zeiss 450	Nidek F10	Canon CX-I	Optos
Excitation wavelength, nm	488	550–605	510–580	490	≅500	532
Barrier filter, nm	500	670–720	695–755	510	>600	>600

niques still predominate, especially in the less developed world (Hee et al., 1998; Shahidi et al., 1994)[5, 6].

Fundus autofluorescence (FAF) is collects the fluorescence emitted by fluorophores of the retina. In particular, to excite lipofuscin, excitation between 470 and 550 nm can be used (Delori et al., 1995)[7].

More than 1 instrument is able to acquire an FAF picture using different wavelengths (table 1).

For visualization of macular edema, however, macular pigment plays a major role. In a normal blue FAF image, the dark spot visible in the central fovea is due to the macular pigment's absorption of the blue light used to excite lipofuscin autofluorescence. In the case of CME, by using blue FAF, it is possible

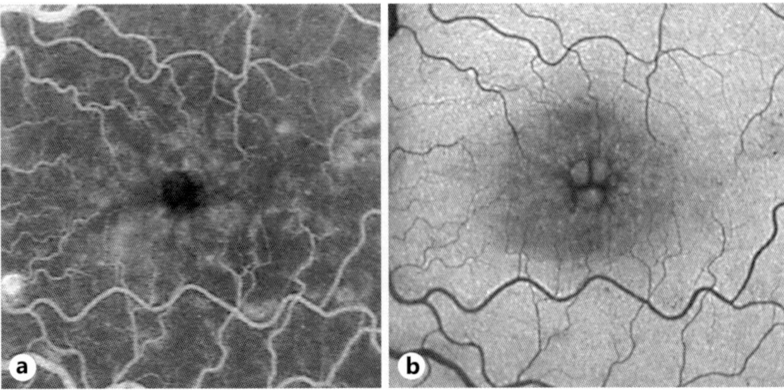

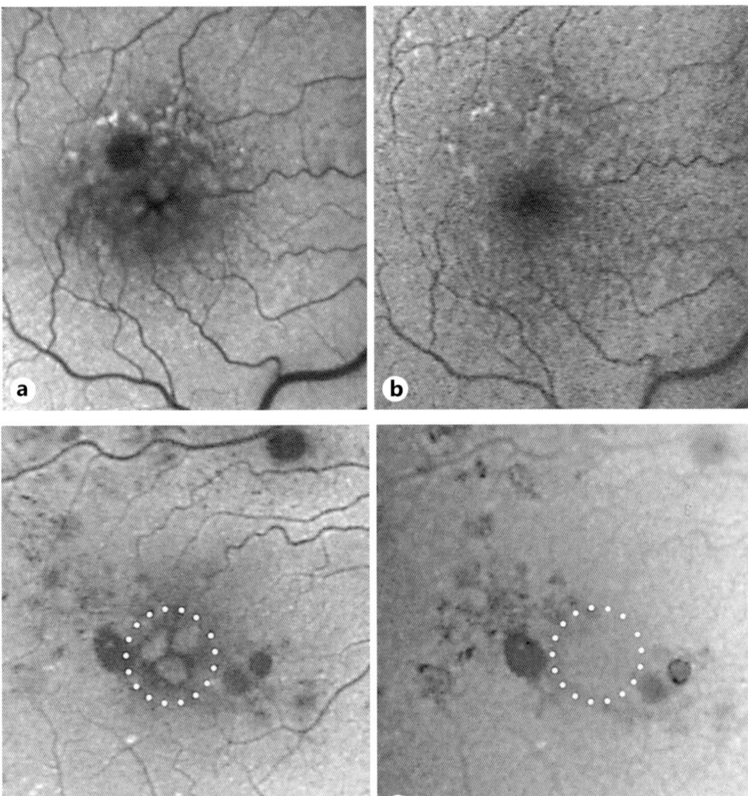

Fig. 3. CME secondary to CRVO visualized in FA (**a**) and 488-nm FAF (**b**).

Fig. 4. CME secondary to Crohn disease, before (**a**) and after (**b**) treatment. The disappearance of CME restored the characteristic darker central area of the macular pigment. **c, d** Patient with diabetic retinopathy and CME. 488-nm FAF (**c**) and 550- to 605-nm FAF (**d**) show the importance of visualization of macular pigment and its displacement for indirect visualization of CME (dotted circles). The inability to visualize macular pigment with green or yellow FAF explains the nonvisualization of CME.

to visualize displacement of macular pigment and consequently the cysts (fig. 3). This tool could be used to evaluate changes during follow-up (fig. 4, 5).

Currently FA is the most common technique used for the diagnosis of macular edema, although it only provides a qualitative assessment of vascular leakage for this pathology. FA illustrates minute dots of fluorescence that correspond to leakage adjacent to the terminal macular vessels. In the case of macular edema, the fluores-

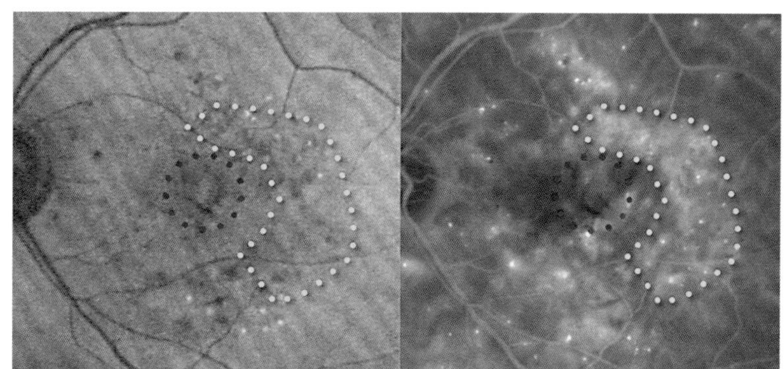

Fig. 5. Diabetic patient with diffuse macular edema and CME. As delimited by yellow dots, an area of diffuse edema is not clearly visible in 488-nm FAF (left). CME is visible in both images (red dotted circle). In contrast, diffuse edema is shown as a decrease in FAF intensity since the fluid under or inside the neurosensory retina is masking the fluorescence coming from the retinal pigment epithelium.

cence appears only in the late phase, becoming visible after 10–15 min. It appears around the fovea and extends centrally and peripherally, involving only a portion of the fovea. If the condition progresses into cyst formation at the macula, fluorescein can be seen to leak into the cysts. The edematous fluid accumulates in the outer plexiform layer of Henle over an area that is seldom more than 2 disk diameters.

Associated findings on FA may help determine the etiology of CME. If leaking microaneurysms are present in the setting of diabetic retinopathy, then diabetes is likely the cause. Vascular collaterals crossing the horizontal raphe on FA can help determine if the etiology of the edema (as well as retinal hemorrhages, if present) is likely due to a vascular occlusion.

Indocyanine green angiography (ICGA) is not considered an effective tool for detecting macular edema. In some cases, however, ICGA can be useful in assisting in or confirming a differential diagnosis.

More recently, a new imaging technique called OCT angiography (OCTA) has been introduced. This tool offers the possibility to quickly assess retinal and choroidal blood flow without the need for any dye injection. In contrast to regular FA and ICGA, which offer a dynamic evaluation of retinal and choroidal pathologies, OCTA is a static imaging technique not influenced by dye leakage, with the main advantage of offering information related to the depth of the lesion.

Considering Macular Edema Based on the Disease

Irvine-Gass Syndrome

The first identification of macular edema occurring after ocular surgery is attributed to Irvine (1953)[8] while its angiographic appearance was described by Gass (1997)[9] 13 years later. When CME develops following cataract surgery and its cause is thought to be directly related to the surgery, it is referred to as Irvine-Gass syndrome. Despite improvement in surgical techniques, this condition still represents one of the most frequent complications of cataract extraction.

When compared with normal postsurgical responses, the patient affected by postsurgical CME usually complains of blurred vision and reduced color perception and contrast sensibility.

The first set of images (fig. 6–13) shows a case of Irvine-Gass syndrome. At fundus examination, this condition usually appears as a blunted or irregular foveal light reflex with prominent cystic formations (fig. 6).

In autofluorescence (fig. 7), the cysts appear as hyperautofluorescent structures due to the shifting of the macular pigments that normally attenuate the autofluorescent signal in the macular region (Johnson, 2009)[1]. The appearance of the fundus alone is not usually enough to make an accurate diagnosis, so further examination is required.

The infrared retinography images (fig. 8) show a nonhomogeneous macular appearance while

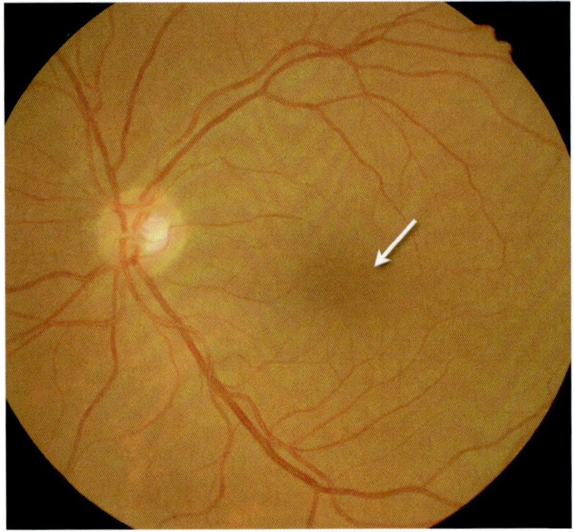

Fig. 6. Irvine-Gass syndrome. Fundus color photo. Arrow = CME.

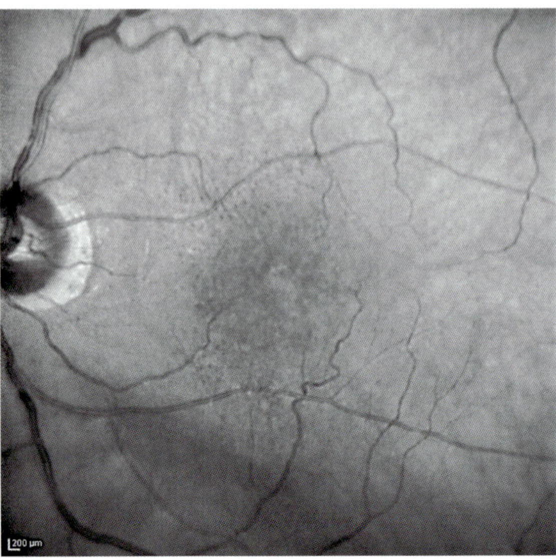

Fig. 8. Irvine-Gass syndrome. Infrared retinography.

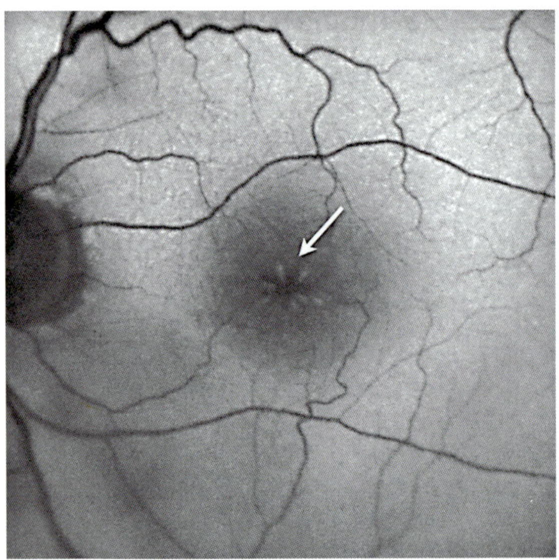

Fig. 7. Irvine-Gass syndrome. Autofluorescence. Arrow = CME.

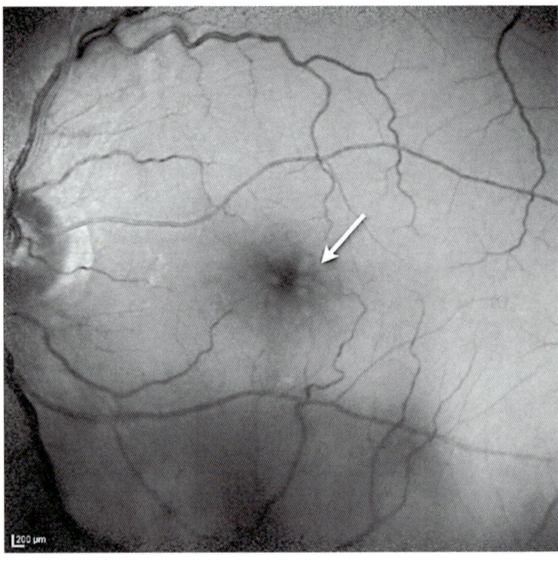

Fig. 9. Irvine-Gass syndrome. Red-free imaging. Arrow = CME.

red-free images (fig. 9) often show bright irregular and almost round shapes in the macular region.

FA (fig. 10) still represents the 'gold standard' test to be performed in this pathology: in early and midphases of the examination, a leakage from parafoveal retinal capillaries can be detected. In the late phases of the fluorescein angiogram, a progressive filling of the cystic spaces leads to a petaloid pattern of pooling in the mac-

Staurenghi · Pellegrini · Invernizzi · Preziosa

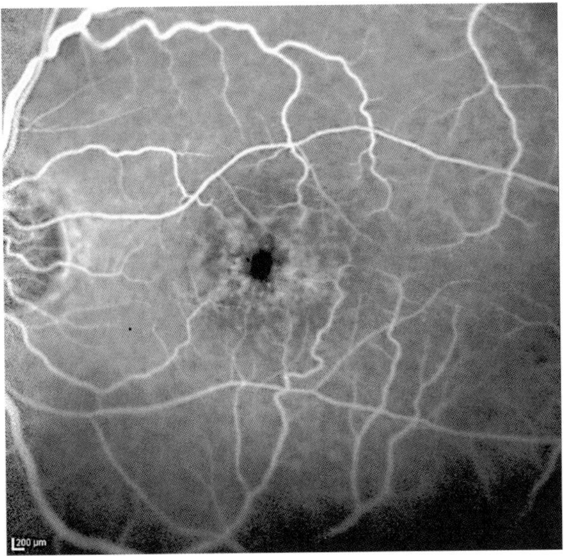

Fig. 10. Irvine-Gass syndrome. FA (early phases).

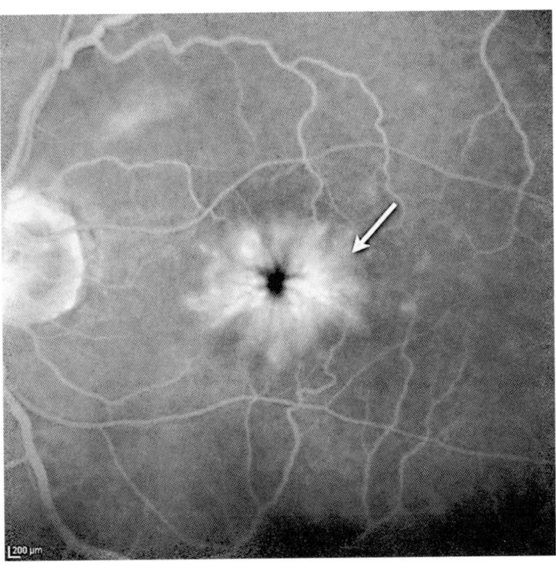

Fig. 11. Irvine-Gass syndrome. FA (late phases). Arrow = CME.

ula. A leakage of the optic disk usually appears in late-phase angiography (fig. 11).

ICGA (fig. 12) does not show any alterations except for a pooling in very late phases (Ray and D'Amico, 2002)[10]. Sometimes the amount of FA leakage does not correlate well with visual acuity; as a result, an important distinction between angiographic and clinically significant CME has to be considered.

Time domain OCT and more recently spectral domain OCT (fig. 13) have enabled this condition to be better defined and permit more accurate follow-up examinations. In addition, the presence of retinal thickening and cystoid spaces can be detected (usually in the foveal region of the outer retina and peripherally to the fovea in the inner retina). Sometimes a detachment of the neurosensory retina occurs which is easily visualized with OCT. No studies have been published yet related to OCTA and Irvine-Gass syndrome.

Irvine-Gass syndrome is often a self-limited pathology, and it can regress spontaneously. In some cases, postsurgical CME can persist for more than 6 months in a chronic form. In

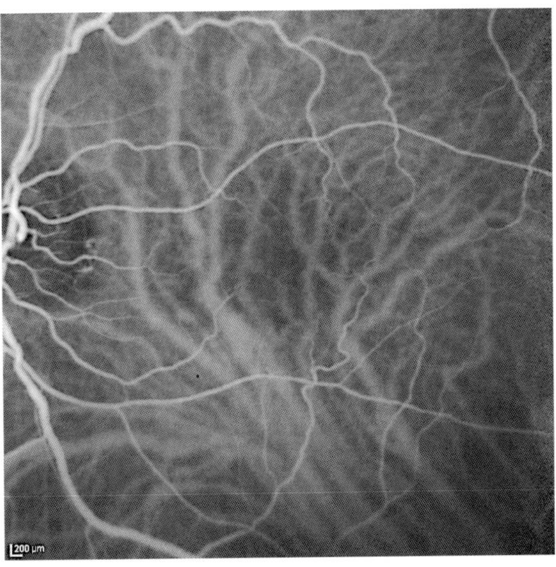

Fig. 12. Irvine-Gass syndrome. ICGA.

the chronic syndrome, cystic spaces can coalesce to develop a foveal macrocyst characterized by photoreceptor disruptions or even evolve with the formation of a lamellar macular hole.

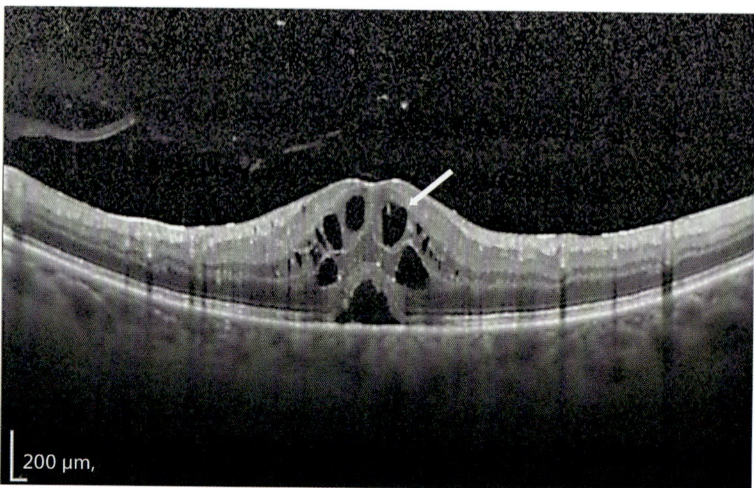

Fig. 13. Irvine-Gass syndrome. Spectral domain OCT. Arrow = CME.

Diabetic Macular Edema

Diabetic macular edema results from the inner blood-retinal barrier being compromised, which leads to leakage of plasma constituents in the surrounding retina. This condition represents the leading cause of legal blindness in the working-age population of most developed countries.

In diabetic retinopathy, at fundus examination (fig. 14), diabetic edema can appear as a localized or diffuse macular thickening depending on the severity of retinopathy. The localization of macular edema can be guided by the presence of characteristic elements such as microaneurysms and hard exudates.

Except for autofluorescence, retinography is not useful for the diagnosis of diabetic macular edema: infrared (fig. 15) and red-free (fig. 16) images can show microaneurysms, hard exudates, or hemorrhages; however, CME can sometimes be detected by infrared as hyperreflectant round areas. The autofluorescence (fig. 17) of cysts looks hyperautofluorescent because of the displacement of macular pigments that naturally attenuate the autofluorescent signal.

FA (fig. 18, 19) allows areas of focal versus diffuse edema to be distinguished: a focal edema consists of a well-defined, focal area of leakage

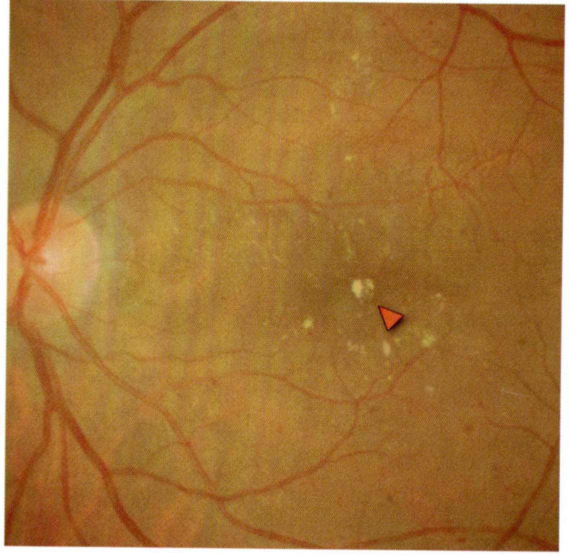

Fig. 14. Diabetic macular edema (arrowhead). Fundus examination.

from microaneurysms or dilated capillaries, whereas diffuse edema appears as a widespread zone of leakage from altered vascular structures. Diffuse cystoid edema can be detected by the presence of diffuse macular leakage accompanied by pooling of dye in cystic spaces (Bhagat et al., 2009)[11].

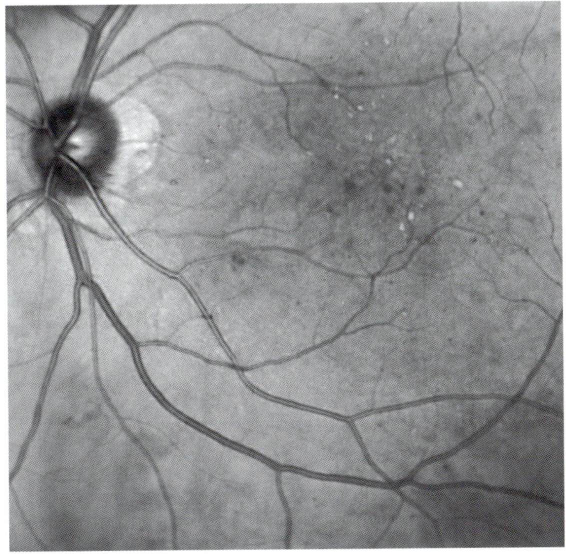

Fig. 15. Diabetic macular edema. Infrared imaging.

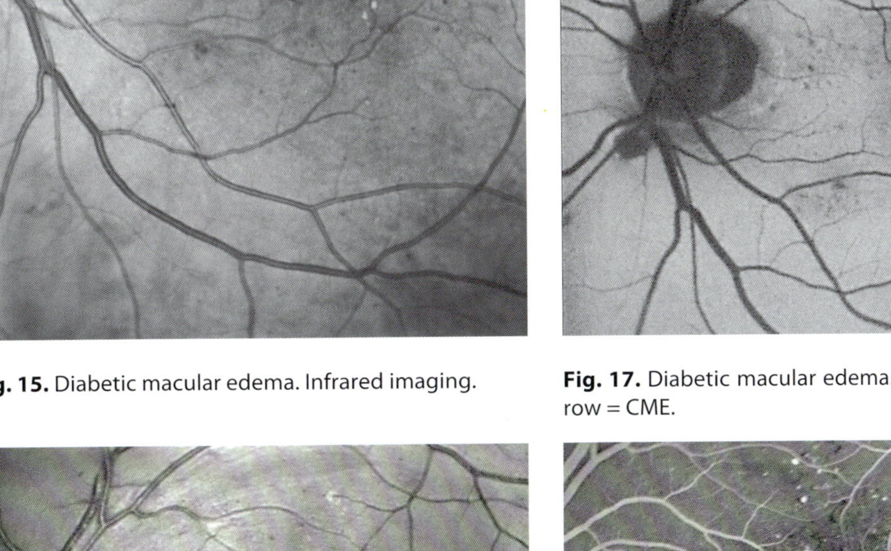

Fig. 17. Diabetic macular edema. Autofluorescence. Arrow = CME.

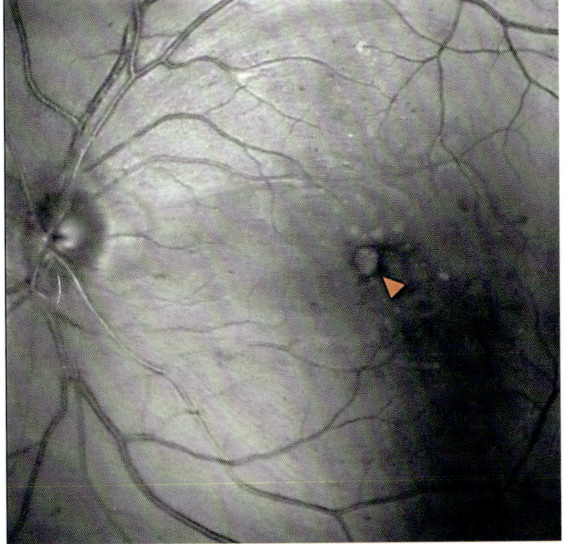

Fig. 16. Diabetic macular edema (arrowhead). Red-free imaging.

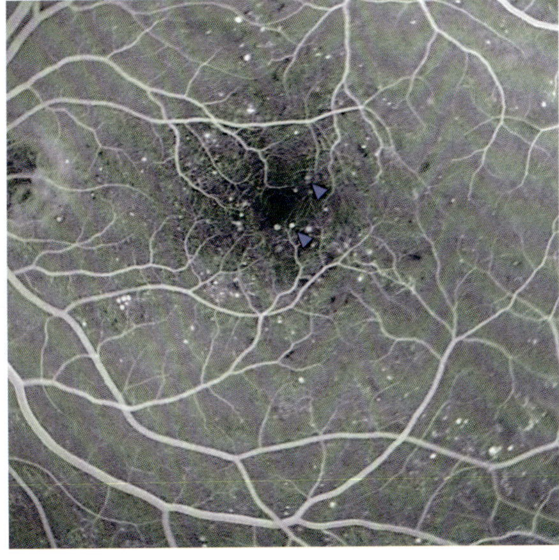

Fig. 18. Diabetic macular edema. FA (early phases). Blue arrowheads = Microaneurysms.

ICGA cannot be used to detect diabetic macular edema, but can reveal the presence and localization of a microaneurysm. Sometimes diabetic edema appears in ICGA, however, as diffuse hyperfluorescence due to a diabetic choroidopathy or due to a breakdown of the blood-retinal barrier (Weinberger et al., 1998)[12].

OCT represents an important tool, helpful both in the diagnosis and follow-up procedure. According to Kim et al. (2006)[13], macular edema

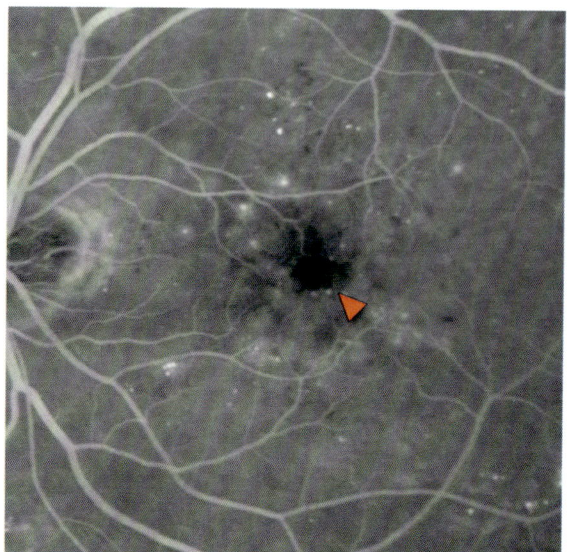

Fig. 19. Diabetic macular edema. FA (late phases). Red arrowhead = Hard exudates.

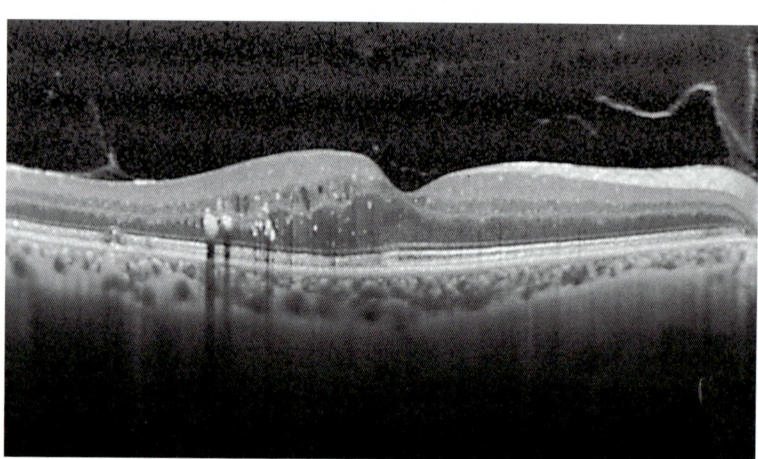

Fig. 20. Diabetic macular edema. Pattern I.

can assume 5 different morphologic patterns at OCT evaluation:

- *Pattern I* is a diffuse retinal thickening, which appears as increased retinal thickness with areas of reduced intraretinal reflectivity, especially in the outer retinal layers (fig. 20)
- *Pattern II* is CME, which appears as oval, only slightly reflective intraretinal cavities, separated by highly reflective septa (fig. 21)
- *Pattern III* shows posterior hyaloidal traction, which appears as a highly reflective band over the retinal surface (fig. 22)
- *Pattern IV* exhibits serous retinal detachment not associated with posterior hyaloidal traction, which appears as a dark accumulation of subretinal fluid beneath a highly reflective and dome-like elevation of detached retina (fig. 23)
- *Pattern V* shows posterior hyaloidal traction and tractional retinal detachment, which appear as a peak-shaped detachment with a highly reflective signal arising from the inner retinal surface and with an area of low signal beneath the highly reflective border of detached retina (fig. 24)

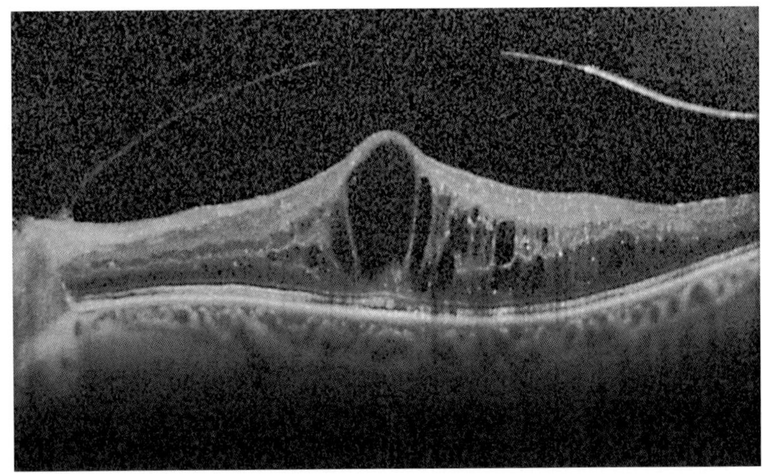

Fig. 21. Diabetic macular edema. Pattern II.

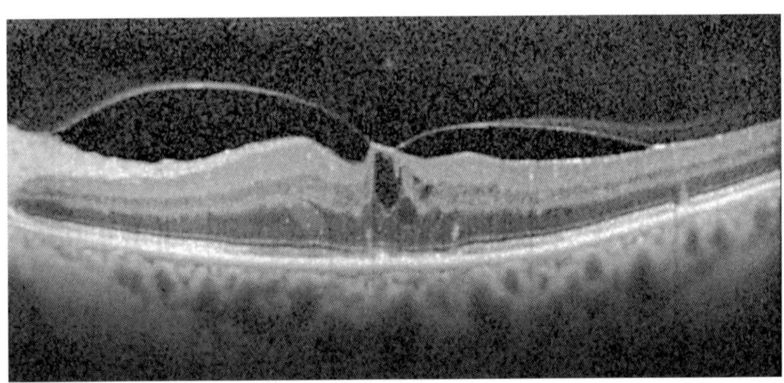

Fig. 22. Diabetic macular edema. Pattern III.

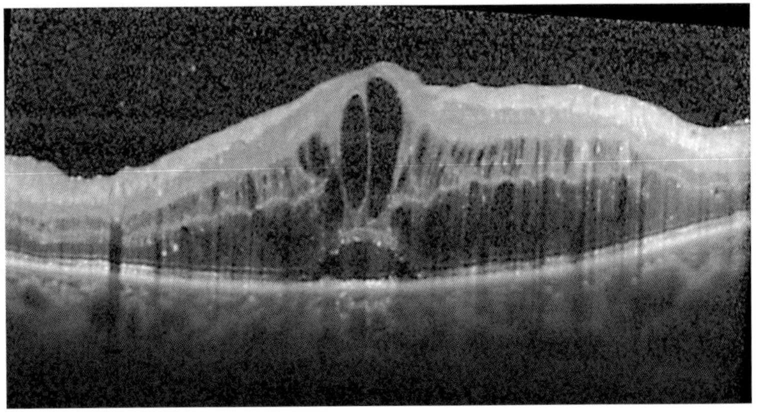

Fig. 23. Diabetic macular edema. Pattern IV.

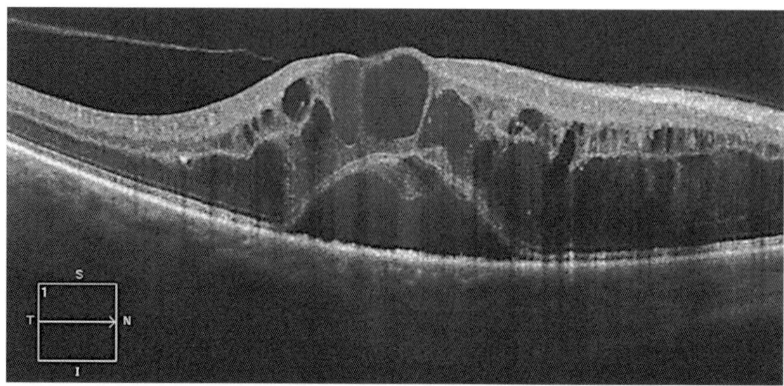

Fig. 24. Diabetic macular edema. Pattern V. S = Superior; N = nasal; I = inferior; T = temporal.

OCTA can visualize microaneurysms and areas of retinal nonperfusion: microaneurysms typically appear as focally dilated saccular or fusiform capillaries of both the superficial and deep capillary plexus. Studies using OCTA in patients with diabetic retinopathy have reported areas with absent or sparse capillaries which correlate with regions of nonperfusion seen on FA. Diabetic eyes were also found to have intraretinal edema appearing as black or grey spaces and irregularity or enlargement of the foveal avascular zone (fig. 25) during central retinal vein occlusion (CRVO; fig. 26, 27), while branch retinal vein occlusion (BRVO) usually involves a limited portion of the posterior pole (fig. 28–30).

In the late phases of the fluorescein angiogram, the pooling of dye into the cystic spaces is clearly visible. In CRVO in the mid-to-late phase there is papillary and vascular leakage (Tranos et al., 2004)[14].

OCT shows retinal thickening and/or CME involving 1 or more quadrants depending on the occlusion site and severity in BRVO (fig. 29), while it is diffuse in CRVO (fig. 27). CME consists of differently sized cysts affecting all the retinal layers and can sometimes be complicated by a neurosensory retinal detachment.

Uveitis

CME represents a common but not specific feature associated with uveitis, and it is the most frequent cause of vision loss in patients affected by this pathology. CME develops most commonly in pars planitis, birdshot retinochoroiditis, idiopathic acute iridocyclitis, and retinal vasculitis. CME also develops in anterior uveitis, HLA-B27-related uveitis, and any chronic uveitis. Since CME is not specific to a typical category of uveitis, global examination of the patient including FA and ICGA, inflammatory indexes, and immunohistochemical analysis should be required (Johnson, 2009)[1].

FA (fig. 31) and ICGA (fig. 32) are useful in order to characterize the vascular involvement and help to classify the vasculitic processes as either occlusive or nonocclusive.

OCT (fig. 33) is helpful to distinguish the retinal thickening and allows the presence of inflammatory epiretinal membranes, alterations in vitreoretinal interfaces, and uveitic macular edema to be detected.

CME associated with uveitis can appear with 3 different patterns depending on its localization and extension (Roesel et al., 2009)[15]: (1) cysts involving the inner layers, (2) cysts involving the outer plexiform layer, and (3) cysts involving all the retinal thickness associated with a disruption or loss of the photoreceptors' inner-outer segment junction. In chronic CME, fluid accumulation is associated with thinning of the retina and fibrosis.

No studies related to OCTA patterns in different uveitis have been published; nevertheless,

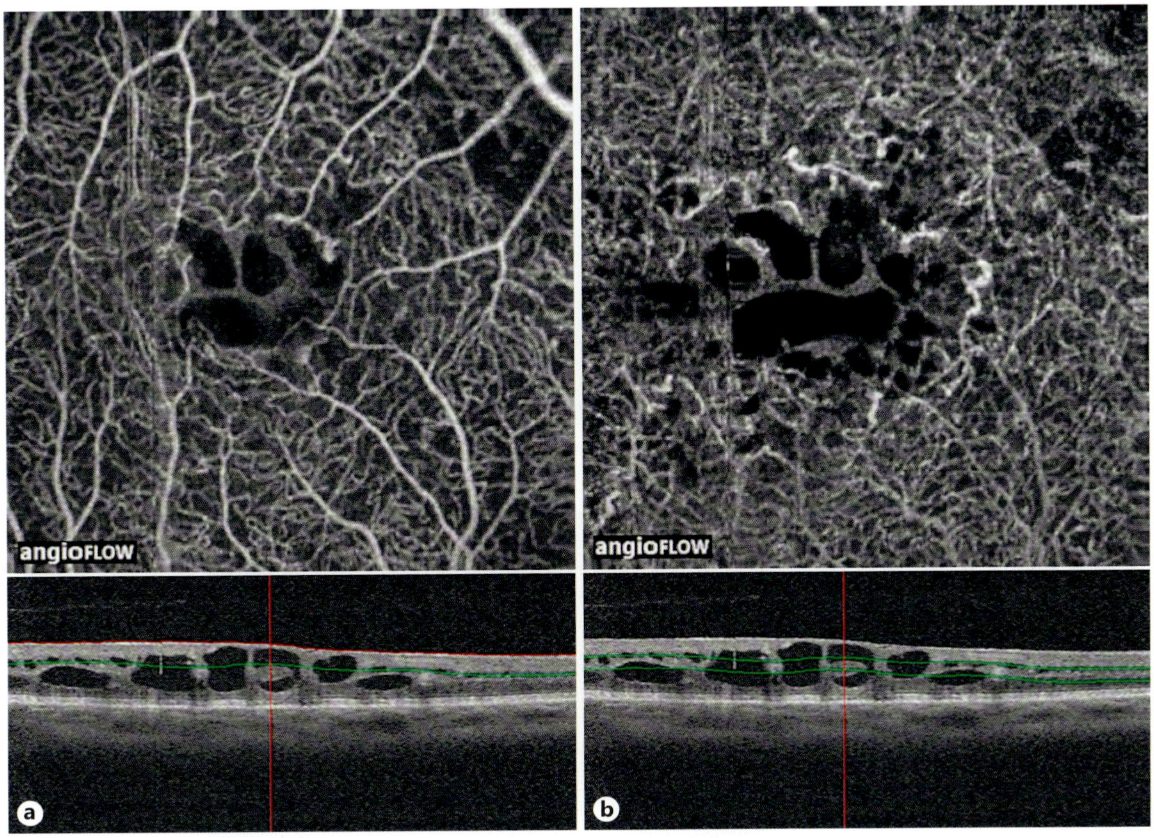

Fig. 25. Diabetic macular edema. OCTA.

this tool may be used to study areas of retinal and choriocapillaris nonperfusion or rule out a possible secondary choroidal neovascularization (CNV).

Vitreoretinal Tractional Conditions
Vitreoretinal tractional conditions can sometimes be characterized by a particular type of CME. At biomicroscopy examination, CME is difficult to detect since the posterior pole appearance is usually subverted by the epiretinal membrane. Retinography or FA does not provide further information about CME features, but both can be useful in visualizing epiretinal membrane traction lines or pooling of dye in the cystic spaces.

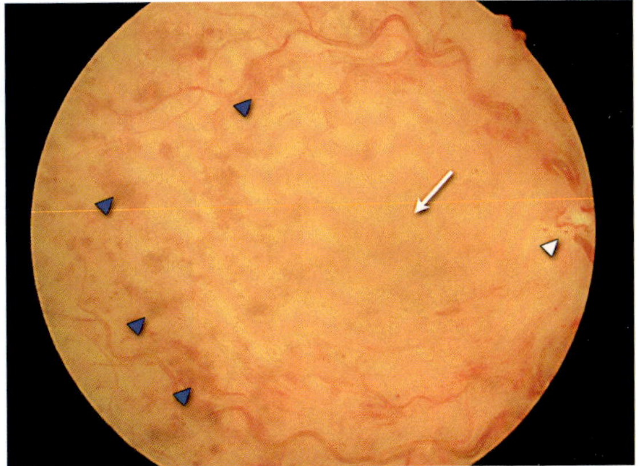

Fig. 26. Fundus CRVO. White arrow = CME; blue arrowheads = hemorrhages; white arrowhead = thrombotic vessel.

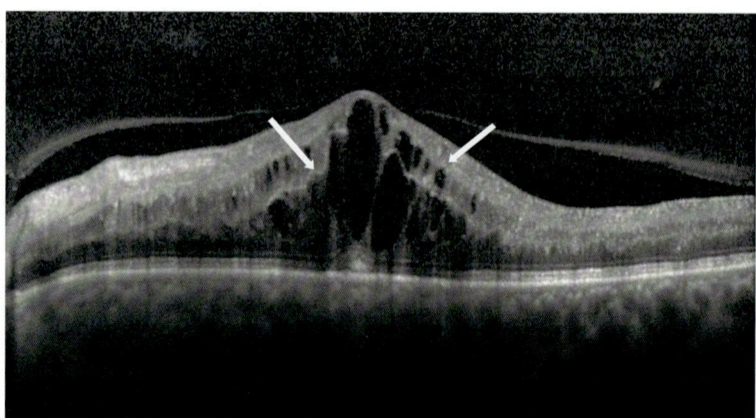

Fig. 27. OCT of CRVO. Arrows = CME.

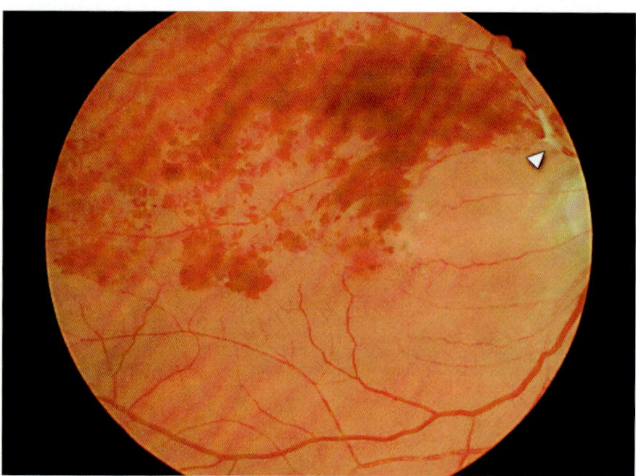

Fig. 28. Fundus BRVO. Arrowhead = Thrombotic vessel.

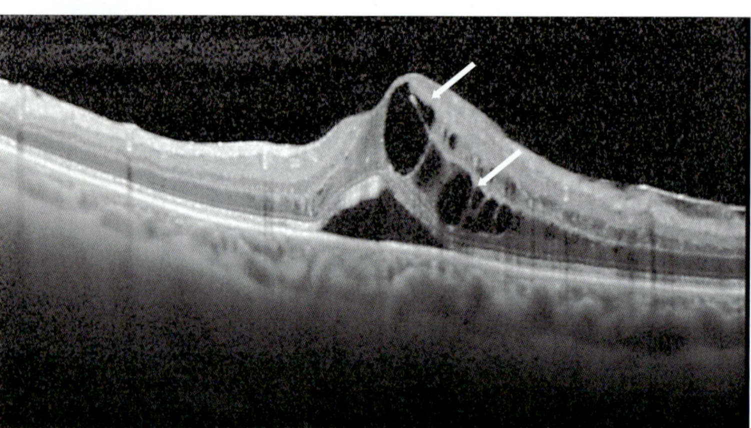

Fig. 29. OCT of BRVO.

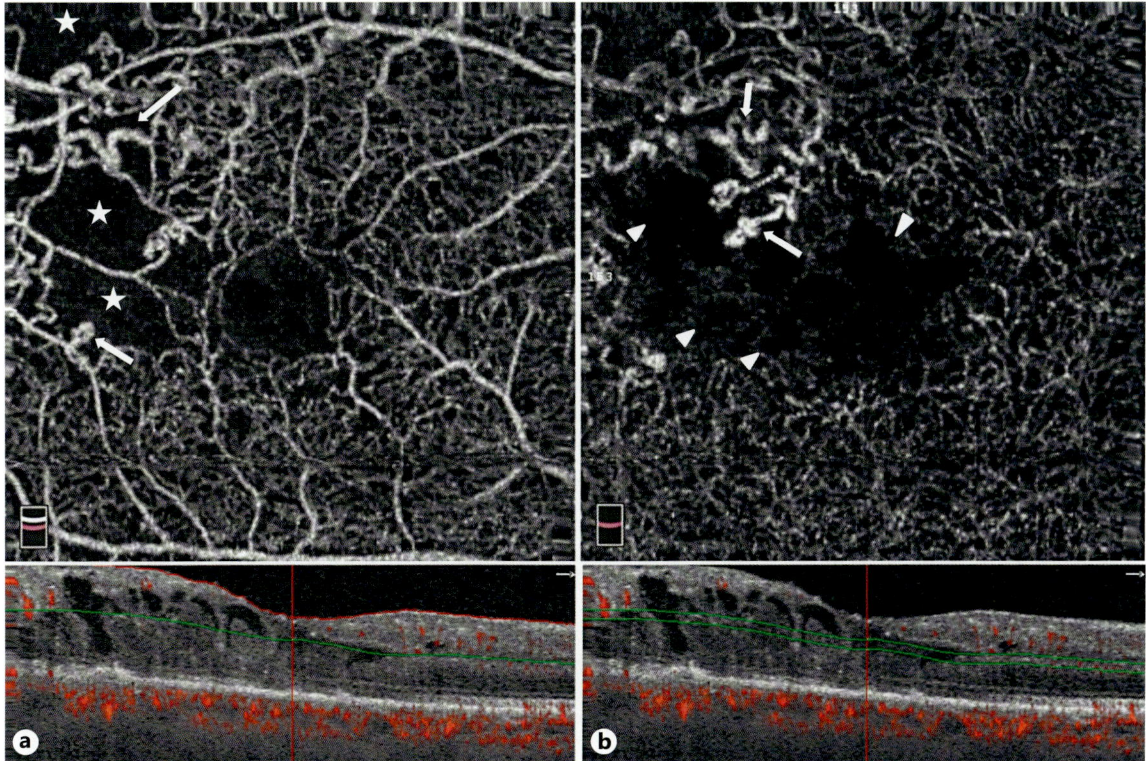

Fig. 30. OCTA of BRVO. Superficial (**a**) and deep (**b**) capillary plexus. Capillary network abnormalities including capillary network disruption and dilation are observed in both the superficial and deep capillary plexus (arrows). Dark areas with reduced capillary density are clearly visible in the superficial capillary plexus and probably correspond to nonperfuse territories (stars); in the deep capillary plexus cystoid spaces appear as well defined, black, circular areas with no flow signal (arrowheads).

OCT represents the most helpful tool for the diagnosis and follow-up of these pathologies. OCT can show perifoveal vitreous detachment, a thickened hyperreflective posterior hyaloid, and epiretinal membranes. CME can appear as multiple cystic spaces (fig. 34) or with a typical pagoda-shaped profile, especially when the edema is caused by an incomplete vitreous detachment, such as a gull-wing posterior vitreous detachment (fig. 35). Sometimes a neurosensory retinal detachment occurs. The macular traction may resolve in the formation of a lamellar macular hole (Tranos et al., 2004)[14].

OCTA, thanks to the possibility to perform high resolution imaging of retinal circulation, may be used to show the amount and direction of vascular dragging and check superficial and deep retinal vascular plexi after surgery.

Idiopathic Macular Telangiectasias
Idiopathic macular telangiectasia is a retinal disorder characterized by the presence of dilated ectasias of retinal capillaries that can lead to chronic macular edema. A recent classification includes two different types of idiopathic macular telangiectasias (Charbel Issa et al., 2008)[16]:
- *Type 1* shows aneurysmal telangiectasia which is visible at fundus examination and affects men in their midlife; this variant usually has a unilateral presentation.

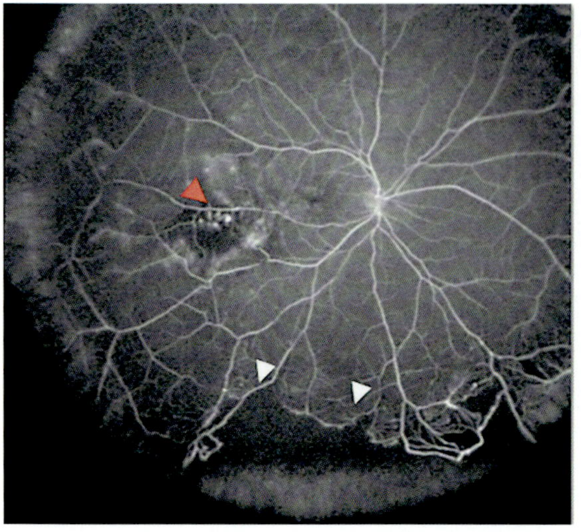

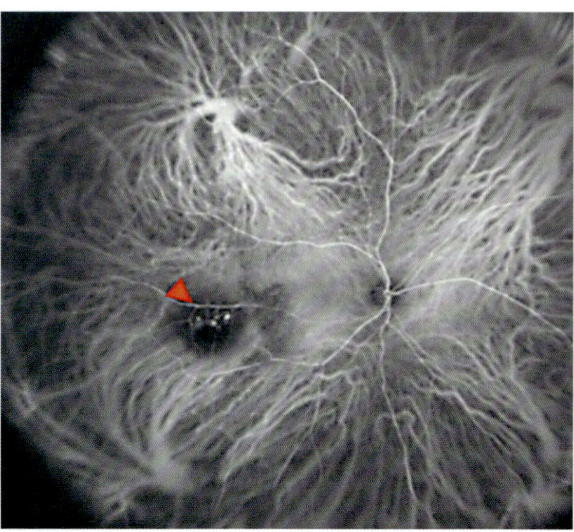

Fig. 31. Uveitis. FA, wide field. Red arrowhead = Vessel abnormalities; white arrowheads = ischemic areas.

Fig. 32. Uveitis. ICGA, wide field. Red arrowhead = Vessel abnormalities.

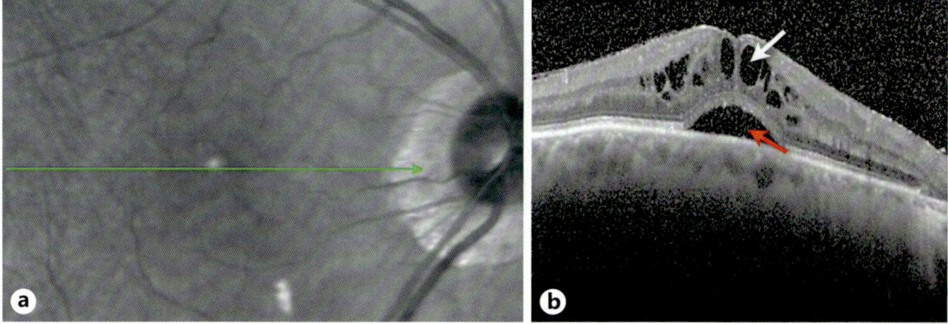

Fig. 33. Uveitis. **a** Site of imaging. **b** OCT. White arrow = CME; red arrow = neuroretinal detachment.

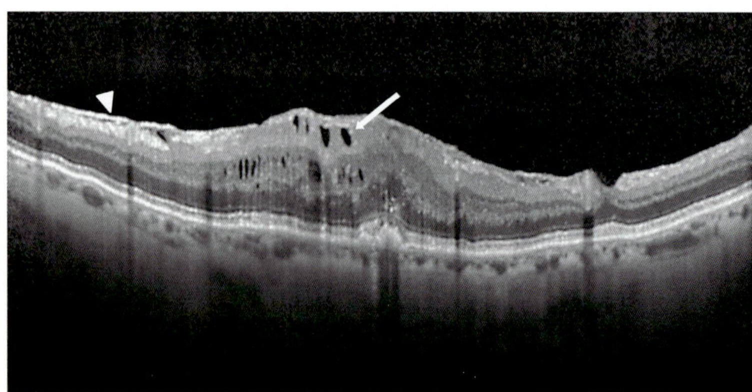

Fig. 34. Vitreoretinal tractional conditions. OCT. Arrow = CME; arrowhead = epiretinal membrane.

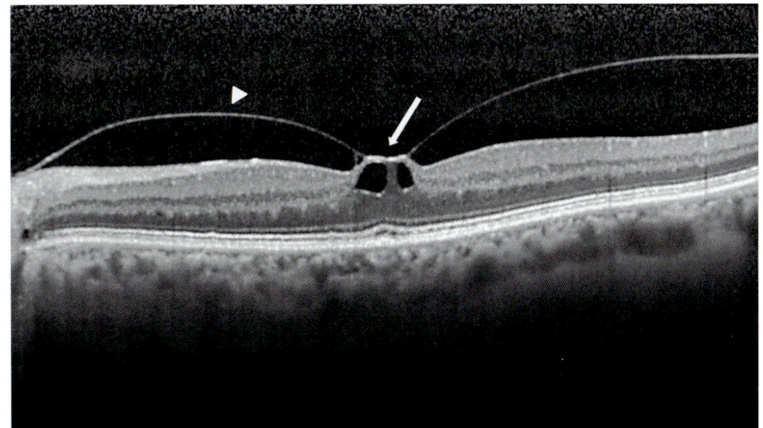

Fig. 35. Vitreoretinal tractional conditions. OCT. White arrow = CME; green arrowhead = gull-wing posterior vitreous detachment.

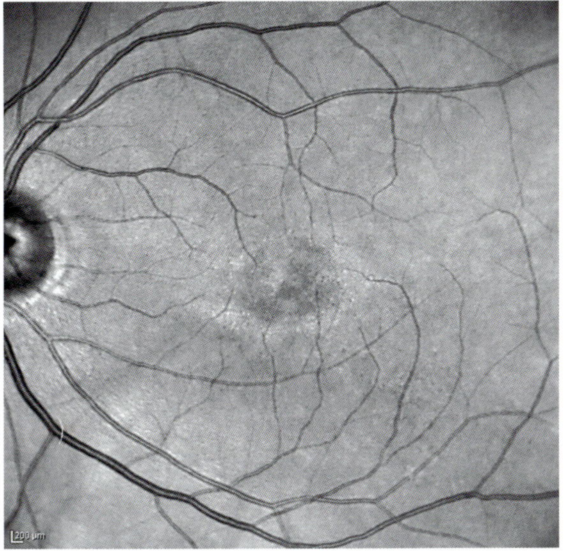

Fig. 36. Idiopathic macular telangiectasias. Infrared retinography.

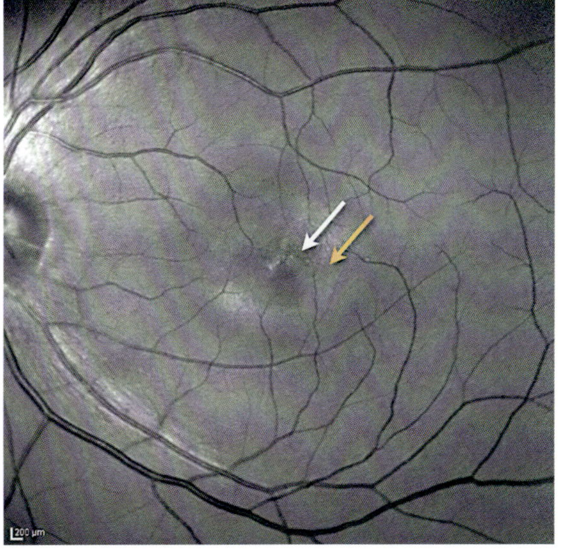

Fig. 37. Idiopathic macular telangiectasias. Red-free imaging. White arrow = CME; orange arrow = areas of macular pigment loss.

- *Type 2* exhibits perifoveal telangiectasia which is not visible at fundus examination; this category is usually bilateral, without sex preference, and affects people between 50 and 60 years of age.

Important information can be acquired from retinal imaging. Regarding retinography, in infrared imaging (fig. 36), macular cystic spaces appear as hyporeflectant, almost round zones. In red-free/confocal blue reflectance imaging (Heidelberg HRA2, 488 nm; fig. 37), a focal or oval hyperreflectance pattern is usually detectable, and it usually appears larger than the hyperfluorescent area characterized in FA images, thus sug-

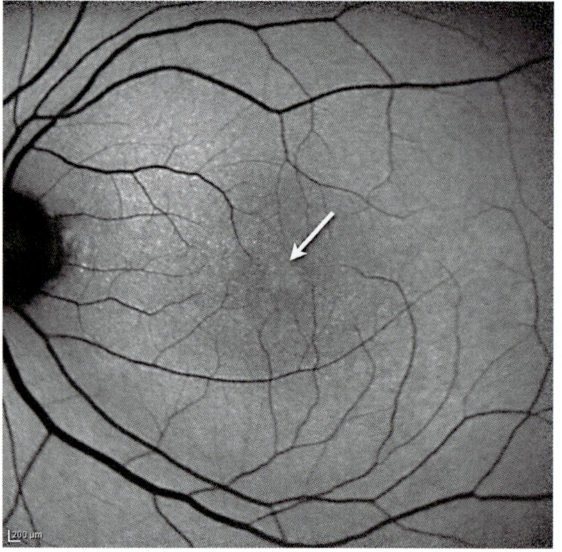

Fig. 38. Idiopathic macular telangiectasias. Autofluorescence. Arrow = CME.

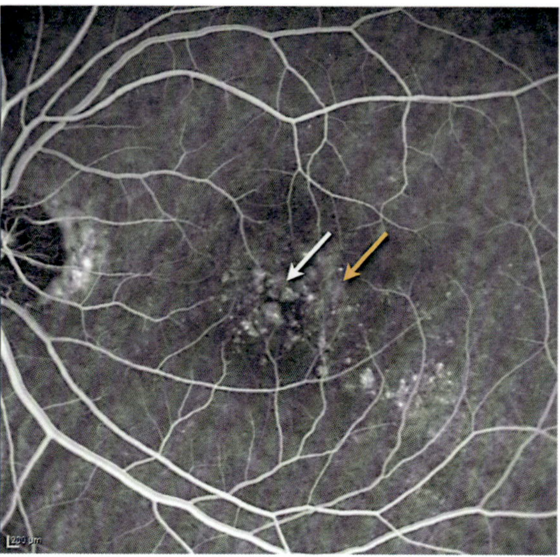

Fig. 39. Idiopathic macular telangiectasias. FA (early phases). White arrow = CME; orange arrow = areas of macular pigment loss.

gesting that the margins of the lesion go beyond the angiographically appearing leakage. Parafoveal deposits appear as spots with increased reflectance. A circle area of hyperreflectance around the macula (due to a lack of macular pigment) can be observed. A correspondence between areas of increased confocal blue reflectance and increased autofluorescence in the perifoveal area can be seen; areas of only increased confocal blue reflectance reveal a normal outer retina in OCT. In autofluorescence (fig. 38), macular cystic spaces appear as hyperautofluorescent almost round zones, and the highest central autofluorescence of longstanding cysts may suggest the loss of foveal macular pigments and photoreceptors. A correlation can be shown between areas of increased confocal blue reflectance and increased autofluorescence in the perifoveal region.

In FA (fig. 39, 40), parafoveal telangiectatic capillaries can be detected in the early angiographic phases (fig. 39). In the mid- to late phases (fig. 40) of the examination, FA images reveal hy-

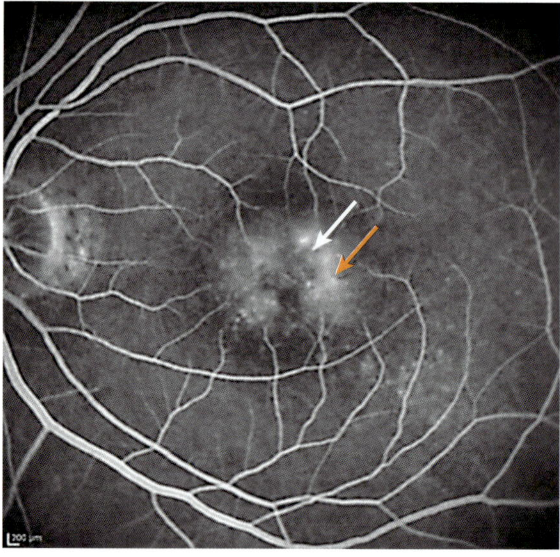

Fig. 40. Idiopathic macular telangiectasias. FA (late phases). White arrow = CME; orange arrow = areas of macular pigment loss.

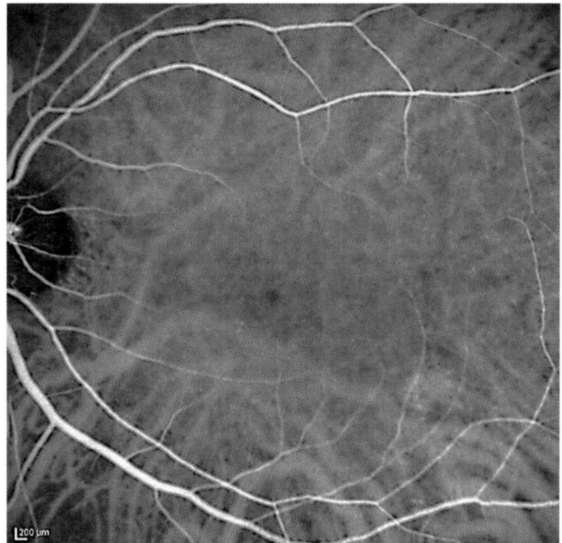

Fig. 41. Idiopathic macular telangiectasias. ICGA.

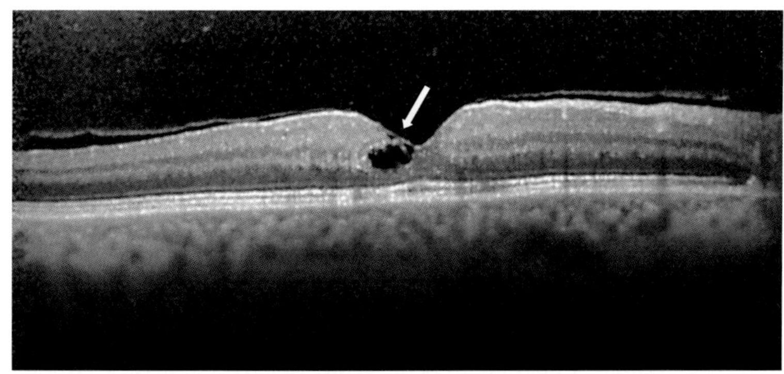

Fig. 42. Idiopathic macular telangiectasias type 2. OCT. Arrow = retinal pseudocyst.

perfluorescent areas corresponding to zones of macular pigment loss in autofluorescence and of increased reflectance in red-free zones. The areas of late hyperfluorescence show abnormalities of the outer retina on OCT examination and do not correspond to intraretinal or subretinal fluid. ICGA (fig. 41) usually shows no choroidal alterations (Bottoni et al., 2010)[17].

OCT (fig. 42) shows the presence of intraretinal foveal cysts localized in the outer retinal layers and abnormalities of the outer plexiform layer with a 'wrinkled' appearance suggesting Müller cell sufferance. One of the main features of idiopathic macular telangiectasias is that strangely intraretinal cysts that can be observed in OCT scans do not appear hyperfluorescent in the late phases of FA, while outer retina abnormalities correspond to the areas of late hyperfluorescence. In macular telangiectasias type I, OCTA reveals a global and focal capillary depletion. The rarefaction of both superficial and deep capillary plexus and abnormal microvascular morphology are better identified by OCTA than by FA. In macular telangiectasias type II, the earliest changes involve the deep capillary plexus, including enlargement of vessels and larger inter-

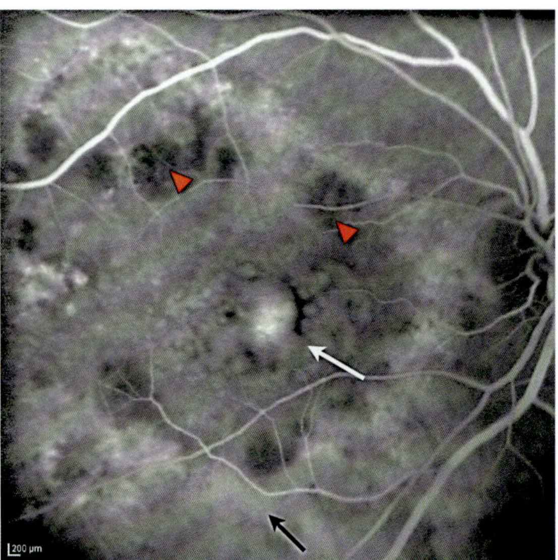

Fig. 43. AMD. FA, advanced CNV. White arrow = CME; red arrowhead = hard exudates; black arrow = retinal pigment epithelium detachment.

vascular spaces, dilated, dendritic appearance of vessels, telangiectasias, reduction and/or loss of capillary density, and the presence of anastomoses toward the superficial capillary plexus.

Age-Related Macular Degeneration
Macular edema represents a common finding in wet age-related macular degeneration (AMD) due to the exudation which characterizes this pathology.

In the early phases of the disease, cystic spaces usually appear small in size and are difficult to observe on biomicroscopic examination, while other features of the lesion-like drusen, such as macular hemorrhages, subretinal fluid, and pigmented epithelium retinal detachments, are predominant.

FA (Macula Photocoagulation Study Group, 1991)[18] is still considered the 'gold standard' test for the diagnosis of wet AMD, and it usually enables detection of mid-to-late phase CME due to the pooling of dye inside the cysts. However, active lesions are characterized by an increase in dye leakage during the test, which causes a masking effect on the subretina. In contrast, old lesions are characterized by a confluence of the cystic spaces and reduced leakage; as a consequence, CME becomes easier to observe both at fundus examination and with FA (fig. 43).

ICGA is a very useful examination to study AMD lesions, such as occult, polypoidal, chorioretinal anastomoses and CNV. However, ICGA is not as helpful in identifying CME. Compared to ICGA, OCTA allows for a direct visualization of the CNV but does not demonstrate dye leakage, and thus recognizing an active lesion may be challenging. Recent studies report how the morphologic appearance of CNV on OCTA could correlate with clinical activity.

Currently the most useful technique to detect and study CME in wet AMD is OCT. With the development of the spectral domain OCT technology, OCTs are able to acquire high-definition images, which allow the operator to identify even extremely small cysts in the earliest phases of the disease and to describe their distribution into the different retinal layers.

Depending on lesion type and in the early phases of the disease, CME shows different patterns of localization: classical lesions usually present intraretinal fluid localized in small cystic spaces primarily disposed into the internal layers (nuclear and plexiform; fig. 44). Occult CNVs are seldom characterized by a huge macular edema: in these lesions, CME, when present, is typically represented by intraretinal small cystic spaces localized to the external retinal layers (nuclear and, more rarely, plexiform; fig. 45).

Retinal angiomatous proliferation lesions represent the type of CNV characterized by the larger amount of CME and often involve both the external and internal retinal layers (fig. 46). The same cyst localization can be observed in polypoidal lesions (fig. 47).

In advanced CNV, CME is characterized by large cystic round spaces surrounded by hyperreflective boundaries; sometimes a single cyst can involve the entire neurosensory retina

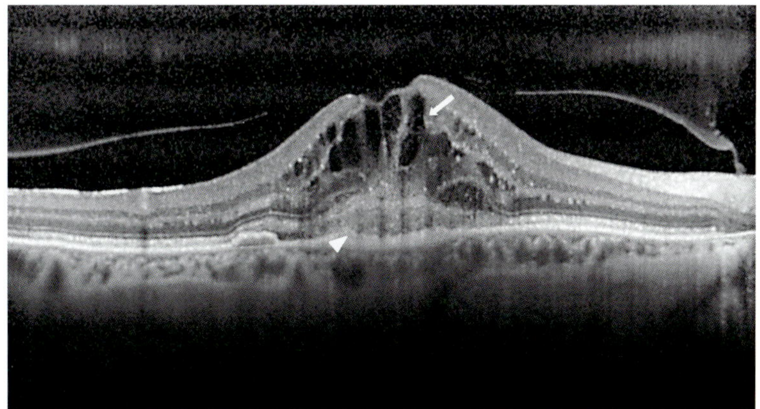

Fig. 44. AMD. OCT, classical lesion. White arrow = CME; white arrowhead = CNV complex.

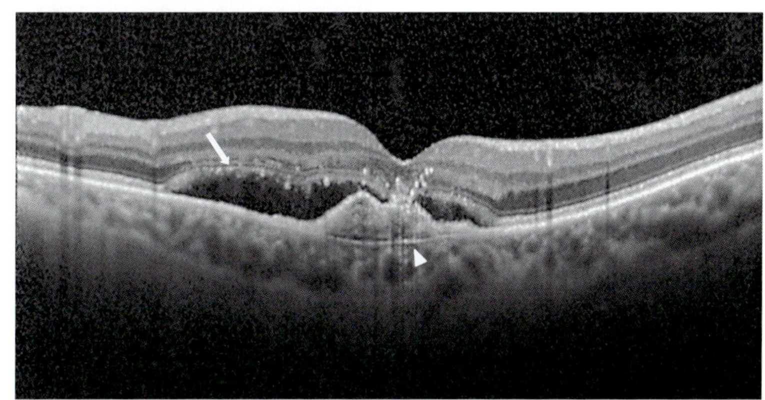

Fig. 45. AMD. OCT, occult lesion. White arrow = serous neuroretinal detachment; arrowhead = retinal pigment epithelium detachment.

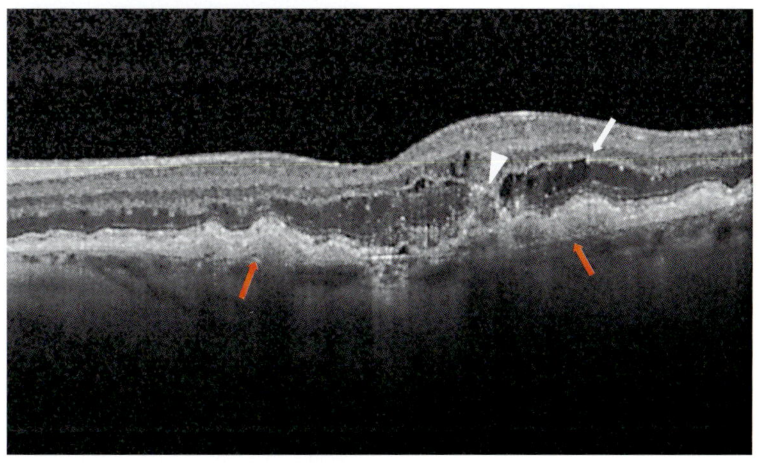

Fig. 46. AMD. OCT, retinal angiomatous proliferation lesion. White arrow = CME; white arrowhead = CNV complex; red arrows = retinal pigment epithelium detachment.

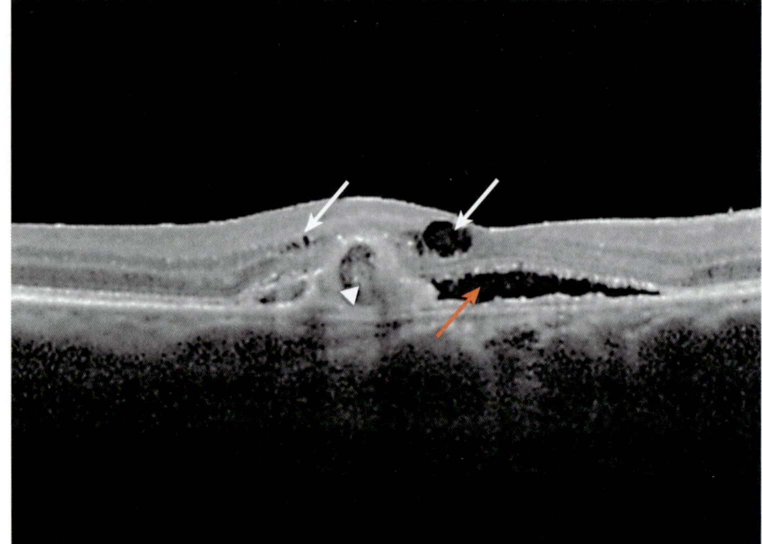

Fig. 47. AMD. OCT, polypoidal lesion. White arrows = CME; white arrowhead = CNV complex; red arrow = neurosensory retinal detachment.

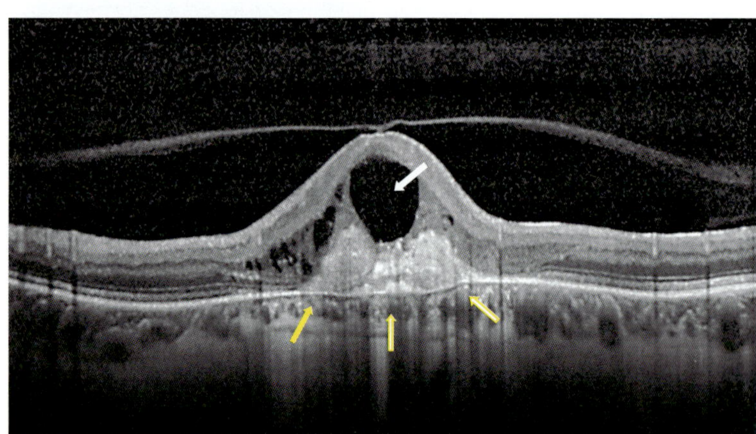

Fig. 48. AMD. OCT, advanced CNV. White arrow = CME; yellow arrows = fibrosis.

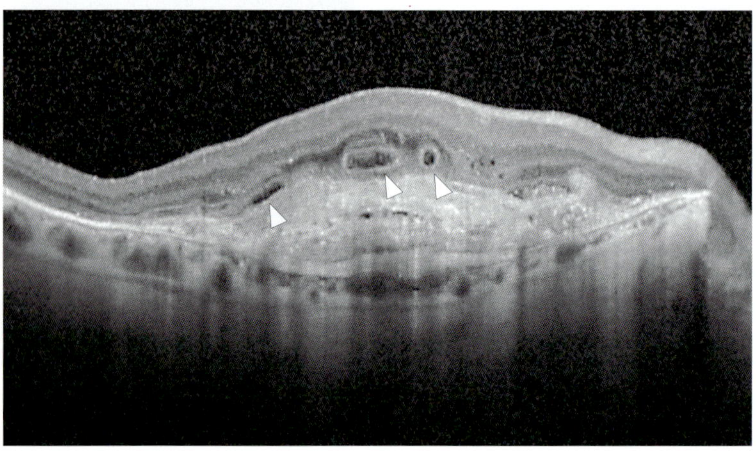

Fig. 49. AMD. OCT, advanced CNV. Arrowheads = Outer retinal tubulations.

	Fundus photography	Retinography	FA	ICGA	OCT
Irvine-Gass syndrome	R	S	U	–	U
Diabetic retinopathy	U	U	U	R	U
Retinal vein occlusions	U	U	U	–	U
Uveitis	U	R	U	U	S
Vitreoretinal tractions	S	U	R	–	U
Idiopathic macular telangiectasias	S	U	S	R	U
AMD	S	S	U	U	U

R = Rarely useful; S = sometimes useful; U = usually useful; – = usually not performed.

(fig. 47, 48). Small round/oval structures with circular midreflectant elements and a central brighter core, which can be observed surrounded by a crown of hyperreflectant spots, can be confused with CME. These formations, called a 'rosette' or 'outer retinal tubulation', represent a stability mark of the lesion (fig. 49) (Zweifel et al., 2009)[19].

Table 2 provides a summary of examination methods discussed in the chapter and estimates the relevance of each diagnostic technique in defining the etiology of CME.

References

1 Johnson MW: Etiology and treatment of macular edema. Am J Ophthalmol 2009; 147:11–21.

2 Early Treatment Diabetic Retinopathy Study Research Group: Photocoagulation for diabetic macular edema. Early Treatment Diabetic Retinopathy Study Report No 1. Arch Ophthalmol 1985; 103:1796–806.

3 Brown JC, Solomon SD, Bressler SB, Schachat AP, Di Bernardo C, Bressler NM: Detection of diabetic foveal edema: contact lens biomicroscopy compared with optical coherence tomography. Arch Ophthalmol 2004;122: 330–335.

4 Sadda SR, Tan O, Walsh AC, Schuman JS, Varma R, Huang D: Automated detection of clinically significant macular edema by grid scanning optical coherence tomography. Ophthalmology 2006; 113:1187.e1–12.

5 Hee MR, Puliafito CA, Duker JS, Reichel E, Coker JG, Wilkins JR, Schuman JS, Swanson EA, Fujimoto JG: Topography of diabetic macular edema with optical coherence tomography. Ophthalmology 1998;105:360–370.

6 Shahidi M, Ogura Y, Blair NP, Zeimer R: Retinal thickness change after focal laser treatment of diabetic macular oedema. Br J Ophthalmol 1994;78:827–830.

7 Delori FC, Dorey CK, Staurenghi G, Arend O, Goger DG, Weiter JJ: In vivo fluorescence of the ocular fundus exhibits retinal pigment epithelium lipofuscin characteristics. Invest Ophthalmol Vis Sci 1995;36:718–729.

8 Irvine SR: A newly defined vitreous syndrome following cataract surgery, interpreted according to recent concepts of the structure of the vitreous. Am J Ophthalmol 1953;36:599–619.

9 Gass JDM: Stereoscopic Atlas of Macular Diseases: Diagnosis and Treatment, ed 4. St Louis, Mosby, 1997.

10 Ray S, D'Amico DJ: Pseudophakic cystoid macular edema. Semin Ophthalmol 2002;17:167–180.

11 Bhagat N, Grigorian RA, Tutela A, Zarbin MA: Diabetic macular edema: pathogenesis and treatment. Surv Ophthalmol 2009;54:1–32.

12 Weinberger D, Kramer M, Priel E, et al: Indocyanine green angiographic findings in nonproliferative diabetic retinopathy. Am J Ophthalmol 1998;126: 238–247.

13 Kim BY, Smith SD, Kaiser PK: Optical coherence tomographic patterns of diabetic macular edema. Am J Ophthalmol 2006;142:405–412.

14 Tranos PG, Wickremasinghe SS, Stangos NT, Topouzis F, Tsinopoulos I, Pavesio CE: Macular edema. Surv Ophthalmol 2004;49:470–490.

15 Roesel M, Henschel A, Heinz C, Dietzel M, Spital G, Heiligenhaus A: Fundus autofluorescence and spectral domain optical coherence tomography in uveitic macular edema. Graefes Arch Clin Exp Ophthalmol 2009;247:1685–1689.

16 Charbel Issa P, Berendschot TT, Staurenghi G, Holz FG, Scholl HP: Confocal blue reflectance imaging in type 2 idiopathic macular telangiectasia. Invest Ophthalmol Vis Sci 2008;49:1172–1177.

17 Bottoni F, Eandi CM, Pedenovi S, Staurenghi G: Integrated clinical evaluation of type 2A idiopathic juxtafoveolar retinal telangiectasis. Retina 2010;30:317–326.

18 Macular Photocoagulation Study Group: Subfoveal neovascular lesions in age-related macular degeneration: guidelines for evaluation and treatment in the Macular Photocoagulation Study. Arch Ophthalmol 1991;109:1242–1257.

19 Zweifel SA, Engelbert M, Laud K, Margolis R, Spaide RF, Freund KB: Outer retinal tubulation: a novel optical coherence tomography finding. Arch Ophthalmol 2009;127:1596–1602.

Prof. Giovanni Staurenghi
Eye Clinic, Department of Biomedical and Clinical Science "Luigi Sacco", Sacco Hospital
Via G.B. Grassi 74
IT-20157 Milan (Italy)
E-Mail giovanni.staurenghi@unimi.it

Staurenghi · Pellegrini · Invernizzi · Preziosa

Coscas G (ed): Macular Edema. 2nd, revised and extended edition.
Dev Ophthalmol. Basel, Karger, 2017, vol 58, pp 63–73 (DOI: 10.1159/000455269)

Optical Coherence Tomography Angiography in Macular Edema

Marco Lupidi[a, c] · Florence Coscas[a, b] · Carlo Cagini[c] · Gabriel Coscas[b]

[a]Centre de l'Odéon, Paris, and [b]Service Universitaire d'Ophtalmologie, Hôpital Intercommunal de Créteil, Créteil, France; [c]Department of Biomedical and Surgical Sciences, Section of Ophthalmology, University of Perugia, S. Maria della Misericordia Hospital, Perugia, Italy

Abstract

OCT angiography is a promising new method to visualize the retinal vasculature and choroidal vascular layers in the macular area and provides depth resolved functional information of the blood flow in the vessels. Given that the main moving elements in the eye fundus are contained in vessels, determining a vascular decorrelation signal enables visualization of 3-dimensional retinal and choroidal vascular network without the administration of intravenous dye and thus reducing the risk of potential adverse events.   © 2017 S. Karger AG, Basel

During the last 50 years, fluorescein angiography (FA) and indocyanine green angiography have provided information about the normal retinal and choroidal anatomy, nearly comparable to histological findings. This has been absolutely fundamental in the evaluation of all retinal and choroidal vascular diseases and has allowed clinicians to define and diagnose several pathological conditions. FA became the *gold standard* in retinal imaging due to the capability to visualize the retinal capillary bed and its changes, particularly in the macular area. However, although the fluorescence of the injected dye enabled improved visualization of retinal capillaries, not all the different layers of the retinal capillary network could be visualized in this bidimensional examination, possibly because of light-scattering phenomena.

Nevertheless, morphological findings such as macular edema (ME) may be clearly evaluated on optical coherence tomography angiography (OCTA). Being confident in detecting the different appearance of ME in OCT angiograms can result in a rapid analysis of the examination and in distinguishing truly decorrelated structures (perfused vessels) from artifacts. *Artifacts* can be due to scan positioning errors caused by normal ocular microsaccades. Active eye tracking (TruTrack™) based on the simultaneous acquisition of fundus and OCT images, presents a very reliable method to acquire OCT volume scans *without motion artifacts* and significantly helps to improve the signal-to-noise ratio.

The authors have experience in a system that allows the use of a *full spectrum amplitude decorrelation algorithm* with a clear differentiation between blood flow and static tissue without sacrificing axial resolution of the OCT images.

Accuracy of layer segmentation is crucial to produce reliable OCTA images which requires high-resolution OCT B-scans. This can be achieved through automated or manual layer segmentation. Moreover, a complete morphofunctional assessment may help in determining both the origin and the clinical activity of a given vascular disease.

OCTA is a promising new method to visualize the retinal vasculature and choroidal vascular layers in the macular area. A key advantage of OCTA over traditional FA is that it provides depth-resolved functional information of the blood flow in the vessels.

Traditional multimodal imaging, such as FA and indocyanine green angiography provided essential dynamic information on the perfusion of different retinal and choroidal vascular layers, including the transit time from the arm to the eye, therefore allowing information about the normal retinal and choroidal anatomy to get obtained, nearly comparable to histological findings (Sulzbacher et al., 2011)[1]. This is absolutely fundamental in the evaluation of all retinal and choroidal vascular diseases and, when added to the morphological data, allows the clinician to detect diseases and define the correct diagnosis.

FA has become the *gold standard* in imaging the fundus due to the fact that FA is the best method to visualize the retinal capillary bed and its changes, particularly in macular area. Moreover, FA allows also the clinician to detect and analyze one main clinical sign: *leakage* from abnormal and/or new vessels.

Although the fluorescence of the injected dye enabled improved visualization of retinal capillaries, not all the different layers of the retinal capillary network could be visualized in this bidimensional examination.

Fluorescein angiographic images of the retina correspond to the anatomical arraignment of the superficial retinal vessels, whereas the deeper retinal capillaries are not visualized in the angiogram (Snodderly et al., 1992; Weinhaus et al., 1995)[2, 3]. Comparative findings suggest the deeper capillary network in the retina is not visualized well by FA, possibly because of light scattering of the retina (Spaide et al., 2015)[4]. Therefore, even if the FA is the gold standard for the visualization of retinal vessels, one of the two major capillary networks do not appear to be imaged well, even though the retina is a nearly transparent structure (Moult et al., 2014)[5].

OCTA allows a clear, depth-resolved visualization of the retinal (Moult et al., 2014)[5] and choroidal microvasculature (Jia et al., 2014)[6] by calculating the decorrelation of the signal between static and nonstatic tissue.

Given that the main moving elements in the eye fundus are contained in vessels, determining a vascular decorrelation signal enables visualization of 3-dimensional retinal and choroidal vascular network (Yannuzzi et al., 1986)[7]. Moreover, OCTA does not require administration of intravenous dye, reducing the risk of potential adverse events (Laser Institute of America, 2007)[8].

The OCTA images in this chapter were obtained by a Spectralis OCT-2 (Heidelberg Engineering, Heidelberg, Germany) that was able to acquire 85,000 A-scans per second with 3.9-μm axial and 6-μm lateral resolutions, and is applicable to a volume scan on a 15×5 or $15 \times 10°$ area (4.3×1.5 or 4.3×2.9 mm), which is composed of a variable number of B-scans (ranging from 131 to 261, respectively) at a distance of 11 μm each. Active eye tracking (TruTrack™, Heidelberg Engineering, Heidelberg, Germany) allows OCT volume scans *without motion artifacts* to be acquired. This eye-tracking system also allows the use of a full-spectrum amplitude decorrelation algorithm and guarantees a clear differentiation between blood flow and static tissue without sacrificing depth resolution of the OCT images. In this way, very thin layers of the vascular network in the C-scan section become distinguishable. The ocular light power exposure was within the American National Standards Institute's safety limit (Bonnin et al., 2015)[9].

The B-scan, in OCTA mode, is generated by computing the decorrelation in between successive standard B-scans that are sequentially acquired at the same location.

C-scan visualization allows the visibility of arteries clearly distinguishable from veins by the presence of a surrounding hypointense halo due to the absence of efferent vessels directly coming out of the walls. The superficial capillary plexus appears as a fine capillary network with a hyperintense signal at the level of the ganglion cell layer, while the deep capillary plexus is shown in the C-scan section taken at the level of the inner nuclear layer.

The superficial capillary plexus and DCP architecture are often disrupted in retinal vascular diseases, and sometimes the presence of ME may be responsible for such vascular impairment.

OCTA has shown promise in identifying intraretinal or subretinal exudation in diabetic retinopathy (Mané et al., 2016)[10], retinal vein occlusion (Coscas et al., 2016)[11], or neovascular age-related macular degeneration (Coscas et al., 2015)[12].

Despite these recent advances, there remains a gap in our diagnostic capabilities for quickly and noninvasively identifying and grading ME in a simple, comparable way. With this new, noninvasive technique, we might be able to analyze progressive vascular changes and provide easily interpretable qualitative pictures of retinal vascularity and ME.

Optical Coherence Tomography Angiography of Exudative Macular Edema

Although ME is mainly a morphological rather than functional feature of different maculopathies, we consider it important to analyze and distinguish ME on an OCT angiogram.

The diagnosis of ME is mainly clinical. The gold standard for diagnosing diabetic macular edema (DME) is stereoscopic color fundus photography. In clinical practice, *contact lens and noncontact fundus biomicroscopy* is often employed, and it can be useful, especially when there is significant retinal thickening. Conventionally, DME is defined as retinal thickening and/or presence of hard exudates within 1 disc diameter of the center of the macula. The term *'clinically significant macular edema'*, initially defined on the base of biomicroscopic examination, was coined to characterize the severity of the disease and to provide a threshold level to apply laser photocoagulation. FA allows visualizing leakage by staining the fluid coming out from the wall of the affected retinal capillaries. It is not, however, sufficient to diagnose ME.

DME can also be classified into focal and diffuse: *cystoid macular edema*, which is often associated with diffuse ME, results from a generalized breakdown of the BRB. *In clinical practice* the distinction between focal and diffuse edema is not always clear and a wide variety of mixed forms can be observed. *In clinical practice* the distinction between focal and diffuse edema is not always clear and a wide variety of mixed forms are observed.

OCT imaging helps in estimating intraretinal modifications and demonstrates an increased retinal thickness and the loss of foveal depression (fig. 1).

On OCTA, ME may show also, as on FA or OCT, different patterns of what should be recognized in order to avoid potential pitfalls and misleading interpretations of the images.

ME may appear on OCTA as:

1 Hypointense intraretinal spaces
2 Grayish intraretinal spaces
3 Focal hyperintense clumps

Hypointense Intraretinal Spaces
Hypointense intraretinal spaces are roundish structures, which may vary in dimension and location depending on the depth of the C-scan section. These findings are due to the presence

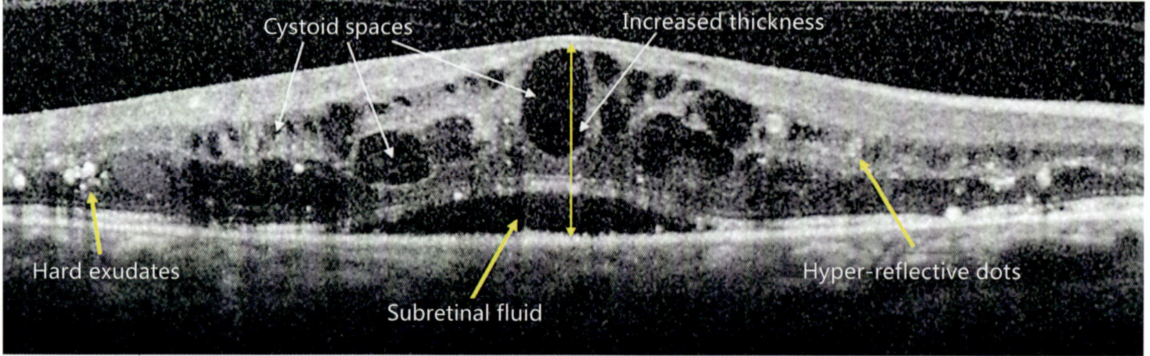

Fig. 1. *OCT B-scan of DME.* OCT imaging may show different features of DME. A thickened retina is visible here with complete loss of the foveal depression. Cystoid spaces are both located at the level of the inner and outer nuclear layers. Hard exudates are visible as highly hyperreflective spots inside the retina and also numerous hyperreflective dots, a sign of inflammatory reaction, are appreciable. This case also shows a serous retinal detachment, which might be due to a potential impairment of the outer retinal barrier.

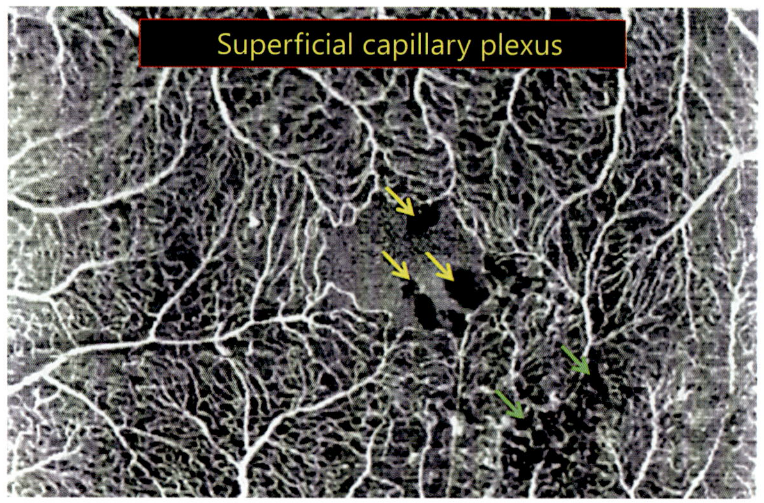

Fig. 2. *OCTA C-scan of the superficial capillary plexus in a case of ME.* The OCT angiogram above may show the superficial capillary plexus of a patient suffering from ME. The enlargement of the foveal avascular zone is associated with focal capillary dilations and small areas of capillary nonperfusion. The presence of large, roundish, hypointense lesions (yellow arrows), which are due to cystoid spaces in the perifoveal area. Smaller cystoid lesions are also visible in the extrafoveal area (green arrows).

of intraretinal cystoid spaces (fig. 2) and they are mainly located in proximity to nonperfused areas.

These findings are generally preceded by focal capillary dilations and zones of capillary nonperfusion. As in structural OCT, their dimension may vary from a lesion that is a few microns in size to large ones that almost involve the entire thickness of the retina. The larger ones are more frequently located in subfoveal and parafoveal area, while smaller ones are more peripheral in the macular and extramacular areas. The latter are often visible at the level of the inner nuclear layer, which is bracketed by the two components of the deep capillary plexus (fig. 3).

Substantial differences of hypointense intraretinal spaces in terms of distribution may be no-

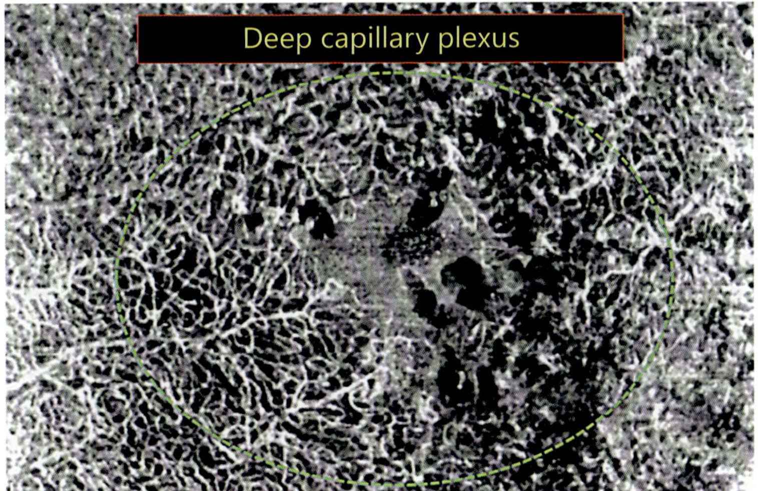

Fig. 3. *OCTA C-scan of the deep capillary plexus in case of ME.* The OCT angiogram taken at the level of the inner nuclear layer clearly shows the deep capillary plexus. A diffuse reduction of the vascularity is visible coupled with an enlargement of the foveal avascular zone, focal capillary dilations, and areas of capillary nonperfusion. Numerous hypointense lesions (cystoid spaces) are appreciable in the macular area (dashed green line).

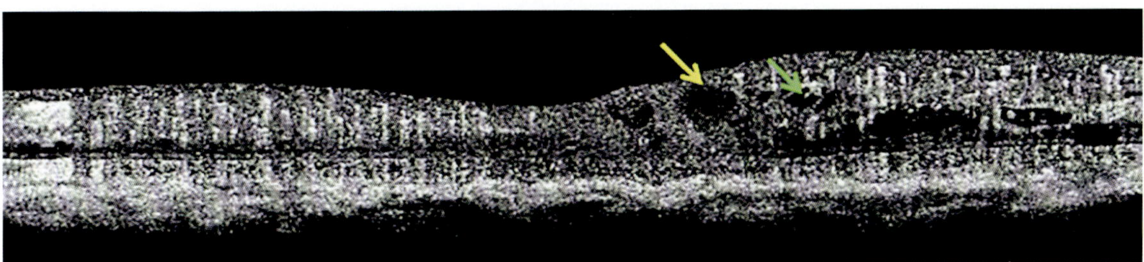

Fig. 4. *OCTA B-scan in a case of ME.* The B-scan OCT angiogram highlights the presence of large cystoid spaces in the perifoveal area (yellow arrow), while the smaller ones are mainly visible at the level of the inner nuclear layer, where the deep capillary plexus is located (green arrow). The hyperintense structures that are shown at the level of the inner retinal layers are referred to as transverse sections of retinal capillaries. It is difficult to visualize the eventual vascular abnormalities with the cross-sectional OCT (B-scan), but it is highly useful to evaluate the morphofunctional correlation with the corresponding structural B-scan.

ticed between the superficial and the deep capillary plexuses. The degree of involvement of the two vascular layers might explain the highly variable appearance. The same findings are visible on the corresponding B-scan OCT angiogram, showing similar features (fig. 4).

Hypointense intraretinal spaces are the most common pattern of ME on OCTA, especially in cases of intraretinal fluid accumulation. This cystoid morphology is quite similar to the one of structural OCT, but in this case borders are not well-demarcated and therefore more difficult to distinguish.

For a comprehensive assessment of a DME patient on OCTA, the imaging approach needs to include a C-scan section taken at the level of the ganglion cell layer (superficial capillary plexus), another one taken at the inner nuclear layer (deep capillary plexus), and the corresponding B-scan passing through the foveal depression (fig. 5). This approach may also be enriched with the structural OCT C-scan (en-face) (fig. 6).

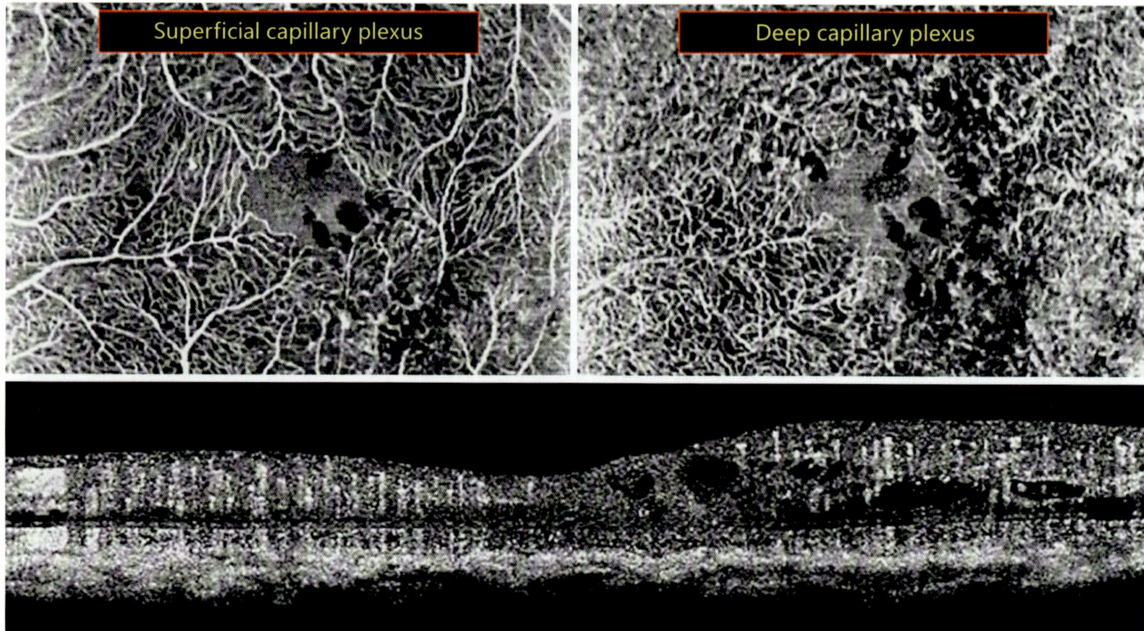

Fig. 5. *Cystoid ME evaluated on OCTA.* Comprehensive assessment of a cystoid ME patient on OCTA. This imaging approach includes a C-scan section taken at the level of the ganglion cell layer (superficial capillary plexus), another one taken at the inner nuclear layer (deep capillary plexus), and the corresponding B-scan passing through the foveal depression.

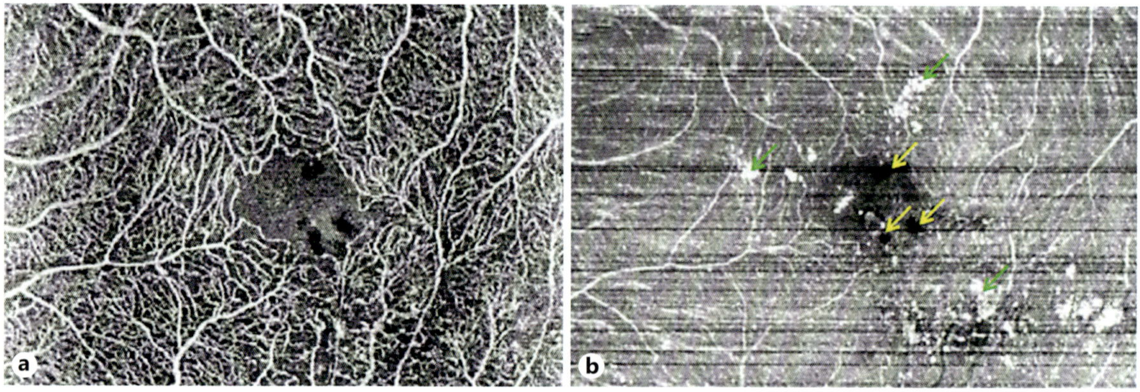

Fig. 6. *ME evaluated on OCTA and on en-face structural OCT.* C-scan section taken at the level of the ganglion cell layer. **a** The entire vascular network of the superficial capillary plexus and some intraretinal cystoid spaces as hypointense intraretinal structures. **b** The corresponding en-face image in which both the cystoid lesions and some hyperreflective spots, due to hard exudates, are visible. The combined analyses of the structural (en-face) and functional (OCTA) images allow a better definition of the degree of involvement in case of exudative maculopathy.

Lupidi · Coscas · Cagini · Coscas

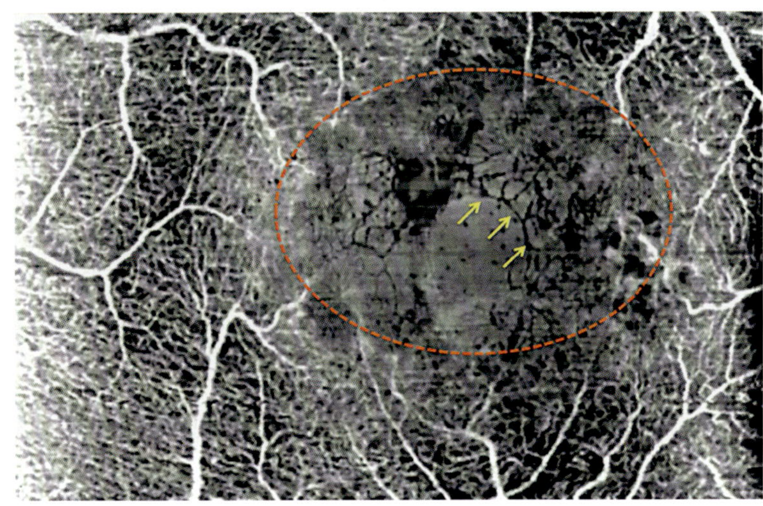

Fig. 7. *Grayish intraretinal spaces as a sign of ME on OCTA.* The C-scan OCT angiogram taken at the level of the ganglion cells layer and therefore showing the superficial capillary plexus. The foveal avascular zone and the macular capillary network are no longer visible due to the severe impairment or retinal vascularity. OCTA shows large areas of vascular nonperfusion partially filled by large grayish intraretinal spaces (dashed red line). This peculiar aspect is given by the Brownian motion of the molecules that are a consequence of an intense intraretinal exudation. Nonperfused vessels, as well-defined dark tubular structures in the intercystoid tissue, are highlighted by the weak decorrelation signal of the cystoid spaces.

Grayish Intraretinal Spaces

Large intraretinal cystoid spaces may sometimes appear with a grayish aspect. This particular pattern may be confusing when interpreting an OCT angiogram, as they share almost the same signal intensity of intervascular spaces. The authors hypothesized that this peculiar aspect might be due to the presence of active motion inside these spaces. This results in a weak decorrelation signal, which has its origin in the Brownian motion of the molecules that are a consequence of an intense intraretinal exudation (Spaide et al., 2015)[13] (fig. 7).

Both C-scan and B-scan visualization allow distinguishing this peculiar phenomenon (fig. 8). This grayish aspect of the large cystoid spaces may sometimes highlight the presence of nonperfused vessels in the intercystoid tissue (fig. 7). These vessels appear as well-defined tubular structures, without any decorrelation signal inside.

Nonperfused vessels are normally not detectable with OCTA since no decorrelation signal comes from flowing blood: the difference in terms of signal intensity between these vessels and the grayish cystoid spaces makes them clearly distinguishable.

Focal Hyperintense Clumps

On C-scan OCT angiograms of a patient with retinal vascular disease, highly decorrelated roundish or fusiform structures that are generally interpreted as microaneurysms or intraretinal vascular abnormalities can often be seen.

This focal hyperintense signal may unfortunately also be related to non-decorrelated lesions such as *hard exudates* (fig. 9). The latter are hyperreflective structures on structural OCT and hyperintense ones on OCTA. Intraretinal hyperreflective material due to hard exudates appears hyperintense on OCTA as it completely reflects the refracted signal coming from the perfused (decorrelated) vessels above. Unlike the RPE and the true perfused lesions (i.e., microaneurysms), these intraretinal clumps are associated on OCTA B-scan (fig. 10) with typical dark back shadowing, implying that the light that hits these deposits is largely reflected (Lupidi et al., 2015)[14].

This phenomenon could also explain the focal lack of signal, corresponding to the lesion area, observed on C-scan OCTA below the same lesion (fig. 11). The peculiar appearance

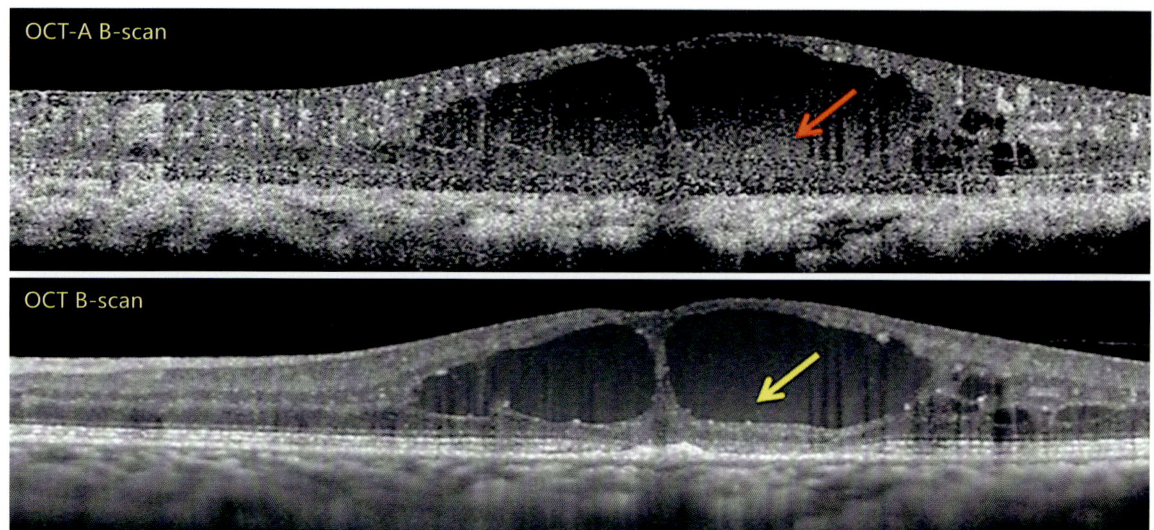

Fig. 8. *Grayish intraretinal spaces as a sign of ME on OCTA and structural OCT B-scans.* The B-scan OCT angiogram (top) shows a weak decorrelation signal inside large cystoid spaces (red arrow). The corresponding structural B-scan (bottom) shows a mild diffuse reflectivity inside the corresponding location inside the cyst.

Fig. 9. *OCTA C-scan of the deep capillary plexus in case of ME showing different types of hyperintense structures.* The OCT angiogram taken at the level of the inner nuclear layer clearly shows the deep capillary plexus. The fusiform hyperintense structure (red square) shows the typical appearance of a microaneurysm. Although sharing some similarities with the previous one, the roundish hyperintense lesion (green box) is due to a focal accumulation of hard exudates. These structures assume this appearance on OCTA since hyperreflective structures are able to reflect the refracted signal coming from the perfused (decorrelated) vessels above.

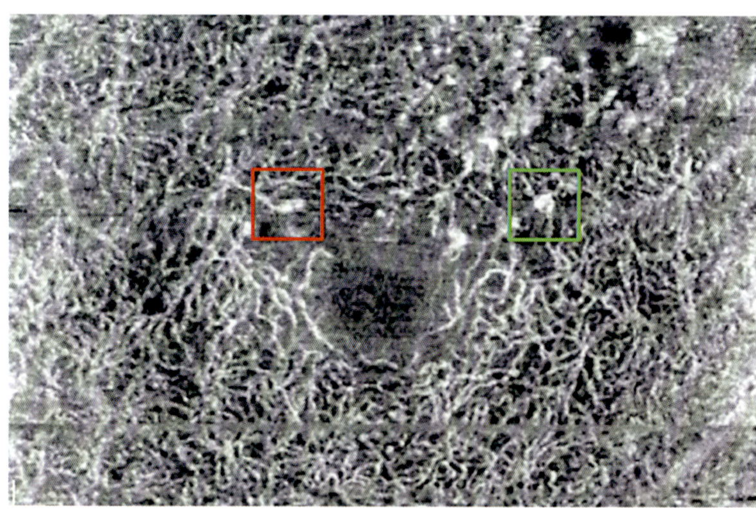

is not due to impaired perfusion of the deeper tissue but rather to a 'shielding effect' caused by the high reflectivity of the clumps above. This particular finding obtained from a simultaneous analysis of the C-scan and the B-scan on OCTA, which is available on the Spectralis OCT-2 automated software, could help to avoid some pitfalls and guide the differential diagnosis.

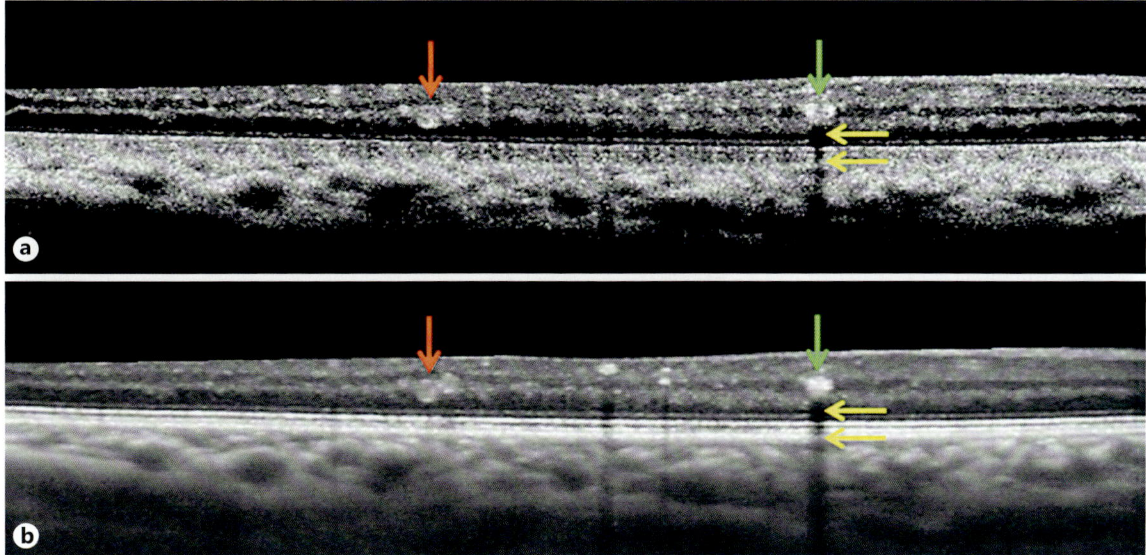

Fig. 10. *Focal hyperintense clumps as a sign of ME on OCTA and structural OCT B-scans.* **a** The B-scan OCT angiogram shows two decorrelated intraretinal structures. One of these (red arrow) does not show any additional findings above or below the lesion itself, while the second one (green arrow) is associated with a dark back shadowing (yellow arrows). This phenomenon is linked to the high reflectivity of the hard exudates. **b** The corresponding structural B-scan highlights the difference in reflectivity of the two intraretinal lesions [microaneurysm (red arrow) versus hard exudates (green arrow)].

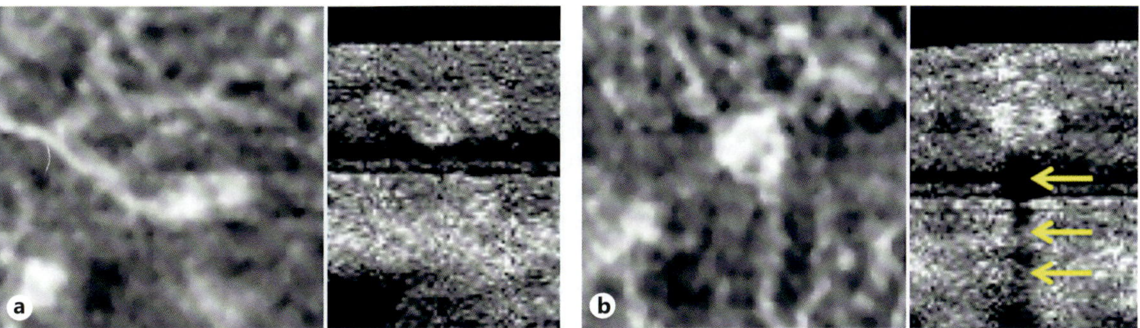

Fig. 11. *Comparative C-scan and B-scan analysis of focal hyperintense clumps in ME.* The simultaneous analysis of the C-scan and the B-scan on OCTA, which is available on the Spectralis OCT-2 automated software, could help to avoid some pitfalls and guide the differential diagnosis between truly perfused lesions (**a**) and artifactual hyperintense structures (**b**). The presence of dark back shadowing (yellow arrows) could help to distinguish these findings and thus ensure an accurate diagnostic process.

OCT Angiography of Ischemic Macular Edema 'Cotton-Wool' Spots

Cotton-wool spots (CWS) are retinal lesions, most commonly seen as manifestations of diabetes mellitus and systemic hypertension. They are also associated with a number of other etiologies including ischemic, embolic, connective tissue, neoplastic, and infectious, but occasionally no underlying cause can be identified.

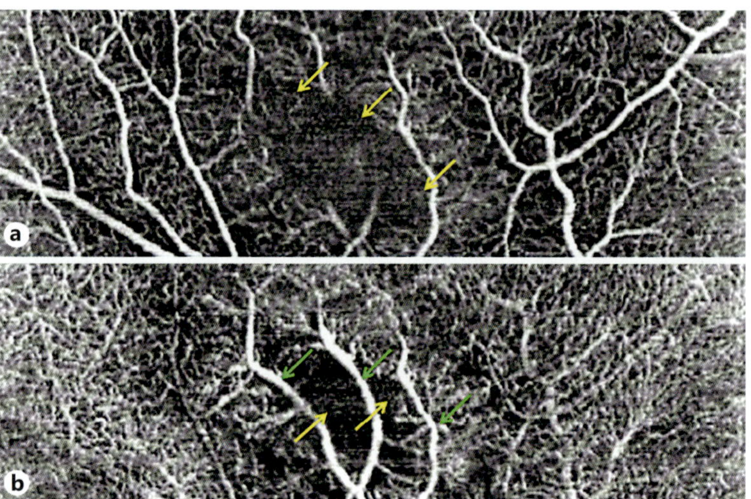

Fig. 12. *Cross-sectional OCT of a CWS.* **a** A structural OCT B-scan reveals a focal thickening of the ganglion cells layer (yellow arrow), partially involving also other inner retinal layers. **b** On the corresponding B-scan OCTA, no hyperintense signals are visible in the involved area (green arrow), while large retinal vessels are displaced deeper in the retina. This phenomenon is due to focal capillary ischemia, and confirmed on morphofunctional analysis.

Fig. 13. *En-face OCTA of a CWS.* **a** The superficial capillary plexus reveals an area of absence of hyperintense signals coming from perfused vessels (yellow arrows). This area almost shares the same features at the level of the deep capillary plexus (**b**), where there is no evidence of decorrelated structures (yellow arrows). Large retinal vessels are visible at this level due to the inward displacement caused by the thickening of the nerve fiber layer, and also because of the absence of a decorrelation signal coming from inner vascular layers.

CWS are thought to represent axoplasmic debris at the level of retinal ganglion cell axons resulting from axoplasmic flow interruption due to vascular or mechanical causes.

At the biomicroscopic examination, CWS appear as whitish, fluffy retinal patches that eventually fade with time. FA may reveal a focal impairment of the blood flow, while OCT (fig. 12) findings are typically characterized by a marked retinal thickening corresponding to the area of the CWS, confined to the level of the retinal nerve fiber layer.

On OCTA a CWS appears as an area of absence of decorrelation signals coming both from the superficial and deep capillary plexus, which may result in being simultaneously involved (fig. 13). Large retinal vessels appear displaced deeper.

Moreover, these large vessels also remain visible at the level of the DCP because of the absence of a decorrelation signal coming from inner vascular layers (Nemiroff et al., 2016)[15].

References

1 Sulzbacher F, Kiss C, Munk M, et al: Diagnostic evaluation of type 2 (classic) choroidal neovascularization: optical coherence tomography, indocyanine green angiography, and fluorescein angiography. Am J Ophthalmol 2011;152: 799–806.e1.

2 Snodderly DM, Weinhaus RS, Choi JC: Neural-vascular relationships in central retina of macaque monkeys (*Macaca fascicularis*). J Neurosci 1992;12:1169–1193.

3 Weinhaus RS, Burke JM, Delori FC, Snodderly DM: Comparison of fluorescein angiography with microvascular anatomy of macaque retina. Exp Eye Res 1995;61:1–16.

4 Spaide RF, Klancnik JM Jr, Cooney MJ: Retinal vascular layers imaged by fluorescein angiography and optical coherence tomography angiography. JAMA Ophthalmol 2015;133:45–50.

5 Moult E, Choi W, Waheed NK, et al: Ultrahigh-speed swept-source OCT angiography in exudative AMD. Ophthalmic Surg Lasers Imaging Retina 2014; 45:496–505.

6 Jia Y, Bailey ST, Wilson DJ, et al: Quantitative optical coherence tomography angiography of choroidal neovascularization in age-related macular degeneration. Ophthalmology 2014;121:1435–1444.

7 Yannuzzi LA, Rohrer KT, Tindel LJ, et al: Fluorescein angiography complication survey. Ophthalmology 1986;93:611–617.

8 American National Standard for Safe Use of Lasers, ANSI Z136. Orlando, Laser Institute of America, 2007.

9 Bonnin S, Mané V, Couturier A, et al: New insight into the macular deep vascular plexus imaged by optical coherence tomography angiography. Retina 2015;35:2347–2352.

10 Mané V, Dupas B, Gaudric A, et al: Correlation between cystoid spaces in chronic diabetic macular edema and capillary nonperfusion detected by optical coherence tomography angiography. Retina 2016;36(suppl 1):S102–S110.

11 Coscas F, Glacet-Bernard A, Miere A, et al: Optical coherence tomography angiography in retinal vein occlusion: evaluation of superficial and deep capillary plexa. Am J Ophthalmol 2016;161:160–171.

12 Coscas GJ, Lupidi M, Coscas F, et al: Optical coherence tomography angiography versus traditional multimodal imaging in assessing the activity of exudative age-related macular degeneration: a new diagnostic challenge. Retina 2015;35:2219–2228.

13 Spaide RF, Fujimoto JG, Waheed NK: Image artifacts in optical coherence tomography angiography. Retina 2015;35:2163–2180.

14 Lupidi M, Coscas G, Cagini C, et al: Optical coherence tomography angiography of a choroidal neovascularization in adult onset foveomacular vitelliform dystrophy: pearls and pitfalls. Invest Ophthalmol Vis Sci 2015;56:7638–7645.

15 Nemiroff J, Kuehlewein L, Rahimy E, et al: Assessing deep retinal capillary ischemia in paracentral acute middle maculopathy by optical coherence tomography angiography. Am J Ophthalmol 2016;162:121–132.

Prof. Gabriel Coscas
Service Universitaire d'Ophtalmologie
Hôpital Intercommunal de Créteil
40, Avenue de Verdun
FR–94000 Créteil (France)
E-Mail gabriel.coscas@gmail.com

Coscas G (ed): Macular Edema. 2nd, revised and extended edition.
Dev Ophthalmol. Basel, Karger, 2017, vol 58, pp 74–86 (DOI: 10.1159/000455275)

Macular Edema – Rationale for Therapy

Thomas J. Wolfensberger

Jules Gonin Eye Hospital, Department of Ophthalmology, University of Lausanne, Lausanne, Switzerland

Abstract

Macular edema represents the end-stage of multiple pathophysiological pathways in a multitude of ocular vascular, inflammatory, and other diseases. The rationale for clinical treatment of macular edema is based on the understanding and the inhibition of these pathophysiological mechanisms. When macular edema is caused by a generalized health problem such as diabetes, high blood pressure, or generalized inflammatory conditions, treatment of these generalized diseases can in many cases cure macular edema directly. In ocular diseases, the local exudation of fluid from blood vessels is governed by Starling's law as well as by intricate cellular mechanisms linked to the tight junctions in the inner and outer blood-retinal barrier. Drugs used in clinical practice, such as non-steroidal anti-inflammatory drugs, corticosteroids, carbonic anhydrase inhibitors, and anti-vascular endothelial growth factor agents, all act in one way or another through these cellular mechanisms. Novel treatments such as neuroprotective agents like nerve growth factors, somatostatins and antiapoptotic agents like calpain, the glutamate blocker memantine, and different caspase inhibitors may in the future inhibit neuronal cell death in the retina by separate pathways. Using dimmed nocturnal illumination may be an additional novel method to reduce hypoxic stress during dark adaptation of the rod photoreceptors in diabetes. Successful surgical treatment of macular edema using vitrectomy and peeling relies, apart from the evident release of vitreomacular traction, on many other cellular and biochemical mechanisms activated by the surgery such as oxygenation of the inner retina, removal of the posterior hyaloid as a growth factor sink, and possible Müller cell remodeling with fluid redirection after internal limiting membrane peeling.

© 2017 S. Karger AG, Basel

Macular edema occurs when the blood-retinal barrier (BRB) breaks down. From a clinical and biological point of view, this can be caused by many different vascular, inflammatory, and other diseases that modulate the integrity of the tight junctions between the retinal vascular endothelial cells as well as at the level of the retinal pigment epithelium (RPE) (fig. 1), and they are governed by a host of different growth factors (Tranos et al., 2004)[1].

Starling's law predicts that macular edema will develop if the hydrostatic pressure gradient between the capillary and retinal tissue is increased (e.g., in the presence of elevated blood pressure) or if the osmotic pressure gradient is decreased

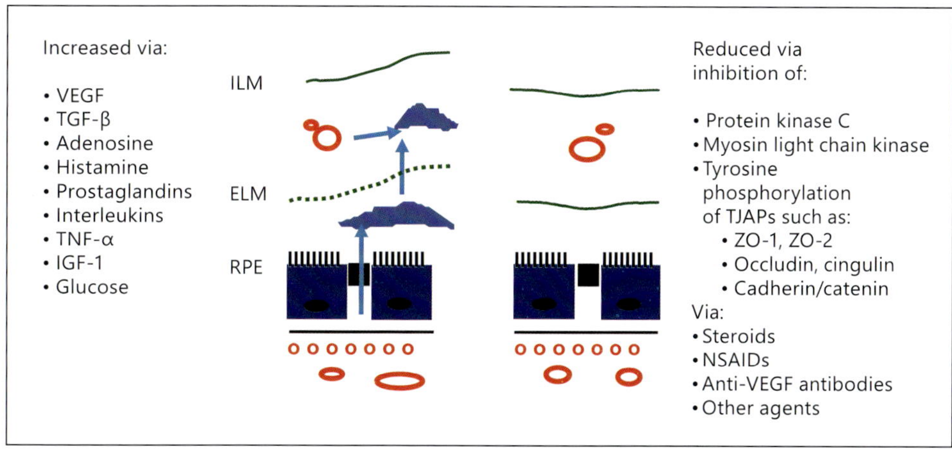

Fig. 1. Schematic diagram of the BRB showing on the left the different growth factors, whose up-regulation can lead to a breakdown of the tight junctions in the retinal endothelial and/or retinal pigment epithelial cells inducing macular edema. On the right hand side of the diagram the different possible therapies are listed, which can reduce the permeability of the BRB. TJAP = Tight junction-associated proteins; ILM = internal limiting membrane; ELM = external limiting membrane.

(e.g., when protein accumulates excessively in the extracellular space within the retina) (Stefánsson, 2009)[2].

The rationale for clinical treatment of macular edema is based on the understanding and the inhibition of these pathophysiological mechanisms.

Rationale for Medical Management

Systemic Medical Therapy

In many cases, macular edema is caused by a generalized health problem such as diabetes, high blood pressure, or inflammatory conditions (Gilles et al., 1997; Gardner and Gabbay, 2009; Aiello et al., 2001)[3–5]. It is evident that these generalized diseases need to be treated first and foremost.

There have been several reports in the literature that such treatments – particularly in diabetes, high blood pressure, and inflammatory diseases – can cure macular edema without any additional specific ocular treatment (Liew et al., 2009)[6].

Nonsteroidal Anti-Inflammatory Drugs

The action of nonsteroidal anti-inflammatory drugs (NSAIDs) is based on the inhibition of the enzyme cyclooxygenase, which in turn inhibits the production of prostaglandins, a degradation product of arachidonic acid in the eye (Colin, 2007)[7] (fig. 2).

Some NSAIDs also act on other mediators. Diclofenac sodium, for example, in high doses inhibits the formation of leukotrienes, which amplify cellular infiltration during an inflammatory reaction (Ku et al., 1986)[8].

NSAIDs have also been shown to modulate chloride movement, and, as a consequence, fluid movement through the RPE (Bialek et al., 1996)[9] (fig. 3).

On the basis of these scientific findings, topical NSAIDs have become the mainstay in the treatment of inflammatory cystoid macular edema (CME) (Wolfensberger and Herbort, 1999)[10]. The clinical efficacy of topical NSAIDs has been shown to be of value both in the prevention (Flach et al., 1990; Almeida et al., 2008; DeCroos and

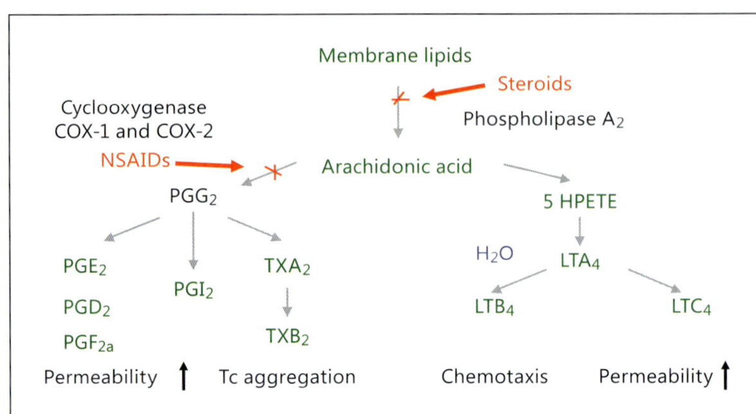

Fig. 2. Schematic diagram of the pharmacological action of corticosteroids and NSAIDs. Note the dual action of steroids both on prostaglandin and leukotriene production.

Afshari, 2008; Rossetti et al., 1998)[11–14] and treatment (Nelson and Martidis, 2003; Sivaprasad et al., 2005; Rojas et al., 1999)[15–17] of inflammatory CME, particularly when related to cataract surgery.

Two double-masked, placebo-controlled studies in which corticosteroids were not used demonstrated that ketorolac 0.5% ophthalmic solution, administered for up to 3 months, improves vision in some patients with chronic CME after cataract surgery (Flach et al., 1987; Flach et al., 1991)[18, 19]. A meta-analysis of the results from several different randomized controlled trials suggests that NSAIDs are beneficial as a medical prophylaxis for aphakic and pseudophakic CME, and as medical treatment for chronic CME (Rossetti et al., 1998)[14].

On the basis of these findings it has been suggested to employ topical NSAIDs in the treatment of inflammatory CME, especially when related to ocular surgery.

Corticosteroids

Corticosteroids have been used in many different ways such as topical, sub-Tenon, and intravitreal administration. Corticosteroids have different potency levels depending on their chemical composition (Haynes and Murad, 1985)[20], and the newer synthetically produced compounds show an up to 25-fold increase of activity as compared to cortisone. These new agents such as triamcinolone, dexamethasone, and fluocinolone acetonide have fluor at the 9α position, which increases corticosteroid receptor binding.

Corticosteroids inhibit the enzyme cyclooxygenase (Fig. 2), but they also have a multitude of other anti-inflammatory effects by acting, among others, on interleukin (IL)-1 and by reducing vascular permeability (Nehmé and Edelman, 2008)[21]. Their additive anti-inflammatory effect to NSAIDs has been shown to be useful in the treatment of various postoperative inflammatory conditions (Othenin-Girard et al., 1992)[22].

One potential mode of action is the increased resorption of fluid through the RPE, although the exact mechanism of this is not as yet clear. Another action of steroids is the downregulation of the production of the vascular endothelial growth factor (VEGF), which, in turn, renders the BRB tighter (fig. 4). Steroids also downregulate VEGF production (Edelman et al., 2005)[23] specifically in the retina (Wang et al., 2008; Zhang et al., 2008)[24, 25], and this explains the clinical observation that the application of steroids both intravitreally and into the sub-Tenon space can reduce macular edema considerably.

Cortisone has also been shown to decreases the phosphorylation of occludin, increasing the

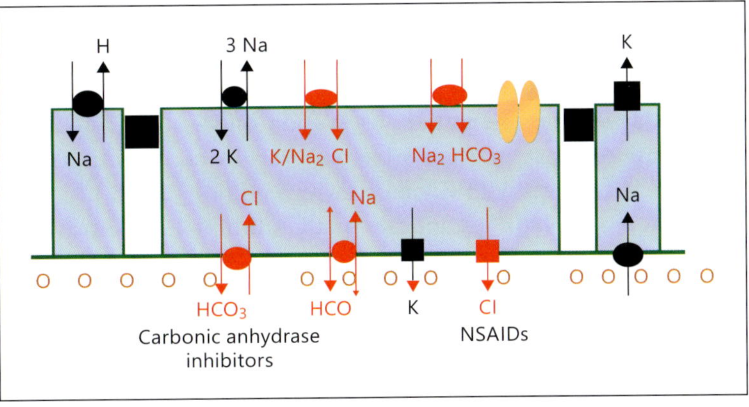

Fig. 3. Schematic diagram showing selected ion channels in the RPE. Note that CA inhibitors act on the bicarbonate/chloride exchange channel in the basal membrane, and NSAIDs have been shown to act on the chloride channel in the basal membrane of the RPE. Both channels are associated with transcellular fluid transport.

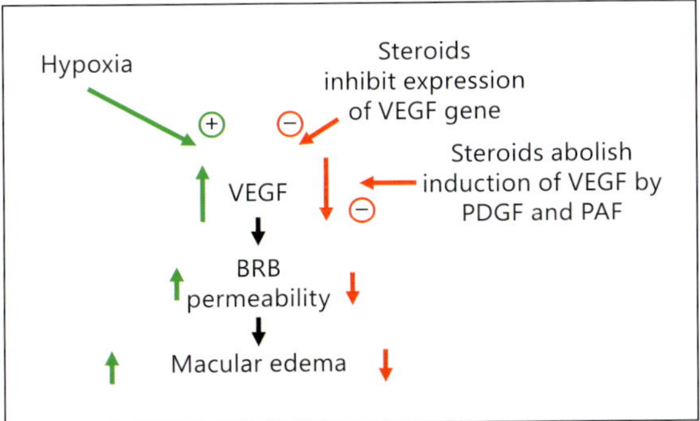

Fig. 4. Schematic diagram showing that hypoxia upregulates VEGF production, which increases BRB permeability with the induction of macular edema. Steroids inhibit not only the expression of the VEGF gene, but also abolish the induction of VEGF by platelet-derived growth factor (PDGF) and platelet-activating factor (PAF).

tightness of the blood-retinal-barrier (Antonetti et al., 2002)[26]. Glucocorticoids induce transactivation of tight junction genes occludin and claudin-5 in retinal endothelial cells via a novel *cis*-element (Felinski et al., 2008)[27].

Furthermore, steroids have been shown to prevent the induction of VEFG production by platelet-activating factor and platelet-derived growth factor (Nauck et al., 1997)[28] (fig. 4). Triamcinolone also inhibits IL-6- and VEGF-induced angiogenesis downstream of the IL-6 and VEGF receptors (Ebrahem et al., 2006)[29].

Leukocyte adhesion plays an important role in macular edema – particularly so in diabetic maculopathy. The endothelial damage resulting from this leukocyte adherence to vessel walls is mediated by nitric oxide, adhesion molecules, and other inflammatory mediators (Leal et al., 2007)[30]. Sub-Tenon triamcinolone inhibits leucocyte-endothelium interactions in the retina and down-regulates adhesion molecules of the retinal vascular endothelium (Mizuno et al., 2007)[31], thus decreasing retinal thickness.

Müller cells represent a further site of action of steroids (Reichenbach et al., 2007)[32]. Macular edema is thought to be partly linked to the down-regulation of the Müller cell protein Kir4.1. The resultant increase in intracellular K^+ leads to the uptake of proteins and osmotic swelling of Müller cells via aquaporin P4 channels. The administration of triamcinolone reduces the production of VEGF, arachidonic acid, and prostaglandins, allowing the reactivation of fluid clearance by Müller cells via endogenous adenosine and the increase in TASK channels. These processes lead to an efflux of potassium, thus correcting the down-regulation of the Kir 4.1 protein (Reichenbach et al., 2007)[32]. It has also been shown that the glucocorticoid triamcinolone acetonide inhibits osmotic swelling of retinal glial cells via stimulation of endogenous adenosine signaling (Uckermann et al., 2005)[33].

Carbonic Anhydrase Inhibitors
Carbonic anhydrase (CA) inhibitors have been used clinically for over 20 years in the treatment of macular edema. The initial observation on its therapeutic efficacy was reported in 1988 in a study of 41 patients with CME of various etiologies (Cox et al., 1988)[34]. It appears that CA inhibitors modulate the polarized distribution of CA at the level of the RPE and thus the fluid resorption from the retina into the choroid.

In the retina, CA is found in the cytoplasm of red/green cones (albeit not in rods) and especially inside Müller cells (Wistrand et al., 1986)[35]. The RPE, however, appears to contain almost exclusively the membrane-bound form of CA (Wolfensberger et al., 1994)[36]. The latter appears to regulate and modulate the extracellular pH gradients created by the metabolic activity of cells and may act as a bicarbonate channel (Wolfensberger et al., 1999; Miller and Steinberg, 1977)[37, 38]. The CA activity in the RPE shows a clear-cut polarized distribution with a large amount of enzymes on the apical surface of the cell, whereas there is less CA activity on the basolateral portion of the cell membrane. Further immunohistochemical differentiation has shown that the isozyme IV is responsible for apical CA activity in the RPE (Wolfensberger et al., 1994)[36]. Under normal conditions, roughly 70% of the subretinal fluid is removed by metabolic transport to the choroid. In an in vivo rabbit model, it could be shown that this fluid transport (which is driven to a large extent by active ion transport through the RPE) can be enhanced by acetazolamide (Marmor and Negi, 1986; Wolfensberger et al., 2000)[39, 40] (fig. 3). Furthermore, experiments in an animal model of iatrogenically induced retinal detachments showed that the disappearance of fluorescein through the RPE increased by 25% after intravenous injection of acetazolamide (Tsuboi and Pederson, 1985)[41]. The same authors also observed a marked increase of resorption of subretinal fluid at a higher dosage of 50–65 mg/kg bodyweight. Further studies on the frog pigment epithelium demonstrated that active chloride and bicarbonate transport probably occurs at the basal surface, which faces the choroidal blood supply, and it was postulated that subretinal fluid absorption occurs at this level (Miller and Steinberg, 1977)[38].

Intravenous injection of acetazolamide has been shown to decrease the pH in the subretinal space in both chicks and cats (Wolfensberger et al., 1999; Yamamoto and Steinberg, 1992)[37, 42]. This acidification was followed immediately by a reduction of the subretinal volume, and it has been postulated that it is the acidification that induces changes in ion and consequent fluid transport through the RPE.

Anti-VEGF Agents
On a cellular level, VEGF has been implicated in many different mechanisms that lead to macular edema. VEGF has, for example, been shown to decrease the occludin protein responsible for the tightness of the intracellular junctions (Antonetti et al., 1998)[43]. VEGF also induces rapid phosphorylation of the tight junction protein occludin and zonula occludens 1, resulting in the breakdown of the BRB (Antonetti et al., 1999)[44]. VEGF-induced BRB breakdown appears to be effected via nitric oxide (Lakshminarayanan et al., 2000)[45]. VEGF also increases paracellular transport without altering the solvent-drag reflection coefficient (DeMaio et al., 2004)[46]. Furthermore, VEGF activation of protein kinase c stimulates occludin phosphorylation and contributes to endothelial permeability (Harhaj et al., 2006)[47].

As discussed above, there are several reports that support the notion that corticosteroids act as indirect anti-VEGF agents (fig. 4). More recently, however, directly acting anti-VEGF agents have come to the forefront as promising treatment options for macular edema of different origins (Cordero Coma et al., 2007; Mason et al., 2006; Rodriguez-Fontal, 2009; Spaide et al., 2009)[48–51]. Several direct antibody compounds, which interfere with the VEGF receptor have been used clinically. Ranibizumab (Lucentis) and bevacizumab (Avastin) are antibodies with high affinity for VEGF, which bind to all VEGF isoforms. These and other drugs have been used widely in age-related macular degeneration for several years, but recently interest has arisen for using these agents in other vascular disease as well. The VEGF aptamer pegaptanib (modified RNA oligonucleotide, which binds and inactivates VEGF165 only) has been shown in animal models to restore BRB in diabetic retinopathy (Starita et al., 2007)[52]. Furthermore, it has been shown that intravitreal injection of bevacizumab potentially reduces not only VEGF but also the stromal cell-derived factor 1α. This suggests that intravitreal bevacizumab may influence intraocular mediators other than VEGF (Arimura et al., 2009)[53].

Other Medical Treatments
Steroid-sparing immunosuppressive drugs are frequently used as additional second-line agents particularly in patients with severe intraocular inflammation and CME (Tranos et al., 2004)[1]. The rationale for these treatments relies on the inhibition of several different proinflammatory cytokines that are specifically involved in causing macular edema by breaking down the BRB in intraocular inflammatory disorders.

Apart from the well-known agents such as VEFG, prostaglandins, and leukotrienes, these cytokines also include insulin-like growth factor-1, IL-6, stromal cell-derived factor-1, and hepatocyte growth factor. Particularly elevated levels of intraocular VEGF and IL-6 have been correlated with the severity of uveitic macular edema (van Kooij et al., 2006; Curnow and Murray, 2006)[54, 55], and treatments directed specifically against these factors have been proposed.

Promising results have also been reported using interferon-α$_2$ (Deuter et al., 2006)[56] as a treatment for long-standing refractory CME in uveitis. In addition, a beneficial effect of interferon on inflammatory CME was noted in a retrospective study of patients with multiple sclerosis-associated intermediate uveitis (Becker et al., 2005)[57].

Others reported comparable efficacy of cyclosporine A to prednisolone in the treatment of macular edema in patients with endogenous uveitis (Nussenblatt et al., 1991)[58]. Anti-tumor necrosis factor (TNF) therapy has also been demonstrated as a promising therapy for uveitic macular edema (Theodossiadis et al., 2007)[59]. Similar effects have been published on diabetic retinopathy in an animal model using etanercept, which could prevent retinal cell death and the upregulation of ICAM-1 (Joussen et al., 2002; Joussen et al., 2009)[60, 61]. However, more recent clinical studies with intravitreal etanercept have shown no benefit of anti-TNF-α therapy in diabetic macular edema disease, and the clinical role of these monoclonal antibodies needs to be reassessed (Tsilimbaris et al., 2007; Wu et al., 2011)[62, 63].

Potential Future Treatments for Diabetic Macular Edema
Several molecular and cellular pathways in the pathophysiology of diabetic macular edema are under investigation by many research groups. The majority of therapies that are in widespread clinical use today are addressing vascular fluid leakage. However, other pathways, which may be equally important, may come to the forefront in the future (Stem and Gardner, 2013)[64]. The following agents are potential future candidates for the treatment of macular edema.

Anti-Inflammatory Agents
It has been described that diabetic retinopathy may be linked to the upregulation of not only VEGF, but also inflammatory cytokines like TNF-α, ICAM-1, and different isoforms of ILs (Koleva-Georgieva et al., 2011)[65]. These cytokines may contribute to leukostasis, and in the long term to ischemia. Any pharmacological agent that can inhibit these factors might potentially play a role in the clinical treatment of diabetic maculopathy.

It has been suggested, for example, that the anti-inflammatory drug aspirin could have a therapeutic effect on diabetic retinopathy (Powell and Field, 1964; Early Treatment Diabetic Retinopathy Study Research Group, 1991)[66, 67], and an animal model has shown that salicylate-based anti-inflammatory drugs reduce cell loss in the ganglion cell layer in the prodromal stages of the disease (Zheng et al., 2007)[68]. Further data of a clinical trial also suggests that nepafenac may reduce the risk of diabetic macular edema after cataract surgery (Stem and Gardner, 2013)[64].

Inhibition of protein kinase C using ruboxistaurin has also been suggested to reduce the progression of macular edema in diabetic retinopathy and the need for macular photocoagulation (Aiello et al., 2006)[69], and others have shown that different isoforms of an atypical class protein kinase C zeta can induce retinal vascular permeability via VEGF and TNF. A specific inhibitor of this enzyme is currently being evaluated for its effectiveness to reduce VEGF-induced retinal vascular leakage (Titchenell et al., 2012)[70].

Another atypical agent with anti-inflammatory properties is minocycline, an antibiotic from the tetracycline family. This drug can inhibit microglial production of TNF-α and IL-1, and it reduces caspase-3 activation (Wang et al., 2005; Krady et al., 2005)[71, 72]. The clinical use of this drug has been evaluated in a phase I/II trial (Cukras et al., 2012)[73], and the result of two further studies have helped to define more clearly the future role of minocycline. Low-dose oral doxycycline has been shown to induce a subclinical improvement in inner retinal function in patients with severe nonproliferative or non-high-risk proliferative diabetic retinopathy (Scott et al., 2014)[74]. However, the same correlation could not be found in a patient group with mild-to-moderate nonproliferative diabetic retinopathy, suggesting that the drug may have a different effect on different stages of diabetic retinal dysfunction (Scott et al., 2014)[75].

A further possible pathway which may be exploited therapeutically is the plasma kallikrein-kinin system. The activation of this system, which is independent of the VEGF pathway, can lead to vascular permeability. Inhibition of the kallikrein-kinin system has been shown to reduce retinal edema in an animal model, and a phase I clinical trial is currently ongoing to assess the role of kallikrein-kinin system inhibitors in clinical practice (Phipps et al., 2012; Abdulaal et al., 2016)[76, 77].

Neuroprotective Agents
It has been shown in different animal models that nerve growth factors such as pigment epithelium-derived factor and brain-derived neurotrophic factor are reduced in diabetes and that the presence of these factors can rescue cell function (Hammes et al., 1995; Seki et al., 2004)[78, 79]. There is experimental evidence that somatostatin, for example, can prevent diabetes-induced retinal neurodegeneration in animals (Beltramo et al., 2016)[80], and its effect has also been evaluated using somatostatin drops to treat the progression of diabetic retinopathy in humans (Cunha-Vaz, 2012)[81]. Somatostatin analogues such as octreotide may also be effective in the treatment of CME by blocking the local and systemic production of growth hormone, insulin-like growth factor, and VEGF (Rothova, 2007)[82]. Treatment with octreotide resulted in marked improvement or even complete resolution of CME in uveitic patients (Kafkala et al., 2006)[83].

Local insulin application to the eye has also been studied in a rat model using hydrogels implanted into the subconjunctival space as a long-term insulin depot. No local side effects were reported, but more studies are needed to ascertain the role of the neuroprotective effect of direct ocular insulin application (Misra et al., 2009)[84].

Antiapoptotic Agents
The inhibition of apoptosis, which is central to cell degeneration in diabetes (Barber et al., 1998)[85], may be a further elegant way to prevent

neural cell death in diabetic retinopathy. Apoptosis can be linked to neurotrophic factor deficiency, hyperglycemia, or glutamate. The action of glutamate is, for example, correlated to caspase-3 and calpain activity (Zhang and Bhavnani, 2006)[86], and inhibiting these proteolytic enzymes may be of use in the future.

Blocking glutamate receptors directly has also been suggested as a strategy to guard the health of the retina in diabetes. It has been shown in diabetic rats that oral memantine therapy could reduce retinal ganglion cell loss, reduce intravitreal VEGF levels, and improve retinal function. This drug has received FDA approval for the treatment of Alzheimer's disease and it may thus potentially be used clinically in the near future for the treatment of diabetic retinopathy (Kusari et al., 2007)[87].

Interestingly, the prostaglandin latanoprost, which is used to increase the transscleral outflow in ocular hypertension, may also have antiapoptotic effects. It has been reported in an animal model that latanoprost drops could reduce glial and neural cell death by inhibiting caspase-3 activity in the ganglion cell layer (Nakanishi et al., 2006)[88].

Further reports have suggested that calpain may also play a role in hypoxia-induced retinal cell damage (Nakajima et al., 2011)[89], and calpain inhibitors have been shown to prevent retinal ganglion cell death in a diabetic retinopathy model in mice, suggesting a future neuroprotective role of these agents (Shanab et al., 2012)[90].

Reduction of Dark Adaption
In the dark adapted state, the rods in the outer retina are subjected to maximal depolarization and glutamate release. This process consumes a very high quantity of oxygen with a potential subsequent hypoxic stress for the retinal tissue (Arden et al., 2005)[91]. It has been hypothesized that the increased metabolic load imposed by dark adaptation cannot be managed as well in the diabetic retina as it would be in a normal retina. Experimental data have shown that this mechanism may thus play a role in exacerbating diabetic retinopathy as retinal hypoxia gives rise to an upregulation of VEGF (Ramsey and Arden, 2015)[92]. A novel method to reduce this metabolic load during dark adaption of the rod photoreceptors would be to use dim nocturnal illumination. A 500-nm light source at night has, for example, been shown to decrease the evolution of early diabetic retinopathy and maculopathy in the short term. The results of a 2-year multicenter clinical trial using a 500 nm light source as a mask over the eyes in patients with noncentral diabetic maculopathy will be available in the near future (Sivaprasad and Arden, 2016)[93].

Rationale for Surgical Management of Macular Edema by Vitrectomy

Although pars plana vitrectomy may be considered as a very simple surgical procedure, its manifold effects on a cellular level are becoming more and more understood (Stefánsson, 2009)[2].

Tractional Origin of Macular Edema

The initial rationale for using vitrectomy in cases of macular edema was entirely structural, i.e., aimed at the removal of vitreous traction on the macula (Fung, 1985; Lewis et al., 1992)[94, 95]. The effect of traction on retinal structures becomes understandable with Newton's third law: to any action there is always an equal reaction in the opposite direction. The force of vitreoretinal traction will thus be met by an equal and opposite force in the retina, resulting in the retinal tissues being pulled apart.

Eventually this results in the lowering of the tissue pressure within the retina, which in turn increases the difference between the hydrostatic pressure in the blood vessels and the tissue, thus contributing to edema formation (Starling's law). Releasing the traction will increase tissue pressure

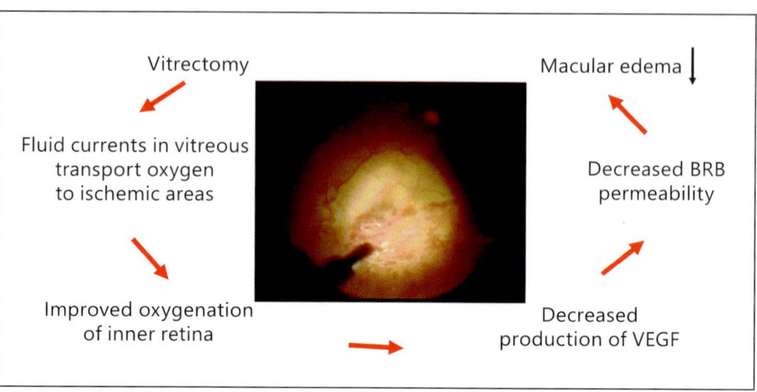

Fig. 5. Schematic diagram showing the effect of a pars plana vitrectomy on intraocular oxygen distribution. Fluid currents during the vitrectomy transport oxygen to the ischemic areas, which creates an improved oxygenation of the inner retina. This in turn reduces VEGF production and BRB permeability, resulting in a decrease in macular edema.

and lower the hydrostatic pressure gradient, reducing the water flux from blood vessels into retinal tissue (Stefánsson, 2009)[2].

Vitreoretinal traction associated with macular edema has been identified in diabetic retinopathy, following complicated cataract surgery (Irvine-Gass syndrome) and in several other disease entities. The removal of such traction by vitreoretinal surgery has been found to be beneficial (Fung, 1985; Lewis et al., 1992; Margherio, 1989)[94–96].

Nontractional Origin of Macular Edema

Recent discoveries have shown that vitrectomy may not only be beneficial in the presence of macular traction, but also in cases where no particular deformation of the macula can be identified. This is particularly true for macular edema of vascular origin, such as diabetes or retinal vein occlusion.

The beneficial effect of the vitrectomy is thought to be based – at least in part – on two mechanisms. Firstly, it has been found, for example, that oxygen transport between the anterior and posterior segments of the eye is increased in the vitrectomized-lentectomized eyes (Stefánsson et al., 1990; Holekamp et al., 2005)[97, 98]. Others have shown that pharmacologic vitreolysis also improves oxygen diffusion within the vitreous cavity (Giblin et al., 2009)[99]. This means that following vitrectomy and/or posterior vitreous detachment, the transport of molecules to and from the retina is increased (fig. 5).

Secondly, it has been shown that several growth factors such as VEGF, IL-6, platelet-derived growth factor, and others are secreted in large amounts into the vitreous during proliferative vasculopathies such as diabetic retinopathy or retinal vein occlusion (Noma et al., 2009; Praidou et al., 2009)[100, 101], and it is conceivable that a complete vitrectomy will remove this excess of growth factors mechanically with the desired effect of a restitution of the BRB. The rapid clearance of VEGF and other cytokines may thus help to prevent macular edema and retinal neovascularization in ischemic retinopathies, such as diabetic retinopathy and retinal vein occlusions. Vitreous clearance of growth factors may indeed have the same effect as the presence of, for example, VEGF antibodies in the vitreous cavity (Stefánsson, 2009; Stefánsson, 2001; Stefánsson, 2006)[2, 102, 103].

A further way of decreasing macular edema through vitrectomy may lie in the peeling of the internal limiting membrane (Park and Kim, 2010)[104], which removes the endplates of the Müller cells. Within those endplates reside both aquaporin 4 and Kir4.1 channels and their removal may remodel the cell in a way that may be beneficial for fluid flow out of the retina.

References

1 Tranos PG, Wickremasinghe SS, Stangos NT, Topouzis F, Tsinopoulos I, Pavesio CE: Macular edema. Surv Ophthalmol 2004;49:470–490.

2 Stefánsson E: Physiology of vitreous surgery. Graefes Arch Clin Exp Ophthalmol 2009;247:147–163.

3 Gillies MC, Su T, Stayt J, Simpson JM, Naidoo D, Salonikas C: Effect of high glucose on permeability of retinal capillary endothelium in vitro. Invest Ophthalmol Vis Sci 1997;38:635–642.

4 Gardner TW, Gabbay RA: Diabetes and obesity: a challenge for every ophthalmologist. Arch Ophthalmol 2009;127:328–329.

5 Aiello LP, Cahill MT, Wong JS: Systemic considerations in the management of diabetic retinopathy. Am J Ophthalmol 2001;132:760–776.

6 Liew G, Mitchell P, Wong TY: Systemic management of diabetic retinopathy. BMJ 2009;338:b441.

7 Colin J: The role of NSAIDs in the management of postoperative ophthalmic inflammation. Drugs 2007;67:1291–1308.

8 Ku EC, Lee W, Kothari HV, Scholer DW: Effect of diclofenac sodium on the arachidonic acid cascade. Am J Med 1986;80:18–23.

9 Bialek S, Quong JN, Yu K, Miller SS: Nonsteroidal anti-inflammatory drugs alter chloride and fluid transport in bovine retinal pigment epithelium. Am J Physiol 1996;270:C1175–C1189.

10 Wolfensberger TJ, Herbort CP: Treatment of cystoid macular edema with non-steroidal anti-inflammatory drugs and corticosteroids. Doc Ophthalmol 1999;97:381–386.

11 Flach AJ, Stegman RC, Graham J, Kruger LP: Prophylaxis of aphakic cystoid macular edema without corticosteroids. A paired-comparison, placebo-controlled double-masked study. Ophthalmology 1990;97:1253–1258.

12 Almeida DR, Johnson D, Hollands H, et al: Effect of prophylactic nonsteroidal antiinflammatory drugs on cystoid macular edema assessed using optical coherence tomography quantification of total macular volume after cataract surgery. J Cataract Refract Surg 2008;34:64–69.

13 DeCroos FC, Afshari NA: Perioperative antibiotics and anti-inflammatory agents in cataract surgery. Curr Opin Ophthalmol 2008;19:22–26.

14 Rossetti L, Chaudhuri J, Dickersin K: Medical prophylaxis and treatment of cystoid macular edema after cataract surgery. The results of a meta-analysis. Ophthalmology 1998;105:397–405.

15 Nelson ML, Martidis A: Managing cystoid macular edema after cataract surgery. Curr Opin Ophthalmol 2003;14:39–43.

16 Sivaprasad S, Bunce C, Patel N: Nonsteroidal anti-inflammatory agents for treating cystoid macular oedema following cataract surgery. Cochrane Database Syst Rev 2005;1:CD004239.

17 Rojas B, Zafirakis P, Christen W, Markomichelakis NN, Foster CS: Medical treatment of macular edema in patients with uveitis. Doc Ophthalmol 1999;97:399–407.

18 Flach AJ, Dolan BJ, Irvine AR: Effectiveness of ketorolac tromethamine 0.5% ophthalmic solution for chronic aphakic and pseudophakic cystoid macular edema. Am J Ophthalmol 1987;103:479–486.

19 Flach AJ, Jampol LM, Weinberg D, et al: Improvement in visual acuity in chronic aphakic and pseudophakic cystoid macular edema after treatment with topical 0.5% ketorolac tromethamine. Am J Ophthalmol 1991;112:514–519.

20 Haynes RC Jr, Murad F: Adrenocorticoropic hormone: adrenocortical steroids and their synthetic analogs: inhibitors of adrenocortical steroid biosynthesis; in Gilman AG, Goodman LS, Rall TW, Murad F (eds): The Pharmacological Basis of Therapeutics. New York, Macmillan, 1985, p 1459.

21 Nehmé A, Edelman J: Dexamethasone inhibits high glucose-, TNF-alpha-, and IL-1beta-induced secretion of inflammatory and angiogenic mediators from retinal microvascular pericytes. Invest Ophthalmol Vis Sci 2008;49:2030–2038.

22 Othenin-Girard P, Borruat X, Bovey E, Pittet N, Herbort CP: Diclofenac-dexamethasone combination in treatment of postoperative inflammation: prospective double-blind study (in French). Klin Monatsbl Augenheilkd 1992;200:362–366.

23 Edelman JL, Lutz D, Castro MR: Corticosteroids inhibit VEGF-induced vascular leakage in a rabbit model of blood-retinal and blood-aqueous barrier breakdown. Exp Eye Res 2005;80:249–258.

24 Wang K, Yanling Wang, Lixin Gao, Xinmin LI, Mingming LI, Jianyou Guo: Dexamethasone inhibits leukocyte accumulation and vascular permeability in retina of streptozotocin-induced diabetic rats via reducing vascular endothelial growth factor and intercellular adhesion molecule-1 expression. Biol Pharm Bull 2008;31:1541–1546.

25 Zhang X, Bao S, Lai D, Rapkins RW, Gillies MC: Intravitreal triamcinolone acetonide inhibits breakdown of the blood-retinal barrier through differential regulation of VEGF-A and its receptors in early diabetic rat retinas. Diabetes 2008;57:1026–1033.

26 Antonetti DA, Wolpert EB, DeMaio L, Harhaj NS, Scaduto RC Jr: Hydrocortisone decreases retinal endothelial cell water and solute flux coincident with increased content and decreased phosphorylation of occludin. J Neurochem 2002;80:667–677.

27 Felinski EA, Cox AE, Phillips BE, et al: Glucocorticoids induce transactivation of tight junction genes occludin and claudin-5 in retinal endothelial cells via a novel cis-element. Exp Eye Res 2008;86:867–878.

28 Nauck M, Roth M, Tamm M, Eickelberg O, Wieland H, Stulz P, Perruchoud AP: Induction of vascular endothelial growth factor by platelet-activating factor and platelet-derived growth factor is downregulated by corticosteroids. Am J Respir Cell Mol Biol 1997;16:398–406.

29 Ebrahem Q, Atsushi Minamoto, George Hoppe, Bela Anand-Apte, Sears JE: Triamcinolone acetonide inhibits IL-6- and VEGF-induced angiogenesis downstream of the IL-6 and VEGF receptors. Invest Ophthalmol Vis Sci 2006;47:4935–4941.

30 Leal EC, Manivannan A, Hosoya K, Terasaki T, Cunha-Vaz J, Ambrosio AF, Forrester JV: Inducible nitric oxide synthase isoform is a key mediator of leukostasis and blood-retinal barrier breakdown in diabetic retinopathy. Invest Ophthalmol Vis Sci 2007;48:5257–5265.

31 Mizuno S, Nishiwaki A, Morita H, Miyake T, Ogura Y: Effects of periocular administration of triamcinolone acetonide on leukocyte-endothelium interactions in the ischemic retina. Invest Ophthalmol Vis Sci 2007;48:2831–2836.

32 Reichenbach A, Wurm A, Pannicke T, Iandiev I, Wiedemann P, Bringmann A: Müller cells as players in retinal degeneration and edema. Graefes Arch Clin Exp Ophthalmol 2007;245:627–636.

33 Uckermann O, Kutzera F, Wolf A, et al: The glucocorticoid triamcinolone acetonide inhibits osmotic swelling of retinal glial cells via stimulation of endogenous adenosine signaling. J Pharmacol Eyp Ther 2005;315:1036–1045.

34 Cox SN, Hay E, Bird AC: Treatment of chronic macular edema with acetazolamide. Arch Ophthalmol 1988;106:1190–1195.

35 Wistrand, PJ, Schenholm M, Lönnerholm G: Carbonic anhydrase isoenzymes CA I and CA II in the human eye. Invest Ophthalmol Vis Sci 1986;27:419–428.

36 Wolfensberger TJ, Mahieu I, Jarvis-Evans J, et al: Membrane-bound carbonic anhydrase in human retinal pigment epithelium. Invest Ophthalmol Vis Sci 1994;35:3401–3407.

37 Wolfensberger TJ, Dmitriev AV, Govardovskii VI: Inhibition of membrane-bound carbonic anhydrase decreases subretinal pH and volume. Doc Ophthalmol 1999;97:261–271.

38 Miller SS, Steinberg RH: Active transport of ions across frog retinal pigment epithelium. Exp Eye Res 1977;25:235.

39 Marmor MF, Negi A: Pharmacologic modification of subretinal fluid absorption in the rabbit eye. Arch Ophthalmol 1986;104:1674–1677.

40 Wolfensberger TJ, Chiang RK, Takeuchi A, Marmor MF: Inhibition of membrane-bound carbonic anhydrase enhances subretinal fluid absorption and retinal adhesiveness. Graefes Arch Clin Exp Ophthalmol 2000;238:76–80.

41 Tsuboi S, Pederson JE: Experimental retinal detachment. X. Effect of acetazolamide on vitreous fluorescein disappearance. Arch Ophthalmol 1985;103:1557–1558.

42 Yamamoto F, Steinberg RH: Effects of intravenous acetazolamide on retinal pH in the cat. Exp Eye Res 1992;54:711–718.

43 Antonetti DA, Barber AJ, Khin S, Lieth E, Tarbell JM, Gardner TW: Vascular permeability in experimental diabetes is associated with reduced endothelial occludin content: vascular endothelial growth factor decreases occluding in retinal endothelial cells. Penn State Retina Research Group. Diabetes 1998;47:1953–1959.

44 Antonetti DA, Barber AJ, Hollinger LA, Wolpert EB, Gardner TW: Vascular endothelial growth factor induces rapid phosphorylation of tight junction proteins occludin and zonula occluden 1. J Biol Chem 1999;274:23463–23467.

45 Lakshminarayanan S, Antonetti DA, Gardner TW, Tarbell JM: Effect of VEGF on retinal microvascular endothelial hydraulic conductivity: the role of NO. Invest Ophthalmol Vis Sci 2000;41:4256–4261.

46 DeMaio L, Antonetti DA, Scaduto RC Jr, Gardner TW, Tarbell JM: VEGF increases paracellular transport without altering the solvent-drag reflection coefficient. Microvasc Res 2004;68:295–302.

47 Harhaj NS, Felinski EA, Wolpert EB, Sundstrom JM, Gardner TW, Antonetti DA: VEGF activation of protein kinase C stimulates occludin phosphorylation and contributes to endothelial permeability. Invest Ophthalmol Vis Sci 2006;47:5106–5115.

48 Cordero Coma M, Sobrin L, Onal S, Christen W, Foster CS: Intravitreal bevacizumab for treatment of uveitic macular edema. Ophthalmology 2007;114:1574–1579.

49 Mason JO 3rd, Albert MA Jr, Vail R: Intravitreal bevacizumab (Avastin) for refractory pseudophakic cystoid macular edema. Retina 2006;26:356–357.

50 Rodriguez-Fontal M, Alfaro V, Kerrison JB, Jablon EP: Ranibizumab for diabetic retinopathy. Curr Diabetes Rev 2009;5:47–51.

51 Spaide RF, Chang LK, Klancnik JM, Yannuzzi LA, Sorenson J, Slakter JS, Freund KB, Klein R: Prospective study of intravitreal ranibizumab as a treatment for decreased visual acuity secondary to central retinal vein occlusion. Am J Ophthalmol 2009;147:298–306.

52 Starita C, Patel M, Katz B, Adamis AP: Vascular endothelial growth factor and the potential therapeutic use of pegaptanib (Macugen) in diabetic retinopathy. Dev Ophthalmol 2007;39:122–148.

53 Arimura N, Otsuka H, Yamakiri K, Sonoda Y, Nakao S, Noda Y, Hashiguchi T, Maruyama I, Sakamoto T: Vitreous mediators after intravitreal bevacizumab or triamcinolone acetonide in eyes with proliferative diabetic retinopathy. Ophthalmology 2009;116:921–926.

54 van Kooij B, Rothova A, Rijkers GT, de Groot-Mijnes JD: Distinct cytokine and chemokine profiles in the aqueous of patients with uveitis and cystoid macular edema. Am J Ophthalmol 2006;142:192–194.

55 Curnow SJ, Murray PI: Inflammatory mediators of uveitis: cytokines and chemokines. Curr Opin Ophthalmol 2006;17:532–537.

56 Deuter CM, Koetter I, Guenaydin I, Stuebiger N, Zierhut M: Interferon alfa-2a: a new treatment option for long lasting refractory cystoid macular edema in uveitis? A pilot study. Retina 2006;26:786–791.

57 Becker MD, Heiligenhaus A, Hudde T, et al: Interferon as a treatment for uveitis associated with multiple sclerosis. Br J Ophthalmol 2005;89:1254–1257.

58 Nussenblatt RB, Palestine AG, Chan CC, Stevens G Jr, Mellow SD, Green SB: Randomized, double-masked study of cyclosporine compared to prednisolone in the treatment of endogenous uveitis. Am J Ophthalmol 1991;112:138–146.

59 Theodossiadis PG, Markomichelakis NN, Sfikakis PP: Tumor necrosis factor antagonists: preliminary evidence for an emerging approach in the treatment of ocular inflammation. Retina 2007;27:399–413.

60 Joussen AM, Poulaki V, Mitsiades N, et al: Nonsteroidal anti-inflammatory drugs prevent early diabetic retinopathy via TNF-alpha suppression. FASEB J 2002;16:438–440.

61 Joussen AM, Doehmen S, Le ML, et al: TNF-alpha mediated apoptosis plays an important role in the development of early diabetic retinopathy and long-term histopathological alterations. Mol Vis 2009;15:1418–1428.

62 Tsilimbaris MK, Panagiotoglou TD, Charisis SK, et al: The use of intravitreal etanercept in diabetic macular oedema. Semin Ophthalmol 2007;22:75–79.

63 Wu L, Hernandez-Bogantes E, Roca JA, et al: Intravitreal tumor necrosis factor inhibitors in the treatment of refractory diabetic macular edema: a pilot study from the Pan-American Collaborative Retina Study Group. Retina 2011;31:298–303.

64 Stem MS, Gardner TW: Neurodegeneration in the pathogenesis of diabetic retinopathy: molecular mechanisms and therapeutic implications. Curr Med Chem 2013;20:3241–3250.

65 Koleva-Georgieva DN, Sivkova NP, Terzieva D: Serum inflammatory cytokines IL-1beta, IL-6, TNF-alpha and VEGF have influence on the development of diabetic retinopathy. Folia Med (Plovdiv) 2011;53:44–50.

66 Powell ED, Field RA: Diabetic retinopathy and rheumatoid arthritis. Lancet 1964;2:17–18.

67 Early Treatment Diabetic Retinopathy Study Research Group: Effects of aspirin treatment on diabetic retinopathy. ETDRS report number 8. Ophthalmology 1991;98:757–865.

68 Zheng L, Howell SJ, Hatala DA, et al: Salicylate-based anti-inflammatory drugs inhibit the early lesion of diabetic retinopathy. Diabetes 2007;56:337–345.

69 Aiello LP, Davis MD, Girach A, et al: Effect of ruboxistaurin on visual loss in patients with diabetic retinopathy. Ophthalmology 2006;113:2221–2230.

70 Titchenell PM, Lin CM, Keil JM, et al: Novel atypical PKC inhibitors prevent vascular endothelial growth factor-induced blood-retinal barrier dysfunction. Biochem J 2012;446:455–467.

71 Wang AL, Yu AC, Lau LT, et al: Minocycline inhibits LPS-induced retinal microglia activation. Neurochem Int 2005; 47:152–158.

72 Krady JK, Basu A, Allen CM, et al: Minocycline reduces proinflammatory cytokine expression, microglial activation, and caspase-3 activation in rodent model of diabetic retinopathy. Diabetes 2005;54:1559–1565.

73 Cukras CA, Petrou P, Chew EY, et al: Oral minocycline for the treatment of diabetic macular edema (DME): results of a phase I/II clinical study. Invest Ophth Vis Sci 2012;53:3865–3874.

74 Scott IU, Jackson GR, Quillen DA, et al: Effect of doxycycline vs placebo on retinal function and diabetic retinopathy progression in patients with severe nonproliferative or non-high-riskproliferative diabetic retinopathy: a randomized clinical trial. JAMA Ophthalmol 2014; 132:535–543.

75 Scott IU, Jackson GR, Quillen DA, et al: Effect of doxycycline vs placebo on retinal function and diabetic retinopathy progression in patients with mild to moderate nonproliferative diabetic retinopathy: a randomized clinical trial. JAMA Ophthalmol 2014;132:1137–1142.

76 Phipps JA, Jobling AI, Greferath U: Alternative pathways in the developement of diabetic retinopathy: the renin-angiotensin and kallikrein-kinin systems. Clin Exp Optom 2012;95:282–289.

77 Abdulaal M, Haddad NM, Sun JK, et al: The role of plasma kallikrein-kinin pathway in the development of diabetic retinopathy: pathophysiology and therapeutic approaches. Semin Ophthalmol 2016;31:19–24.

78 Hammes HP, Federoff HJ, Brownlee M: Nerve growth factor prevents both neuroretinal programmed cell death and capillary pathology in experimental diabetes. Mol Med 1995;1:527–534.

79 Seki M, Tanaka T, Nawa H, et al: Involvement of brain-derived neurotrophic factor in early retinal neuropathy of streptozotocin-induced diabetes in rats: therapeutic potential of brain-derived neurotrophic factor for dopaminergic amacrine cells. Diabetes 2004;53:2412–2419.

80 Beltramo E, Lopatinia T, Mazzeo A, et al: Effects of the neuroprotective drugs somatostatin and brimonidineon retinal cell models of diabetic retinopathy. Acta Diabetol 2016;53:957–964.

81 Cunha-Vaz J: Neurodegeneration as an early event in the pathogenesis of Diabetic Retinopathy: A multicentric, prospective, phase II-III, randomised controlled trial to assess the efficacy of neuroprotective drugs administered topically to prevent or arrest Diabetic Retinopathy. EUROCONDOR – EU FP7 Project. Acta Ophthalmol 2012;90:0.

82 Rothova A: Inflammatory cystoid macular edema. Curr Opin Ophthalmol 2007; 18:487–492.

83 Kafkala C, Choi JY, Choopong P, Foster CS: Octreotide as a treatment for uveitic cystoid macular edema. Arch Ophthalmol 2006;124:1353–1355.

84 Misra GP, Singh RS, Aleman TS, et al: Subconjunctivally implantable hydrogels with degradable and thermoresponsive properties for sustained release of insulin to the retina. Biomaterials 2009; 30:6541–6547.

85 Barber AJ, Lieth E, Khin SA, et al: Neural apoptosis in the retina during experimental and human diabetes. Early onset and effect of insulin. J Clin Invest 1998; 102:783–791.

86 Zhang Y, Bhavnani BR: Glutamate-induced apoptosis in neuronal cells is mediated via caspase-dependent and independent mechanisms involving calpain and caspase-3 proteases as well as apoptosis inducing factor (AIF) and this process is inhibited by equine estrogens. BMC Neurosci 2006;7:49.

87 Kusari J, Zhou S, Padillo E, et al: Effect of memantine on neuroretinal function and retinal vascular changes of streptozotocin-induced diabetic rats. Invest Ophth Vis Sci 2007;48:5152–5159.

88 Nakanishi Y, Nakamura M, Mukuno H, et al: Latanoprost rescues retinal neuroglial cells from apoptosis by inhibiting caspase-3, which is mediated by p44/p42 mitogen-activated protein kinase. Exp Eye Res 2006;83:1108–1117.

89 Nakajima E, Hammond KB, Rosales JL, et al: Calpain, not caspase, is the causative protease for hypoxic damage in cultured monkey retinal cells. Invest Ophthalmol Vis Sci 2011;52:7059–7067.

90 Shanab AY, Nakazawa T, Ryu M, et al: Metabolic stress response implicated in diabetic retinopathy: the role of calpain, and the therapeutic impact of calpain inhibitor. Neurobiol Dis 2012;48:556–567.

91 Arden GB, Sidman RL, Arap W, et al: Spare the rod and spoil the eye. Br J Ophthalmol 2005;89:764–769.

92 Ramsey DJ, Arden GB: Hypoxia and dark adaptation in diabetic retinopathy: interactions, consequences, and therapy. Curr Diab Rep 2015;15:118.

93 Sivaprasad S, Arden G: Spare the rods and spoil the retina: revisited. Eye (Lond) 2016;30:189–192.

94 Fung WE: Vitrectomy for chronic aphakic cystoid macular edema. Results of a national, collaborative, prospective, randomized investigation. Ophthalmology 1985;92:1102–1111.

95 Lewis H, Abrams GW, Blumenkranz MS, et al: Vitrectomy for diabetic macular traction and edema associated with posterior hyaloidal traction. Ophthalmology 1992;99:753–759.

96 Margherio RR, Trese MT, Margherio AR, et al: Surgical management of vitreomacular traction syndromes. Ophthalmology 1989;96:1437–1445.

97 Stefánsson E, Novack RL, Hatchell DL: Vitrectomy prevents retinal hypoxia in branch retinal vein occlusion. Invest Ophthalmol Vis Sci 1990;31:284–289.

98 Holekamp NM, Shui YB, Beebe DC: Vitrectomy surgery increases oxygen exposure to the lens: a possible mechanism for nuclear cataract formation. Am J Ophthalmol 2005;139:302–310.

99 Giblin FJ, Quiram PA, Leverenz VR, et al: Enzyme-induced posterior vitreous detachment in the rat produces increased lens nuclear pO_2 levels. Exp Eye Res 2009;88:286–292.

100 Noma H, Funatsu H, Mimura T, et al: Vitreous levels of interleukin-6 and vascular endothelial growth factor in macular edema with central retinal vein occlusion. Ophthalmology 2009;116:87–93.

101 Praidou A, Klangas I, Papakonstantinou E, et al: Vitreous and serum levels of platelet-derived growth factor and their correlation in patients with proliferative diabetic retinopathy. Curr Eye Res 2009;34:152–161.

102 Stefánsson E: The therapeutic effects of retinal laser treatment and vitrectomy. A theory based on oxygen and vascular physiology. Acta Ophthalmol Scand 2001;79:435–440.

103 Stefánsson E: Ocular oxygenation and the treatment of diabetic retinopathy. Surv Ophthalmol 2006;51:364–380.

104 Park DH, Kim IT: Long-term effects of vitrectomy and internal limiting membrane peeling for macular edema secondary to central retinal vein occlusion and hemiretinal vein occlusion. Retina 2010;5:1089–1093.

Prof. Thomas J. Wolfensberger, MD, MBA
Jules Gonin Eye Hospital, Department of Ophthalmology, University of Lausanne
Avenue de France 15
CH–1000 Lausanne 7 (Switzerland)
E-Mail thomas.wolfensberger@fa2.ch

Coscas G (ed): Macular Edema. 2nd, revised and extended edition.
Dev Ophthalmol. Basel, Karger, 2017, vol 58, pp 87–101 (DOI: 10.1159/000455276)

Drug Delivery to the Posterior Segment of the Eye

Elad Moisseiev · Anat Loewenstein

Division of Ophthalmology, Tel Aviv Sourasky Medical Center, Sackler Faculty of Medicine, Tel Aviv University, Tel Aviv, Israel

Abstract

Drug delivery into the posterior segment of the eye is complicated by the existence of the blood-ocular barrier. Strategies for delivering drugs to the posterior segment include systemic administration, modification of the barrier, and local drug delivery (including transcorneal, transscleral, and intravitreal). The most commonly used method for drug delivery into the posterior segment is by intravitreal injection. Other routes that can be used to achieve therapeutic drug levels in the posterior segment include topical, iontophoretic, and juxtascleral delivery. Extended-release intravitreal drug delivery systems can achieve sustained therapeutic levels with the goal of providing a prolonged clinical benefit with significantly fewer interventions. © 2017 S. Karger AG, Basel

The Posterior Segment of the Eye and the Blood-Ocular Barrier

The blood-ocular barrier (BOB) has three key functions: it maintains tissue/fluid composition, produces aqueous humor, and keeps pathogens out of the eye. The barrier consists of tight junctions at the level of the iris vascular epithelium and nonpigmented ciliary epithelium, where they form the blood-aqueous barrier, and at the level of the retinal vascular endothelium and retinal pigment epithelium (RPE), where they form the blood-retinal barrier. In addition to preventing pathogens from entering the eye, the BOB also restricts drugs from entering the eye (Hughes et al., 2005; Urtti, 2006)[1,2].

This barrier can be damaged by surgery; conditions such as uveitis, diabetes, and ocular infection; and by certain treatments such as photocoagulation and cryopexy. When the BOB breaks down, drugs can enter and leave the eye more easily; a shift in Starling forces (forces controlling the fluid balance) can occur, resulting in macular edema; and serum can also leak into the eye, leading to cellular proliferation, and there can be aqueous hyposecretion.

Strategies for Delivering Drugs to the Posterior Segment

Conceptually, there are three approaches to delivering drugs to the eye:

1 *Deliver large amounts of drugs systemically.* Traditionally drugs are administered systemically in amounts that are theoretically large enough to achieve therapeutic levels in the eye. In practice, however, the amounts of drugs actually reaching the posterior segment are limited by the BOB, which therefore requires very high doses to be administered systemically in order to achieve even borderline therapeutic retinal drug levels. The limiting factor to this approach is frequently the systemic toxicity associated with the relatively high systemic drug levels needed to overcome the BOB.

2 *Modify the BOB.* The second approach to drug delivery is to modify the permeability of the BOB to allow greater drug penetrance and allow access to certain drugs and compounds [e.g., histamines, bradykinin agonists, and vascular endothelial growth factor (VEGF)] that can increase vascular permeability. This approach is rarely used.

3 *Local delivery of drugs to the eye.* The third strategy involves delivering drugs locally to the target tissues. There is evidence to suggest that local delivery of drugs to the posterior segment is the most effective approach to the management of posterior segment diseases, and this approach is the one most commonly used in clinical practice.

Local Therapy

There are numerous approaches of local drug delivery to the posterior segment, which can be very different from one another. These span a spectrum starting from topical administration of drops to bypassing the BOB entirely via intravitreal injection of drugs directly into the eye.

Topical therapy is the most common mode of drug delivery into the eye, but it is mostly ineffective for posterior segment diseases due to low penetrance. The concept of transcorneal iontophoresis has been under extended development for years but has not yet been adapted for any indication. Periocular approaches and intravitreal injections have long been used and can be extremely effective. This chapter will discuss the various approaches of posterior segment drug delivery, and the recent advances in their research.

Topical Drug Delivery

Penetration and distribution of a drug into the posterior tissues of the eye after topical administration can occur by diffusion into the iris root and subsequently into the posterior chamber and segment, or through the pars plana, without encountering the blood-retinal barrier (Hughes et al., 2005)[1]. The drugs can also enter the sclera by lateral diffusion followed by penetration of Bruch's membrane and the RPE. To a lesser extent, the drug can be absorbed into the systemic circulation either through the conjunctival vessels or via the nasolacrimal duct and gain systemic access to the retinal vessels.

Topically applied drugs reach the posterior segment via the transcorneal or transconjunctival pathways (Urtti, 2006; Chiou and Watanabe, 1982; Ahmed and Patton, 1985; Geroski and Edelhauser, 2000)[2–5]. Transcorneal penetration involves crossing the corneal epithelial barrier, across into the anterior chamber, and then through the lens or the iris root. Transscleral or transconjunctival penetration is either across the sclera, choroid, choriocapillaris, and the RPE to the retina, or indirectly into the retrobulbar space and the optic nerve head (Ahmed and Patton, 1985)[4].

Although topical administration of drugs for the treatment of posterior segment pathology is not commonly utilized, one should remember this can be a very safe and effective means of therapy. For example, topical administration of steroid and non-steroidal anti-inflammatory drops is widely used for the management of pseudophakic cystoid macular edema with excellent results (Guo et al., 2015)[6]. The main limitations of this simple method of drug administration are ocular surface irritation (usually due to preservatives in drop formulations) and its dependence on patient compliance.

Transcorneal Route

The cornea is a unique tissue which has an aqueous phase (stroma) sandwiched by 2 lipid layers (epithelium and endothelium). As a result, a drug that is both hydrophobic and hydrophilic can penetrate corneal tissue freely. If a drug is a pure polar or a pure nonpolar compound, it cannot penetrate the cornea effectively. The corneal barrier is formed upon maturation of the epithelial cells. The apical corneal epithelial cells form tight junctions that limit paracellular drug permeation. Therefore, lipophilic drugs typically have at least an order of magnitude higher permeability through the cornea than hydrophilic drugs. Despite the tightness of the corneal epithelial layer, transcorneal permeation is the main route of drug entrance from the lacrimal fluid to the aqueous humor. The amount of drug that penetrates does not depend on the volume of the drop once it is above 10 μl (Maurice, 2002)[7]. The maximum concentration in the aqueous humor occurs between 0.5 and 3 h after instillation and there is a ×150,000 dilution of the drop for a hydrophilic drug and a ×1,500 dilution for a lipophilic drug (Maurice, 2002)[7].

Transscleral/Transconjunctival Route

The sclera has a large and accessible surface area and a high degree of hydration that renders it conducive to water-soluble substances. It is relatively devoid of cells. Moreover, the sclera has few proteolytic enzymes or protein-binding sites that can degrade or sequester drugs. Scleral permeability does not appreciably decline with age (Olsen et al., 1995)[8]. Mechanically blocking off the corneal surface has little effect on drug penetration into the posterior tissues, suggesting that the transscleral/transconjunctival route is more important for posterior segment drug delivery.

Subconjunctival injection of a lipophobic tracer results in a ×1/100,000 decrease in retinal and vitreous levels. For a very lipophilic tracer, these quantities are about 10 times greater (Maurice, 2002)[7].

New Topical Therapies for Retinal and Choroidal Diseases

Although several topical therapies for retinal and choroidal diseases are under development, none are currently available for clinical use. The following are a few examples of such drugs.

TargeGen 801 VEGF Receptor/src Kinase Inhibitor

The TargeGen 801 VEGF receptor/src kinase inhibitor acts against VEGF receptor/PDGF receptor/Src family kinases resulting in antipermeability, antiangiogenic, and anti-inflammatory effects. Pharmacokinetic data across multiple species have shown that the drug moves from the front to the back of the eye via a transscleral route. The drug is delivered as a prodrug, with a molecular weight of 580 kDa, which is then converted to an active agent with a molecular weight of 476 kDa.

A phase I trial has been completed in 42 healthy volunteers who were given high- and low-dose TG100801 twice daily for 14 days. The drug was well tolerated at both doses. A phase II trial was initiated in patients with choroidal neovascularization due to age-related macular degeneration (AMD). While some clinical benefit was seen, the study was halted due to the formation of corneal deposits (unpubl. data).

Othera OT-551

Othera OT-551 is a small prodrug molecule which gets converted to TEMPOL (4-hydroxy-2,2,6,6-tetramethylpiperidine-N-oxyl) hydroxylamine. The multiple modes of action include antioxidant, antiangiogenic, and anti-inflammatory properties. It suppresses photo-oxidative damage in the RPE and photoreceptors, and also down-regulates disease-induced overexpression of NF-κB. It also inhibits angiogenesis stimulated by VEGF and other factors, and is synergistic/additive with ranibizumab. Othera OT-551 penetrates the cornea and sclera, and distributes to the retina. Results of phase II clinical trials of this drug in geographic atrophy and neovascular AMD reported good tolerability but no significant beneficial effect in visual outcome measures. Therefore, this drug has not been explored further as a potential treatment (Ni and Hui, 2009; Wong et al., 2010)[9, 10].

Pazopanib

Pazopanib (GW786034) is a potent multitargeted receptor tyrosine kinase inhibitor against VEGF receptors 1, 2, and 3; platelet-derived growth factor receptors α and β, and the stem cell factor receptor (c-kit) (Kumar, 2007)[11]. It has shown significant activity in preclinical models of ocular neovascularization and tumor angiogenesis. Pazopanib eye drops were well-tolerated by patients with AMD; however, their use did not have a significant effect on visual acuity and did not reduce the need for intravitreal ranibizumab injections (Singh et al, 2014; Csaky et al., 2015)[12, 13]. Overall, this drug did not result in therapeutic benefit beyond that obtained with ranibizumab alone, and therefore it is not used in clinical practice.

Iontophoresis for Drug Delivery

A number of chemical and physical enhancement techniques have been developed in an attempt to compromise epithelial barrier function in a reversible manner. Ocular iontophoresis was first investigated in 1908 by the German investigator Wirtz. Iontophoresis involves the application of a small electric potential to maintain a constant current, which allows controlled drug delivery (Wirtz, 1908)[14].

The amount of compound delivered is directly proportional to the quantity of charge passed. The basic electrical principle that oppositely charged ions attract and same charged ions repel is the central tenet of iontophoresis. The ionized substances are driven into the tissue by electrorepulsion at either the anode (for positive drugs) or the cathode (for negatively charged drugs) (Guy, 2000)[15]. This ionic-electric field interaction, also called the Nernst-Planck effect, is the largest contributor to flux enhancement for small ions.

Other advantages include an improved onset time as well as a more rapid offset time, such that once the current is switched off, there is no further transport. Moreover, the current profile can be customized to achieve the desired drug input kinetics depending on whether continuous or pulsatile delivery is required. The electromigration of a molecule depends on the concentration of the drug, the magnitude of current, and the pH value.

Several investigators conducted clinical studies using transscleral iontophoresis of the anti-inflammatory corticosteroid, methylprednisolone hemisuccinate SoluMedrol®. Halhal et al. (2003)[16] presented the results of a study of patients with acute corneal graft rejection. Iontophoretic treatment of methylprednisolone using 1.5 mA (3 mA/cm^2) for 4 min was performed once daily for 3 consecutive days, with no need for analgesia. Of the eyes treated, 88% demonstrated complete reversal of the rejection processes with no significant side effects.

Periocular/Sub-Tenon/Juxtascleral Drug Delivery

The posterior juxtascleral depot method delivers drugs into the sub-Tenon space onto bare sclera in a depot in the region of the macula.

This method of drug delivery avoids the risk of intraocular damage and endophthalmitis posed by an intravitreal injection. Much like subconjunctival injections, there is an increased risk of systemic drug exposure due to drug contact with orbital tissue when compared with intravitreal injections, though there is much less systemic exposure than occurs with either topical or systemic therapy.

Sub-Tenon Triamcinolone Acetonide

The sub-Tenon administration of triamcinolone acetonide is commonly practiced in clinical ophthalmology. This method provides two important goals. First it specifically delivers the drug to the site of desired activity while avoiding most systemic side effects secondary to systemic drug absorption. Second, the drug is slowly released while contained in a closed sub-Tenon compartment, thus local tissue levels of the drug are constant for a relatively long duration of time. The drug can be delivered in various methods, such as by cannula to the posterior sub-Tenon space or to the orbital floor. The commonly used dose is 40 mg in 1 ml. This method of administration may cause a rise in intraocular pressure (IOP) and cataract progression; however, this risk appears to be relatively low (Byun and Park, 2009)[17], and these complications are related to the steroids and not the injection procedure.

Sub-Tenon triamcinolone has been reported to be effective in the treatment of selected cases of refractory diabetic macular edema or intermediate uveitis (Bakri and Kaiser, 2005; Venkatesh et al., 2007)[18, 19].

Juxtascleral (Modified Sub-Tenon) Anecortave Acetate

Anecortave acetate (Retaane, Alcon) was formulated after removal of the 11β-hydroxyl group and the addition of the 21-acetate group in a typical steroid. Conceptually, the goal was to maintain the therapeutic benefit of the steroid but eliminate the likelihood of steroid-related ocular side effects, primarily glaucoma and cataract. Anecortave inhibits vascular proliferation by decreasing extracellular protease expression and inhibiting endothelial cell migration. It is administered as a posterior juxtascleral depot of 15 mg/0.5 ml every 6 months using the 19-gauge, 56° posterior juxtascleral cannula. The clinical trials of anecortave acetate in wet AMD and primary open-angle glaucoma have been discontinued since they failed to show efficacy in phase III trials after initially showing benefit in phase II trials (Russell et al., 2007)[20], and this drug is not currently used.

Drug Delivery to the Suprachoroidal Space

The suprachoroidal space (SCS) is a potential space between the choroid and the sclera, and recent advances in optical coherence tomography technology have made it possible to image it in patients (Moisseiev et al., 2016)[21]. The SCS is an attractive new route for drug delivery to the posterior segment, as it bypasses the sclera without the risk of intraocular penetration and can accommodate up to 1 ml of fluid. Also, although it does not bypass the blood-retinal barrier, it may be the method of choice for administration of drugs targeted at the RPE. It has been shown that drug delivery from the SCS to the vitreous declines with an increase in drug lipophilicity and molecular weight (Kadam et al., 2013)[22], but as it may hold a relatively large volume these limitations can be overcome. Specialized short small-gauge microneedles have been developed to allow safe in-office injections into the SCS. Administration of corticosteroids via this route was shown to reduce intraocular inflammation, and administration of antiglaucoma agents was shown to reduce IOP in animal models (Gilger et al., 2013; Patel et al., 2012)[23, 24].

A phase I/II study evaluating the safety and tolerability of 4 mg/100 µl triamcinolone acetonide administered to the SCS in patients with noninfectious uveitis has been performed (clinicaltrials.gov NCT01789320; data unpublished as of print).

Intravitreal Injections

Intravitreal injections have a long history of use in clinical practice. This method provides maximum drug concentrations within the vitreal cavity with minimal systemic absorption. Once used primarily to deliver antibiotic agents to treat endophthalmitis and retinitis, and later used to deliver steroids to treat macular edema of various causes, this method is now widely used for the treatment of a multitude of posterior segment pathologies, most notably neovascular AMD and macular edema secondary to vascular occlusive disease and diabetes. At present, intravitreal injections are the most commonly used route of drug delivery to the posterior segment.

The introduction of a needle through the sclera may be the port of entry of bacteria into the eye. The feared complication of bacterial endophthalmitis does not seem to be as common as once believed. Large-scale clinical trials have yielded low rates of endophthalmitis after intravitreal injections done utilizing topical povidone-iodine, sterile speculum, and topical anesthesia, and currently the estimated risk is under 0.1% (Bhavsar et al., 2009)[25].

Other ocular complications that can be caused by intravitreal injections include cataract formation, elevated IOP and glaucoma, choroidal hemorrhage, endophthalmitis, vitreous hemorrhage, retinal breaks, and retinal detachment (Prasad et al., 2007)[26].

A variety of drugs can be administered via intravitreal injection, the most common being anti-VEGF agents such as ranibizumab, bevacizumab, and aflibercept. This route is also frequently used for the administration of steroids (e.g., triamcinolone) as well as antibiotics. It is widely agreed that the maximal volume of drug that can be injected intravitreally is 0.1 ml (Doshi et al., 2011)[27]; therefore, most formulations of anti-VEGF require injection of only 0.05 ml. While each drug has its own pharmacokinetic and pharmacodynamics profiles, it should be remembered that their clearance rates are increased in previously vitrectomized eyes so their effect may be shortened.

Posterior segment pathologies that are treated by intravitreal injections typically require repeated injections, as they are chronic conditions, while the effects of the drugs wear off after 1–3 months. Therefore, considerable efforts have been made towards developing longer-lasting intravitreal drug delivery systems.

Intravitreal Drug Delivery by Long-Lasting Implants

Another way of delivering drugs to the posterior segment is through implants that allow the release of controlled amounts of drugs over time (sustained release). This allows for a longer duration of drug effect in the eye, with a reduced number of interventions.

The ganciclovir implant (Vitrasert®) was the first intravitreal implant to be approved by the FDA in 1996 for the treatment of cytomegalovirus retinitis. Subsequently, by using a similar technology containing fluocinolone acetonide, the Retisert® implant was approved in 2005 by the FDA for the treatment of uveitis. Both of these require a surgical procedure for their implantation.

Later on, the Ozurdex™ implant, which is biodegradable and contains dexamethasone, was approved by the FDA in 2009 for the treatment of macular edema caused by retinal vein occlusion, and was later approved for the treatment of non-infectious uveitis and diabetic macular edema. Recently, the Iluvien® implant containing fluocinolone has been approved by the FDA in 2014 for the treatment of diabetic macular edema. Other implants are either under development or being tested in clinical trials.

Vitrasert® Ganciclovir Implant (Bausch and Lomb)

The ganciclovir implant has a drug core surrounded by two membranes, one of which is permeable (polyvinyl alcohol) and the other imper-

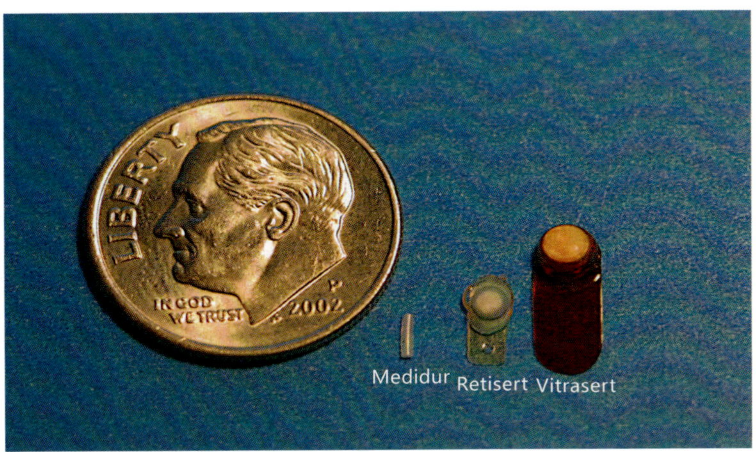

Fig. 1. Comparative sizes of Iluvien®, Retisert®, and Vitrasert® (left to right order).

meable (ethylene vinyl acetate). The impermeable ethylene vinyl acetate membrane is discontinuous at the posterior aspect of the implant and releases the drug in a circular ring-like fashion. This structure is similar to that of the Retisert® fluocinolone acetonide implant, although it is bigger (fig. 1). Insertion of the ganciclovir and fluocinolone implants requires a surgical incision of 5.5 and 3.5 mm, respectively, of the pars plana, and both implants are sutured to the eye wall. Neither one is biodegradable. Although an empty implant can remain indefinitely in the eye, these are usually removed if another implant is to be inserted.

Local delivery of ganciclovir with the reservoir implant has been shown to be a much more effective way of delivering the drug to the vitreous than intravenous administration (the most efficient systemic drug delivery route). Clinical trials showed that the mean time to reactivation of cytomegalovirus retinitis was 210 days for eyes treated with a ganciclovir implant compared to 70 days for eyes treated with intravenous ganciclovir. The difference in drug quantities is remarkable and demonstrates the power of local therapy for chorioretinal disease. For example, when treating a 70-kg male patient, the ganciclovir implant containing 5 mg of ganciclovir typically lasts for 8 months and achieves an intravitreal drug level of 4 µg/ml (Hughes et al., 2005)[1]. For the same treatment duration of 8 months, approximately 100,000 mg of drug would have been administered intravenously to control the disease (assuming induction doses of 5 mg/kg twice daily for 4 weeks to achieve quiescence followed by 6 weeks of maintenance therapy of 5 mg/kg once daily, with recurrence requiring resumption of induction therapy and a repeat of the cycle of 4 weeks induction/6 weeks maintenance throughout an 8-month period). Importantly, the intravenous therapy achieves an intravitreal drug level of only 1 µg/ml (Urtti, 2006)[2]. Thus, with 20,000 times more drug, the level of intravitreal ganciclovir achieved with intravenous injections is 4 times less than that achieved with the reservoir implant. These differences in drug levels may also be critical to ensure the efficacy of other therapeutic agents (Kuppermann et al., 1993; Martin et al., 1994)[28, 29].

Retisert® Fluocinolone Acetonide Implant (Bausch and Lomb)

Retisert® (Bausch and Lomb, Rochester, NY, USA) is an intraocular implant containing fluocinolone acetonide which has been approved for the treatment of chronic noninfectious uveitis affecting the posterior segment of the eye.

Retisert® is implanted into the eye via a surgical procedure entailing a 3.5-mm circumferential incision through the pars plana, and the implant is sutured to the eye wall. The implant is not biodegradable. The fluocinolone implant investigated in the uveitis study has also been studied in a multicenter, randomized, controlled clinical trial for the treatment of diabetic macular edema. Patients in the study were randomized 2:1 to receive either a 0.59-mg fluocinolone implant or standard of care, defined as repeat laser treatment or observation. Pearson et al. (2011)[30] reported that at 36 months the implant resolved edema at the center of the macula and produced a 3-line or more improvement in visual acuity in a significant proportion of eyes studied (n = 197). At 36 months, no evidence of edema was present in 58% of implanted eyes compared with 30% of eyes that received the standard of care (p < 0.001). Visual acuity improvements of 3 lines or more occurred more frequently in implanted eyes (28 vs. 15%, p < 0.05). The most common serious adverse events in the implanted eyes were cataract development requiring extraction and an increase in IOP. Of the phakic implanted eyes, 95% required cataract surgery, and 35% experienced increased IOP. A filtering procedure was necessary in 28% of implanted eyes, and explantation was performed in 5% of eyes to manage IOP.

Iluvien® Fluocinolone Acetonide Implant (Alimera)

A second fluocinolone acetonide sustained-delivery device has been developed. The injectable Iluvien® fluocinolone acetonide implant (Alimera Sciences Inc., Alpharetta, Ga., USA/pSivida, Watertown, Mass., USA) does not require sutures and can be inserted in an ophthalmologist's office. This drug delivery pellet is injected through a 25-gauge needle and floats freely in the vitreous cavity, typically embedding itself in the inferior vitreous base. The Iluvien® implant is not biodegradable and contains roughly half the amount of fluocinolone acetonide of the Retisert® implant.

It has been shown that a single injection of Iluvien® resulted in sustained intraocular levels of fluocinolone acetonide in patients with diabetic macular edema, and they also had significantly improved visual acuity and reduced edema (Campochiaro et al., 2010)[31]. Fluocinolone Acetonide in Diabetic Macular Edema (FAME) were phase III studies that evaluated the Iluvien® implant in patients with diabetic macular edema. These included 956 patients in the USA, Canada, Europe, and India, and evaluated 2 doses of fluocinolone (0.2 and 0.5 µg per day) compared to standard of care (which was macular laser at the time). The top-line 2-year primary efficacy and safety data (pSivida Corporation, 2009)[32] demonstrated both safety and efficacy, paving the way for the FDA approval of the drug. These results included 26.8% of subjects in the low-dose group, and 26.0% of those receiving a high dose had a 3-line improvement in best corrected visual acuity (BCVA); 30.6 and 31.2% of subjects in the low- and high-dose group, respectively, had an increase in BCVA; the percentage of eyes with IOP greater than 30 mm Hg at any time point was 16.3% in the low-dose and 21.6% in the high-dose group; surgical trabeculectomy was performed in 2.1% of low-dose patients and 5.1% of high-dose patients by 24 months. Based on these results, the lower dose was the one approved by the FDA and is now available for the treatment of diabetic macular edema.

Ozurdex™ Dexamethasone Biodegradable Implant (Allergan)

The Ozurdex™ dexamethasone implant contains dexamethasone (350 or 700 µg) and polylactic-co-glycolic acid, which is a biodegradable copolymer. It hydrolyzes to lactic and glycolic acids, and the lactic acid produced is further metabolized to H_2O and CO_2. Glycolic acid is either excreted or enzymatically converted to other me-

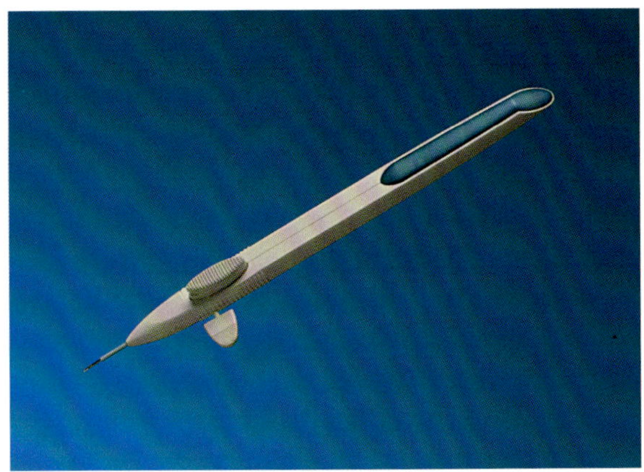

Fig. 2. The Ozurdex™ dexamethasone implant.

tabolized species. It is injected in a biplanar manner through the pars plana in an office setting by a customized, single-use 22-gauge applicator (fig. 2). Like the Iluvien® implant, the Ozurdex™ implant floats freely in the vitreous cavity and typically embeds itself in the inferior vitreous base. However, unlike the Iluvien® implant, which even when emptied of drug leaves a husk permanently in the eye, the Ozurdex™ implant completely biodegrades in the eye once drug delivery is complete.

Two doses of dexamethasone in this biodegradable drug delivery system were evaluated in a 6-month multicenter randomized clinical trial. The 315 patients in this phase II trial had persistent macular edema due to diabetic retinopathy (n = 172), retinal vein occlusion (n = 102), Irvine-Gass syndrome (n = 27), or uveitis (n = 14). In each patient, 1 eye was randomized either to treatment with a 350-μg dose of dexamethasone, a 700-μg dose of dexamethasone (both implants inserted into the vitreal cavity via a small pars plana incision), or observation. Implantation with Ozurdex™ resulted in a statistically significant increase in patients gaining 2 and 3 lines or more of visual acuity in a dose-dependent fashion at 90 and 180 days compared with observation (p < 0.025). The percentages of patients who gained 2

lines or more of visual acuity 180 days after implantation were 32.4% in the 700-μg group, 24.3% in the 350-μg group, and 21% in the observation group (p = 0.06). The percentages of patients who gained 3 lines or more of visual acuity 180 days after implantation were 18.1% in the 700-μg group, 14.6% in the 350-μg group, and 7.6% in the observation group (p = 0.02). The visual acuity improvements achieved with the 700-μg implant were consistent across all subgroups at day 90. In addition, at the primary endpoint, 2% of the patients who were implanted with Ozurdex™ containing either 350 or 700 μg of dexamethasone had an increase in IOP of 10 mm Hg or more from baseline, compared with 1% of patients in the observation arm. All were successfully managed with either observation or topical IOP-lowering medication. Cataracts were present in 15% of the 350-μg group, 17.8% of the 700-μg group, and 12.4% of the observation group (p < 0.001 vs. observation) (Kuppermann, 2007)[33].

Based on the results of this successful phase II trial, several additional clinical trials evaluating the Ozurdex™ implant have been performed. As the 700-μg dose proved more effective than the 350-μg dose with a similar safety profile, it has been chosen as the optimal dose for the Ozurdex™ implant (in contrast with Iluvien®, where the lower dose has been chosen). Multiple large-scale randomized controlled trials have established the efficacy of Ozurdex™ for the treatment of cystoid macular edema caused by retinal vein occlusions, noninfectious uveitis, and diabetic macular edema (Haller et al., 2011; Lowder et al., 2011; Boyer et al., 2011; Boyer et al., 2014)[34–37], and it is currently approved by the FDA for all these indications. It has been demonstrated that high concentrations of dexamethasone are sustained in the retina and vitreous during the first 2 months after the injection, and lower concentrations are sustained up to 6 months (Chang-Lin et al., 2011)[38]. However, in clinical reality many patients require reinjection before 6 months.

Brimonidine Biodegradable Implant (Allergan)
Brimonidine tartrate has been shown to have neuroprotective effects on the optic nerve and retina in preclinical studies. A brimonidine implant containing 200 or 400 mg brimonidine tartrate was developed by Allergan using the same biodegradable platform as the Ozurdex™ dexamethasone implant. This implant is designed to release the drug for 6 months, then the polylactic-co-glycolic acid polymer subsequently biodegrades to lactic acid and carbon dioxide over a period of a few additional months. A phase II trial has been completed in which patients with bilateral geographic atrophy were treated with the brimonidine implant (200 or 400 mg vs. sham), and were followed for 6 months (NCT00658619). No significant changes in progression of geographic atrophy of BCVA were noted. Although the safety profile was good, this implant did not demonstrate enough therapeutic benefit and is therefore not currently in use.

Renexus (Neurotech)
Encapsulated cell technology utilizes a unique cell-based approach for drug delivery. A surgically implanted pellet, which is sutured to the eye wall, contains modified RPE cells in an immune protected capsule. The RPE cells are programmed to produce therapeutic levels of ciliary neurotrophic factor (CNTF), a neuroprotective agent, for 3 years. The RPE cells, however, can be programmed to produce almost any complex molecule, including bevacizumab and ranibizumab. This technology addresses a key problem of long-term drug delivery of complex molecules – how to manage long-term stability of proteins and other complex molecules at the physiologic intravitreal temperature of 37°C. In this case, since the drug-eluting RPE cells are producing the molecules continuously, no long-term stability issues occur.

Renexus (formerly NT-501; Neurotech) is a semipermeable hollow-fiber membrane capsule which surrounds a scaffold of polyethylene strands that can be loaded with cells. The semipermeable membrane allows for outward diffusion of CNTF, while also allowing inward diffusion of nutrients necessary to support the cells while protecting them from exposure to the immune system. Data from two phase I studies showed that Renexus was well tolerated in patients with retinitis pigmentosa and macular telangiectasia (Chew et al., 2015; Sieving et al., 2006)[39, 40]. In a phase II study (Zhang et al., 2011)[41], patients with geographic atrophy were randomized in a 2:1:1 ratio to receive high-dose CNTF (20 ng/day), low-dose CNTF (5 ng/day), or sham. At 12 months, there was a statistically significant difference in the change in total macular volume in the study eye compared with baseline in the high- or low-dose CNTF groups but not in the sham group, with increased macular volume demonstrated in the treated eyes accompanied by increased width of the outer layer complex on optical coherence tomography. Additionally, stable BCVA was reported in the high-dose group while there was a trend toward greater decline in BCVA in patients with better baseline vision in eyes treated with the low dose or sham. In patients with baseline vision better than 20/63, at 12 months the mean BCVA in the high-dose group was 10.5 and 10.0 letters better than the low-dose and sham groups, respectively. Also, the growth rate of the geographic atrophy area was reduced in CNTF-treated eyes compared with fellow eyes at 12 and 18 months. The safety profile was good and no group had an increased rate of complications. These results may indicate that the higher dose of Renexus may be preferable.

Sustained Intravitreal Drug Delivery Systems
Triamcinolone Acetonide I-vation Sustained Drug Delivery System (SurModics)
This implant has a helical design and is implanted through a 25-gauge incision by surgical conjunctival cutdown. The surface area for drug delivery is increased by this novel helical design. This

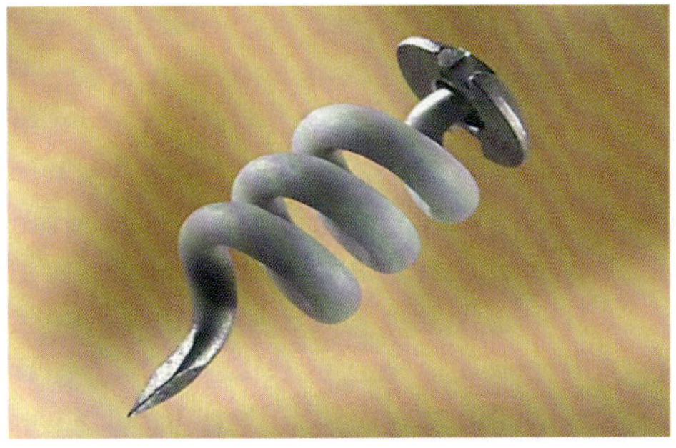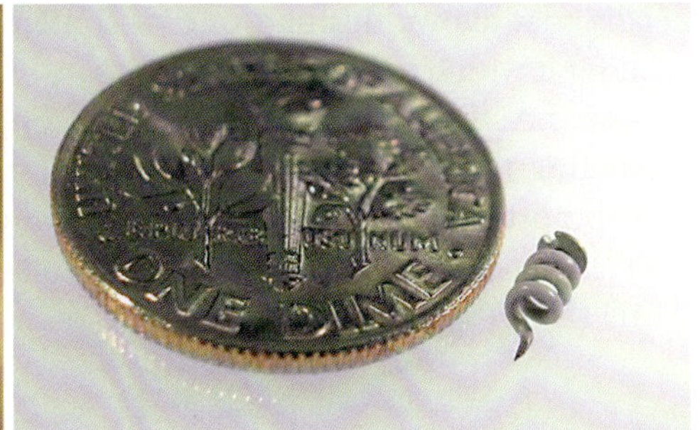

Fig. 3. The I-vation sustained drug delivery system.

device is self-anchoring within the sclera and is removable (fig. 3). It is nonbiodegradable. The SurModics polymer coating technology has adjustable drug elution rates. The I-vation device contains triamcinolone acetonide as the therapeutic agent.

The prospective, randomized, double-masked Sustained Triamcinolone Release for Inhibition of Diabetic Macular Edema (STRIDE) trial assessed the safety and tolerability of the I-vation triamcinolone acetonide (SurModics, Irvine, Calif., USA) in 30 patients. In this study, patients were randomized to either a slow-release or fast-release implant, each containing 925 µg of triamcinolone. They were also stratified by baseline visual acuity and by presence or absence of prior laser treatment. From screening to 6 months, the proportion of patients with visual acuity of at least 70 ETDRS (Early Treatment Diabetic Retinopathy Study) letters (in the study eye) increased from 14 to 46% in the slow group and from 18 to 41% in the fast group. A gain of more than 15 letters occurred in 8% of patients in the slow group and in 18% of patients in the fast group. Both implant formulations were associated with improvements in macular thickness. However, every phakic eye in the study developed a visually significant cataract. Also, increases in IOP occurred in 50% of eyes, though none required surgery to treat the IOP increase. Based on these preliminary results, further studies with I-vation triamcinolone acetonide have been suspended.

Micropump™ (Replenish Inc.)
The Micropump™ is a drug delivery device designed for the treatment of chronic conditions that at present require numerous repeated interventions. It includes a reservoir that is surgically implanted in the subconjunctival space, and has a flexible cannula that can be placed in the anterior or posterior segment. The device also includes a battery which can power electrolysis to drive the drug from the reservoir into the eye through the cannula, and this can be controlled electronically after implantation. It is refillable and designed to last at least 5 years before replacement is required.

One study reported a ranibizumab-loaded Micropump™ has been well-tolerated in 11 patients with diabetic macular edema (Humayun et al., 2014)[42]. Further studies will establish the long-term efficacy of this device.

Port Drug Delivery System (Genentech/ForSight VISION4 Inc.)
Genentech is currently evaluating another implantable refillable drug delivery system that is designed to elute ranibizumab over a long period of time. The device is implanted surgically, and has a reservoir that is accessible by a special

needle that allows flushing out its contents and refilling it with a fresh dose of drug.

The LADDER study is currently ongoing, evaluating the efficacy and safety of the ranibizumab port delivery system for its sustained delivery in patients with subfoveal neovascular AMD (NCT02510794).

Nanoparticles

'Nano' is a prefix that means very small or microscopic. The term 'nanotechnology' generally applies to dealing with objects smaller than 100 nm, and is broadly used in medicine, engineering, and other fields of science. Recent technological advances have led to several approaches of posterior segment drug delivery based on microscopic particles. Although none of these is clinically available at the present, they are expected to develop in the future and will be briefly discussed in this section.

Intraocular Self-Reporting Nanocrystals (Smart Dust) for Intraocular Drug Delivery

These nanocrystals are small porous particles made from drug-laden porous silicone photonic crystals. Spectral properties of these crystals (empty vs. drug-laden) permit in vivo monitoring of residual drug in the crystals. The nanostructure allows control of the temporal release profile, and they can be loaded with any drug of choice. The porous silicon photonic crystals have been shown to be biocompatible with no toxicity, and are therefore a suitable intraocular drug-delivery system (Cheng et al., 2008)[43]. It has also been shown that alkylating their surface increases their intravitreal stability and slowed their rate of degradation, making them capable of having long-term effects (Cheng et al., 2008)[43].

Nanoparticles

Drug-laden nanoparticles can also be used as long-term reservoirs that slowly release active drugs. These do not enable monitoring of their drug levels as above. Also, nanoparticles are not only intended for intravitreal injection.

1.5% dexamethasone γ-cyclodextrin nanoparticle eye drops have been demonstrated to achieve similar effects on visual acuity and macular thickness as a posterior sub-Tenon triamcinolone injection in patients with diabetic macular edema who were followed for 12 weeks (Ohira et al., 2015)[44]. This attests to their potential clinical value, which is impressive given the fact they were administered topically.

Additionally, polymethylmethacrylate nanoparticles loaded with carboplatin administered by posterior sub-Tenon injection in patients with retinoblastoma achieved transscleral transport of nanoparticle carboplatin, with a sustained-release behavior and no short-term ocular or systemic side effects (Kalita et al., 2014)[45].

Lipid Nanoparticles

Solid lipid nanoparticles are spherical elements about 10–1,000 nm in diameter, which are composed of a solid lipid core matrix that can solubilize lipophilic molecules. These can be used to deliver drugs to the cornea or to the retina (Wang et al., 2015)[46].

The liposome protamine/DNA lipoplex is another type of lipid nanoparticle, which is electrostatically assembled from cationic liposomes and an anionic complex of protamine and DNA. It is composed of a lipid bilayer with a diameter of about 100 nm, and contains condensed DNA (Wang et al., 2015)[46]. These properties make it particularly suitable to serve as a vector for gene therapy delivery to the posterior segment. Successful gene transfer to the retina using this approach has been shown in a murine model of X-linked retinoschisis (Apaolaza et al., 2015)[47]. As advances are made in gene therapy, these lipid nanoparticles may become a frequently used platform for their administration.

Conclusion

In conclusion, many ocular diseases still need improved pharmacological solutions. First- generation drug delivery technology exists and is being further refined. Present research is focused on both developing new drug delivery approaches as well as improving the existing ones. Future devices will allow longer drug duration, increased target specificity and possibly even real-time monitoring of active drug levels and reciprocal dose adjustments. Technological developments allow for longer-acting drug delivery and good long-term control of disease, but have the potential for drug or suppressive side effects; however, these issues may be remedied with refillable and dose-adjustable devices. Different approaches may be used in different diseases to achieve maximum benefit with minimal risks. As the therapeutic options for posterior segment diseases increase, future comparative studies will be needed to establish the optimal treatment patterns for them.

References

1 Hughes PM, Olejnik O, Chang-Lin JE, Wilson CG: Topical and systemic drug delivery to the posterior segments. Adv Drug Deliv Rev 2005;57:2010–2032.
2 Urtti A: Challenges and obstacles of ocular pharmacokinetics and drug delivery. Adv Drug Deliv Rev 2006;58:1131–1315.
3 Chiou GC, Watanabe K: Drug delivery to the eye. Pharmacol Ther 1982;17:269–278.
4 Ahmed I, Patton TF: Importance of the noncorneal absorption route in topical ophthalmic drug delivery. Invest Ophthalmol Vis Sci 1985;26:584–587.
5 Geroski DH, Edelhauser HF: Drug delivery for posterior segment eye disease. Invest Ophthalmol Vis Sci 2000;41:961–964.
6 Guo S, Patel S, Baumrind B, Johnson K, Levinsohn D, Marcus E, Tannen B, Roy M, Bhagat N, Zarbin M: Management of pseudophakic cystoid macular edema. Surv Ophthalmol 2015;60:123–137.
7 Maurice DM: Drug delivery to the posterior segment from drops. Surv Ophthalmol 2002;47(suppl 1):S41–S52.
8 Olsen TW, Edelhauser HF, Lim JI, Geroski DH: Human scleral permeability. Effects of age, cryotherapy, transscleral diode laser, and surgical thinning. Invest Ophthalmol Vis Sci 1995;36:1893–1903.
9 Ni Z, Hui P: Emerging pharmacologic therapies for wet age-related macular degeneration. Ophthalmologica 2009;223:401–410.
10 Wong WT, Kam W, Cunningham D, Harrington M, Hammel K, Meyerle CB, Cukras C, Chew EY, Sadda SR, Ferris FL: Treatment of geographic atrophy by the topical administration of OT-551: results of a phase II clinical trial. Invest Ophthalmol Vis Sci 2010;51:6131–6139.
11 Kumar R, Knick VB, Rudolph SK, Johnson JH, Crosby RM, Crouthamel MC, Hopper TM, Miller CG, Harrington LE, Onori JA, Mullin RJ, Gilmer TM, Truesdale AT, Epperly AH, Boloor A, Stafford JA, Luttrell DK, Cheung M: Pharmacokinetic-pharmacodynamic correlation from mouse to human with pazopanib, a multikinase angiogenesis inhibitor with potent antitumor and antiangiogenic activity. Mol Cancer Ther 2007;6:2012–2021.
12 Singh R, Wurzelmann JI, Ye L, Henderson L, Hossain M, Trivedi T, Kelly DS: Clinical evaluation of pazopanib eye drops in healthy subjects and in subjects with neovascular age-related macular degeneration. Retina 2014;34:1787–1795.
13 Csaky KG, Dugel PU, Pierce AJ, Fries MA, Kelly DS, Danis RP, Wurzelmann JI, Xu CF, Hossain M, Trivedi T: Clinical evaluation of pazopanib eye drops versus ranibizumab intravitreal injections in subjects with neovascular age-related macular degeneration. Ophthalmology 2015;122:579–588.
14 Wirtz R: Die Ionentherapie in der Augenheilkunde. Klin Monbl Augenheilkd 1908;46:543–549.
15 Guy J: New therapies for optic neuropathies: development in experimental models. Curr Opin Ophthalmol 2000;11:421–429.
16 Halhal M, Renard G, Bejjani RA, Behar-Cohen F: Corneal graft rejection and corticoid iontophoresis: 3 case reports (in French). J Fr Ophtalmol 2003;26:391–395.
17 Byun YS, Park YH: Complications and safety profile of posterior subtenon injection of triamcinolone acetonide. J Ocul Pharmacol Ther 2009;25:159–162.
18 Bakri SJ, Kaiser PK: Posterior subtenon triamcinolone acetonide for refractory diabetic macular edema. Am J Ophthalmol 2005;139:290–294.
19 Venkatesh P, Abhas Z, Garg S, Vohra R: Prospective optical coherence tomographic evaluation of the efficacy of oral and posterior subtenon corticosteroids in patients with intermediate uveitis. Graefes Arch Clin Exp Ophthalmol 2007;245:59–67.

20 Russell SR, Hudson HL, Jerdan JA; Anecortave Acetate Clinical Study Group: Anecortave acetate for the treatment of exudative age-related macular degeneration – a review of clinical outcomes. Surv Ophthalmol 2007;52(suppl 1):S79–S90.

21 Moisseiev E, Loewenstein A, Yiu G: The suprachoroidal space: from potential space to a space with potential. Clin Ophthalmol 2016;10:173–178.

22 Kadam RS, Williams J, Tyagi P, Edelhauser HF, Kompella UB: Suprachoroidal delivery in a rabbit ex vivo eye model: influence of drug properties, regional differences in delivery, and comparison with intravitreal and intracameral routes. Mol Vis 2013;19:1198–210.

23 Gilger BC, Abarca EM, Salmon JH, Patel S: Treatment of acute posterior uveitis in a porcine model by injection of triamcinolone acetonide into the suprachoroidal space using microneedles. Invest Ophthalmol Vis Sci 2013;54: 2483–2492.

24 Patel SR, Berezovsky DE, McCarey BE, Zarnitsyn V, Edelhauser HF, Prausnitz MR: Targeted administration into the suprachoroidal space using a microneedle for drug delivery to the posterior segment of the eye. Invest Ophthalmol Vis Sci 2012;53:4433–4441.

25 Bhavsar AR, Googe JM Jr, Stockdale CR, Bressler NM, Brucker AJ, Elman MJ, Glassman AR; Diabetic Retinopathy Clinical Research Network: Risk of endophthalmitis after intravitreal drug injection when topical antibiotics are not required: the diabetic retinopathy clinical research network laser-ranibizumab-triamcinolone clinical trials. Arch Ophthalmic 2009;127:1581–1583.

26 Prasad AG, Schadlu R, Apte RS: Intravitreal pharmacotherapy: applications in retinal disease. Compr Ophthalmol Update 2007;8:259–269.

27 Doshi RR, Bakri SJ, Fung AE: Intravitreal injection technique. Semin Ophthalmol 2011;26:104–113.

28 Kuppermann BD, Quiceno JI, Flores-Aguilar M, Connor JD, Capparelli EV, Sherwood CH, Freeman WR: Intravitreal ganciclovir concentration after intravenous administration in AIDS patients with cytomegalovirus retinitis: implications for therapy. J Infect Dis 1993;168:1506–1509.

29 Martin DF, Parks DJ, Mellow SD, Ferris FL, Walton RC, Remaley NA, Chew EY, Ashton P, Davis MD, Nussenblatt RB: Treatment of cytomegalovirus retinitis with an intraocular sustained-release ganciclovir implant. A randomized controlled clinical trial. Arch Ophthalmol 1994;112:1531–1539.

30 Pearson PA, Comstock TL, Ip M, Callanan D, Morse LS, Ashton P, Levy B, Mann ES, Eliott D: Fluocinolone acetonide intravitreal implant for diabetic macular edema: a 3-year multicenter, randomized, controlled clinical trial. Ophthalmology 2011;118:1580–1587.

31 Campochiaro PA, Hafiz G, Shah SM, Bloom S, Brown DM, Busquets M, Ciulla T, Feiner L, Sabates N, Billman K, Kapik B, Green K, Kane F; Famous Study Group. Sustained ocular delivery of fluocinolone acetonide by an intravitreal insert. Ophthalmology 2010;117:1393–1399.

32 pSivida Corporation: Form 8-K document submitted to the Securities and Exchange Commision (SEC). December 23, 2009.

33 Kuppermann BD, Blumenkranz MS, Haller JA, Williams GA, Weinberg DV, Chou C, Whitcup SM; Dexamethasone DDS Phase II Study Group: Randomized controlled study of an intravitreous dexamethasone drug delivery system in patients with persistent macular edema. Arch Ophthalmol 2007;125: 309–317.

34 Haller JA, Bandello F, Belfort R, Blumenkranz MS, Gillies M, Heier J, et al: Dexamethasone intravitreal implant in patients with macular edema related to branch or central retinal vein occlusion. Ophthalmology 2011;118:2453–2460.

35 Lowder C, Belfort R Jr, Lightman S, Foster CS, Robinson MR, Schiffman RM, et al: Dexamethasone intravitreal implant for noninfectious intermediate or posterior uveitis. Arch Ophthalmol 2011;129: 545–553.

36 Boyer DS, Faber D, Gupta S, Patel SS, Tabandeh H, Li XY, Liu CC, Lou J, Whitcup SM; Ozurdex CHAMPLAIN Study Group: Dexamethasone intravitreal implant for treatment of diabetic macular edema in vitrectomized patients. Retina 2011;31:915–923.

37 Boyer DS, Yoon YH, Belfort R Jr, Bandello F, Maturi RK, Augustin AJ, Li XY, Cui H, Hashad Y, Whitcup SM; Ozurdex MEAD Study Group: Three-year, randomized, sham-controlled trial of dexamethasone intravitreal implant in patients with diabetic macular edema. Ophthalmology 2014;121:1904–1914.

38 Chang-Lin JE, Attar M, Acheampong AA, et al: Pharmacokinetics and pharmacodynamics of a sustained-release dexamethasone intravitreal implant. Invest Ophthalmol Vis Sci 2011;52:80–86.

39 Chew EY, Clemons TE, Peto T, Sallo FB, Ingerman A, Tao W, Singerman L, Schwartz SD, Peachey NS, Bird AC; MacTel-CNTF Research Group: Ciliary neurotrophic factor for macular telangiectasia type 2: results from a phase 1 safety trial. Am J Ophthalmol 2015;159: 659–666.

40 Sieving PA, Caruso RC, Tao W, Coleman HR, Thompson DJ, Fullmer KR, Bush RA: Ciliary neurotrophic factor (CNTF) for human retinal degeneration: phase I trial of CNTF delivered by encapsulated cell intraocular implants. Proc Natl Acad Sci USA 2006;103: 3896–3901.

41 Zhang K, Hopkins JJ, Heier JS, Birch DG, Halperin LS, Albini TA, Brown DM, Jaffe GJ, Tao W, Williams GA: Ciliary neurotrophic factor delivered by encapsulated cell intraocular implants for treatment of geographic atrophy in age-related macular degeneration. Proc Natl Acad Sci USA 2011;108: 6241–6245.

42 Humayun M, Santos A, Altamirano JC, Ribeiro R, Gonzalez R, de la Rosa A, Shih J, Pang C, Jiang F, Calvillo P, Huculak J, Zimmerman J, Caffey S: Implantable MicroPump for drug delivery in patients with diabetic macular edema. Transl Vis Sci Technol 2014;3: 5.

43 Cheng L, Anglin E, Cunin F, Kim D, Sailor MJ, Falkenstein I, Tammewar A, Freeman WR: Intravitreal properties of porous silicon photonic crystals: a potential self-reporting intraocular drug-delivery vehicle. Br J Ophthalmol 2008; 92:705–711.

44 Ohira A, Hara K, Jóhannesson G, Tanito M, Ásgrímsdóttir GM, Lund SH, Loftsson T, Stefánsson E: Topical dexamethasone γ-cyclodextrin nanoparticle eye drops increase visual acuity and decrease macular thickness in diabetic macular oedema. Acta Ophthalmol 2015;93:610–615.

45 Kalita D, Shome D, Jain VG, Chadha K, Bellare JR: In vivo intraocular distribution and safety of periocular nanoparticle carboplatin for treatment of advanced retinoblastoma in humans. Am J Ophthalmol 2014;157:1109–1115.

46 Wang Y, Rajala A, Rajala RV. Lipid nanoparticles for ocular gene delivery. J Funct Biomater 2015;6:379–394.

47 Apaolaza PS, Del Pozo-Rodríguez A, Torrecilla J, Rodríguez-Gascón A, Rodríguez JM, Friedrich U, Weber BH, Solinís MA: Solid lipid nanoparticle-based vectors intended for the treatment of X-linked juvenile retinoschisis by gene therapy: in vivo approaches in Rs1h-deficient mouse model. J Control Release 2015;217:273–283.

Elad Moisseiev, MD
Division of Ophthalmology, Tel Aviv Sourasky Medical Center
6, Weizman St.
Tel Aviv 64239 (Israel)
E-Mail elad_moi@netvision.net.il

Coscas G (ed): Macular Edema. 2nd, revised and extended edition.
Dev Ophthalmol. Basel, Karger, 2017, vol 58, pp 102–138 (DOI: 10.1159/000455277)

Diabetic Macular Edema

Francesco Bandello[a] · Maurizio Battaglia Parodi[a] · Paolo Lanzetta[b] ·
Anat Loewenstein[c] · Pascale Massin[d] · Francesca Menchini[b] · Daniele Veritti[b]

[a]Department of Ophthalmology, University Vita-Salute, Scientific Institute San Raffaele, Milan, and [b]Department of Medical and Biological Sciences – Ophthalmology, University of Udine, Udine, Italy; [c]Department of Ophthalmology, Tel Aviv Medical Center, Tel Aviv, Israel; [d]Department of Ophthalmology, Lariboisière Hospital, Paris, France

Abstract

Diabetic macular edema (DME), defined as a retinal thickening involving or approaching the center of the macula, represents the most common cause of vision loss in patients affected by diabetes mellitus. In the last few years, many diagnostic tools have proven to be useful in the detection and the monitoring of the features characterizing DME. On the other hand, several therapeutic approaches can now be proposed on the basis of the DME-specific characteristics. The aim of the present chapter is to thoroughly delineate the clinical and morphofunctional characteristics of DME and its current treatment perspectives. The pathogenesis and the course of DME require a complex approach with multidisciplinary intervention both at the systemic and local levels.

© 2017 S. Karger AG, Basel

Despite continued improvement in diagnostic screening techniques and the proven efficacy of pharmacologic and laser treatments in preventing visual loss, diabetic retinopathy (DR) remains the leading cause of legal blindness in working-age populations of industrialized countries.

Future perspectives are not encouraging: the World Health Organization estimates that more than 180 million people worldwide have diabetes. Fueled by increased life expectancy, sedentary lifestyle, and obesity, this number is expected to rise to epidemic proportions within the next 20 years (King et al., 1998)[1]. Although our understanding of biochemical and hemodynamic stimuli and mediators that ultimately lead to microvascular changes in diabetic patients has progressively improved, and despite a substantial body of scientific evidence that underlies current treatment recommendations for DR, this disease remains a *major public health problem* with significant socioeconomic implications, affecting approximately 50% of diabetic subjects.

Vision loss due to DR may result from several mechanisms. Macular edema or capillary nonperfusion may directly impair central vision. Retinal and/or disk neovascularization in the course of proliferative diabetic retinopathy (PDR) can cause severe and often irreversible visual loss due to vitreous/preretinal hemorrhage and tractional retinal detachment. While complications of PDR lead more frequently to severe visual loss, the *most common cause* of visual impairment among diabetic patients is diabetic macular edema (DME), accounting for about three fourths of cases of visual loss.

The development of macular edema is not limited to diabetic patients but represents a common response to a broad spectrum of potential problems caused by retinal disease. The predilection of the edema to the macular region is probably secondary to the higher susceptibility of the macula to both ischemic and oxidative stress and to its peculiar anatomical features, for example, loose intercellular adhesion and an absence of Müller cells in the fovea.

The pathogenesis of DME is complex and multifactorial, and mainly results from the disruption of the blood-retinal barrier (BRB), leading to accumulation of fluid and serum macromolecules in the intercellular space (Antonetti et al., 1999)[2]. Accelerated apoptosis of pericytes and endothelial cells, acellular capillaries, basement membrane thickening, and capillary occlusion all contribute to endothelial damage and breakdown of the inner BRB.

Significant variations in the incidence and prevalence of DME have been reported in various epidemiologic studies, depending on the type of diabetes (type I or II), the treatment modality (insulin, oral hypoglycemic agents, or diet only), and the mean duration of diabetes. DME can develop at any stage of DR, but it occurs more frequently as the duration of diabetes and the severity of DR increase. In the Wisconsin Epidemiologic Study of Diabetic Retinopathy (WESDR), the 10-year rate of developing DME was 20.1% in patients with type I diabetes, 13.9% in patients with type II diabetes not using insulin, and 25.4% in type II diabetes patients using insulin. DME prevalence increases with the severity of DR: it affects 3% of eyes with mild nonproliferative diabetic retinopathy (NPDR), rises to 38% of eyes with moderate to severe NPDR, and reaches 71% of eyes with PDR.

The natural history of DME is characterized by a slow progression of *retinal thickening* until the center of the macula is involved, causing visual acuity deterioration. Spontaneous resolution of DME is rare and usually secondary to improvement in systemic risk factors, such as glycemic control, hypertension, or hypercholesterolemia. If untreated, 29% of eyes with DME and foveal involvement experience moderate visual loss (doubling of the visual angle) after 3 years. Spontaneous visual recovery is also unusual, with improvement of at least 3 Early Treatment Diabetic Retinopathy Study (ETDRS) lines occurring in 5% of cases.

Definition and Classification

The diagnosis of macular edema is clinical. Traditionally, the gold standard for diagnosing DME is stereoscopic fundus photography. In clinical practice, noncontact fundus biomicroscopy is often employed, and it can be useful, especially when there is significant retinal thickening. In early or borderline cases, however, contact lens biomicroscopy is considered more sensitive.

Fluorescein angiography is not necessary for diagnosing DME, but it provides a qualitative assessment of vascular leakage, helps in identifying treatable lesions, and is essential for assessing the presence of an enlargement of the foveal avascular zone (FAZ), which may be associated with poor visual prognosis (Antonetti et al., 1999)[2].

Conventionally, DME is defined as retinal thickening or the presence of hard exudates within 1 disk diameter of the center of the macula. The term 'clinically significant macular edema' (CSME) was coined to characterize the severity of the disease and to provide a threshold level to apply laser photocoagulation (table 1) (Early Treatment Diabetic Retinopathy Study Research Group, 1985)[3].

In addition to this ophthalmoscopic classification, DME can be classified into focal and diffuse.

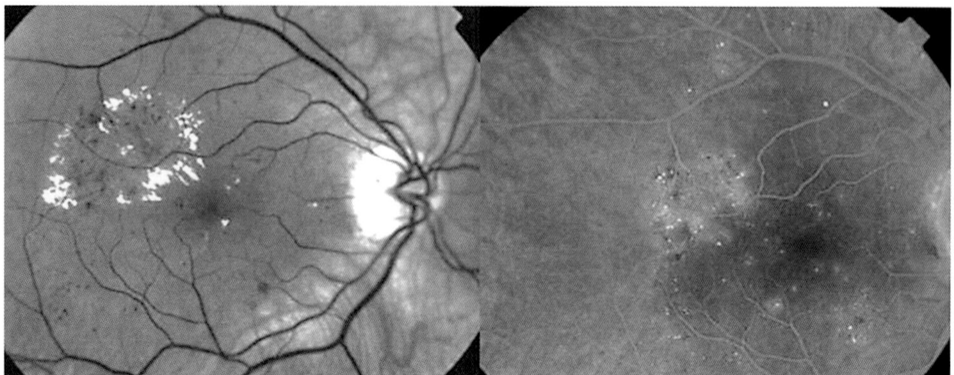

Fig. 1. Focal DME. Left: red-free photograph shows circinate ring of hard exudates surrounding microaneurysms. Right: fluorescein angiography reveals leakage from hyperfluorescent punctate lesions corresponding to microaneurysms.

Table 1. ETDRS definition of CSME

Thickening of the retina at or within 500 μm of the center of the macula
Hard exudates at or within 500 μm of the center of the macula, if associated with thickening of adjacent retina
A zone or zones of retinal thickening at least 1 disk area in extent, any part of which is within 1 disk diameter of the center of the macula

Focal macular edema is characterized by the presence of localized areas of retinal thickening, derived from focal leakage of individual microaneurysms or clusters of microaneurysms. Fluorescein angiography clearly demonstrates that microaneurysms are the major source of dye leakage (fig. 1). Areas of focal leakage are often demarcated by a partial or complete ring of hard exudates with a circinate appearance.

Diffuse macular edema is derived from extensively damaged capillaries, microaneurysms, and arterioles, and it is characterized by a more widespread thickening of the macula secondary to generalized abnormal permeability of the retinal capillary bed that appears to be diffusely dilated (fig. 2). Diffuse macular edema tends to be symmetric and without significant exudation. Ocular and systemic risk factors for the development and progression of diffuse DME are an increasing microaneurysm count, advanced retinopathy, vitreomacular traction, adult-onset diabetes, renal disease, and severe hypertension.

Cystoid macular edema, often associated with diffuse macular edema, results from a generalized breakdown of the BRB with fluid accumulation in a petaloid pattern, primarily in the outer plexiform and inner nuclear layers. The presence or absence of cystoid appearance, however, does not directly influence the prognosis and management of DME.

In clinical practice, the distinction between focal and diffuse edema is not always clear, and a wide variety of *mixed forms* are observed. These two patterns of leakage can be clearly visualized

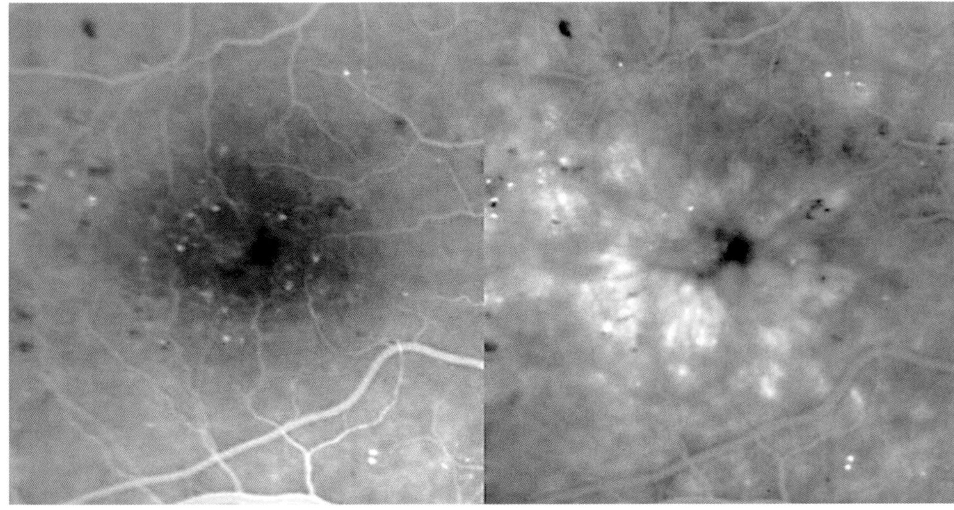

Fig. 2. Diffuse DME. Fluorescein angiography (left: early phase; right: late phase) shows leakage throughout the posterior pole with late dye pooling at the macula in a petaloid pattern.

by fluorescein angiography. It is important to note that leakage on fluorescein angiography is not always synonymous with retinal edema since it does not necessarily indicate retinal thickening.

Once the diagnosis of CSME and the decision to treat have been made, fluorescein angiography is extremely useful in helping to decide on the treatment strategy and in determining the vascular perfusion. Ischemic or nonperfused macular edema is an important variant of DME, and it can be revealed by fluorescein angiography.

Ischemic maculopathy is defined by the presence of rarefaction and occlusion of the perifoveal capillary network, with doubling of the extension of the FAZ (fig. 3). Normally the FAZ is approximately 350–750 μm in diameter. Even in the absence of macular edema in diabetic eyes, abnormalities of the FAZ are often seen, and include irregular margins and widening of the intercapillary spaces.

On a pathogenic basis, DME can be further classified into prevalently retinovascular or nonretinovascular, the latter definition including different clinical entities, such as diabetic retinal pigment epitheliopathy, tractional macular edema,

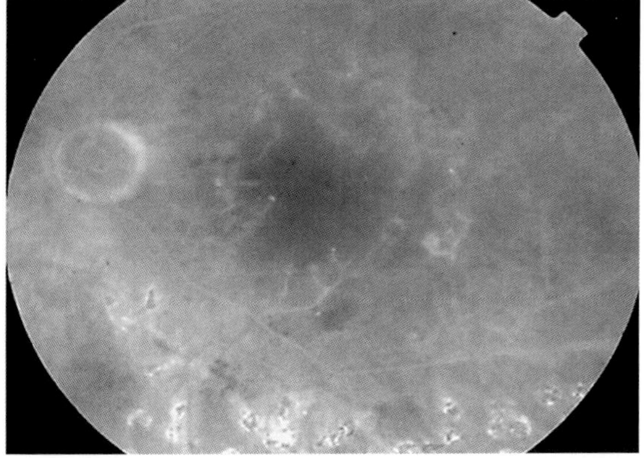

Fig. 3. Ischemic maculopathy. Fluorescein angiography shows extensive capillary nonperfusion at the macula, with enlargement and irregularity of the FAZ.

and macular edema with taut, attached posterior hyaloid. In most cases, different pathogenic components are combined, making it difficult to decide which component is prevalent and what treatment is the most indicated.

The common pathway that results in DME is *disruption of the BRB*. The mechanism of the BRB breakdown is multifactorial: it is caused by chang-

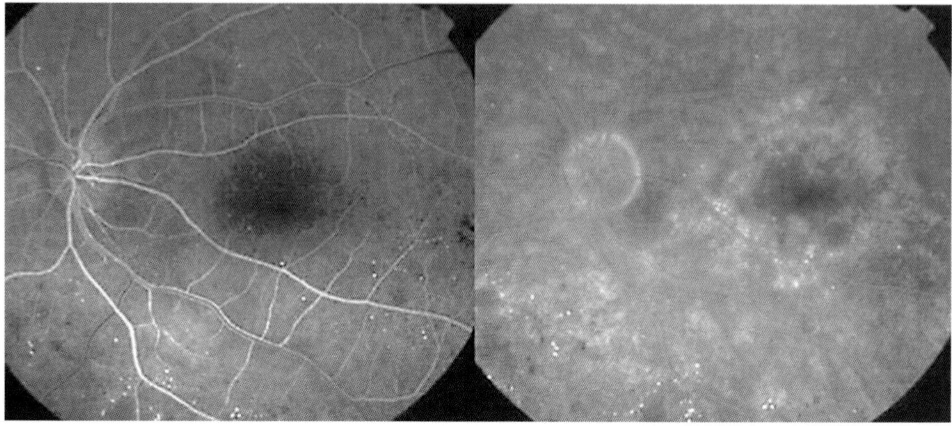

Fig. 4. Macular edema associated with taut, attached posterior hyaloid. In early (left) angiographic phases, hypofluorescence and minimal diabetic changes are evident. In the late (right) phase, fluorescein angiography shows diffuse leakage around the macular area.

es in the tight junction, pericyte loss, endothelial cell loss, retinal vessel leukostasis, upregulation of vesicular transport, retinal vessel dilation, imbalance in the water and ion homeostasis control by retinal Müller glial cells, and vitreoretinal traction.

Prevalently retinovascular DME is characterized by abnormal permeability of retinal capillaries, and it includes previously described focal or diffuse DME caused by pathological changes primarily of retinal vascular origin, including pericyte dropout, microaneurysm formation, and generalized breakdown of the inner BRB. Fluorescein angiography is indispensable to distinguish between prevalently retinovascular and nonretinovascular macular edema. In prevalently retinovascular macular edema, early fluorescein angiograms clearly define microvascular abnormalities as the major source of late dye leakage.

In 1995, an unusual form of diabetic maculopathy was described for the first time, in which the retinal pigment epithelium (RPE) and the subretinal space played a main role (Weinberger et al., 1995)[4]. Fluorescein angiograms of 1,850 patients with NPDR were examined, and 1% of cases exhibited an area of diffuse RPE leakage spread around the macular region in the late phase; no cystic changes or cystoid macular edema were present in any of the eyes. This condition was named *diabetic retinal pigment epitheliopathy.*

DME may be caused or exacerbated by persistent *vitreomacular traction* by residual cortical vitreous on the macula following posterior vitreous detachment, macular traction due to tractional proliferative membrane, and a thickened and taut posterior hyaloid that may exert tangential macular traction and cause edema (Lewis et al.,1992; Harbour et al., 1996)[5, 6]. On biomicroscopy, a thick, taut, glistening posterior hyaloid is visible, while fluorescein angiography exhibits a characteristic early hypofluorescence, and deep, diffuse round late leakage, often from vascular arcade to arcade (fig. 4). Unlike what occurs in prevalently retinovascular DME, in these cases there is no topographic correspondence between microvascular abnormalities visible in the early phase of the angiography and late leakage.

Optical coherence tomography (OCT) is a noninvasive, noncontact instrument, which provides cross-sectional, high-resolution images of

Bandello · Battaglia Parodi · Lanzetta · Loewenstein · Massin · Menchini · Veritti

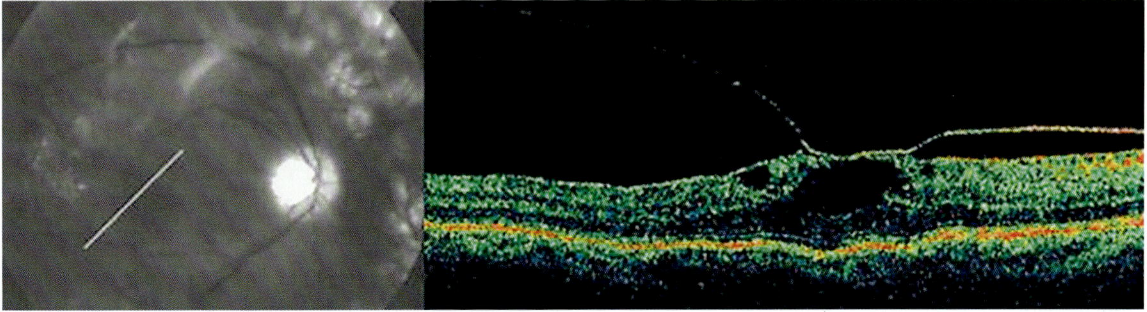

Fig. 5. Localized vitreous traction. Red-free photograph (left) shows the presence of a vitreous strand adherent to the macula. The presence of a focal traction, causing loss of physiologic foveal depression, is clearly visualized by OCT (right).

the retina and a quantitative assessment of retinal thickness with a high degree of accuracy and reproducibility. The advantage of OCT in diagnosing CSME as compared to fundus biomicroscopy is its ability to provide an objective, quantitative, measure of retinal thickness as well as additional morphological details.

Correlation between OCT and fluorescein angiography findings in the course of CSME is fairly good: about 60% of patients with foveal thickening and homogeneous intraretinal optical reflectivity on OCT have focal leakage on fluorescein angiography, while more than 90% of patients with diffuse cystoid leakage exhibit foveal thickening with decreased optical reflectivity in the outer retinal layers or foveal thickening with subretinal fluid accumulation on OCT (Kang et al., 2004)[7]. Furthermore, OCT clearly visualizes the vitreoretinal interface and reveals the presence and extent of vitreomacular traction and epiretinal membrane (fig. 5). More recently, a new OCT-based diagnostic tool has been developed. OCT angiography is a new noninvasive imaging technique that employs motion contrast imaging to high-resolution volumetric blood flow data, producing angiographic images.

An *international clinical disease severity scale* has been developed for DR and DME (table 2). This scale, based on the ETDRS classification of DR and on the data collected in clinical trials and epidemiologic studies of DR, was proposed with the aim to improve communication between ophthalmologists and primary care physicians involved in diabetic patient care. According to the International Clinical Diabetic Retinopathy and Diabetic Macular Edema Disease Severity Scales, eyes with apparent DME are separated from those with no apparent thickening or lipid in the macula (DME present and absent); an additional division is based on the distance of retinal thickening and/or lipid from the fovea (mild, moderate, and severe) (Wilkinson et al., 2003)[8].

Epidemiology

DME occurs in approximately 14% of diabetics and can be found in both type I and type II patients (Girach and Lund-Andersen, 2007)[9]. The reported risk factors for occurrence and progression of DME, most of which are derived from large studies such as the WESDR and the UK Prospective Diabetes Study, are duration of diabetes, degree of metabolic control, elevated glycosylated hemoglobin A_{1c}, severity of DR, hypertension, low socioeconomic status, and older age (Girach and Lund-Andersen, 2007; Williams et al., 2004)[9, 10].

Table 2. International clinical DME disease severity scale (Wilkinson et al., 2003)[8]

Proposed disease severity level	Findings on dilated ophthalmoscopy
DME apparently absent	No apparent retinal thickening or hard exudates in posterior pole
DME apparently present	Some apparent retinal thickening or hard exudates in posterior pole
If DME is present, it can be classified into: DME present	• Mild DME: some retinal thickening or hard exudates in posterior pole but distant from the center of the macula
	• Moderate DME: retinal thickening or hard exudates approaching the center of the macula but not involving the center
	• Severe DME: retinal thickening or hard exudates involving the center of the macula

Additional risk factors for progression of DME have been reported including dyslipidemia, microalbuminuria, and proteinuria. (Among the WESDR patients with gross proteinuria at baseline, 95% had an increased risk for progression to DME.) Pregnancy may cause progression of DME and PDR with postpartum regression in some patients and persistent edema in others. Elevated plasma levels of IL-6 were also strongly related to the severity of macular edema (Girach and Lund-Andersen, 2007)[9].

Prevalence

Prevalence studies on type II diabetes show that 2–8.2% of diabetic patients had macular edema 5 years after the diagnosis, while 28% had the condition 20 years after the diagnosis. For type I diabetic patients, 0.0% had macular edema 5 years after the diagnosis, while 29% had the condition 20 years after the diagnosis (Williams et al., 2004)[10]. A study of a mixed population in the United States found a slightly different prevalence of macular edema: 36.7% of diabetic Afri-

can Americans had DR and 11.1% had macular edema; 37.4% of diabetic Hispanics had DR and 10.7% had macular edema; 24.8% of diabetic Caucasians had DR and 2.7% had macular edema, and 25.7% of diabetic Chinese had DR and 8.9% had macular edema (Varma et al., 2004)[11]. Patients treated with insulin were found to have a higher prevalence of macular edema. Fifteen years after the diagnosis, 18% of type I and 20% of type II diabetic patients treated with insulin had macular edema, while only 12% of type I and type II diabetic patients not treated with insulin had macular edema. The prevalence of CSME varies worldwide. Among American Caucasians, CSME was found in 6% of type I diabetic patients and in 2–4% of type II diabetic patients. The African-American population shows a prevalence of 8.6% of CSME in type II and in the mixed cohort, and the Hispanic population shows a prevalence of 6.2% in the mixed cohort (Williams et al., 2004; Varma et al., 2004)[10, 11]. The prevalence of CSME in the type II diabetic population in South America is 3.4–5.5%, while 5.4% of type II diabetics in Europe had CSME. In the UK specifically, 2.3–6.4% of type I diabetics and 6.4–6.8% of the mixed cohort had CSME. The prevalence of CSME in the type II diabetic population of South Asia was 6.4–13.3%, and 2.3% specifically in China. With regard to the duration of the disease, the prevalence of CSME was 5% in type I and 2% in type II during the first years after diagnosis and an increase to 20% in type I patients over 25 years was noted (Williams et al., 2004)[10].

Incidence

The incidence of CSME is reported to be correlated with the increase in the number of retinal microaneurysms (Girach and Lund-Andersen, 2007)[9] and the duration of the disease. In American Caucasians with diabetes duration of over 10 years, the incidence of CSME has been reported to be 20.1% in type I patients and 13.9% in type II patients. In a study among a mixed cohort of the Australian population, an incidence rate of 7% per year was reported. In the Scandinavian population, the incidence of CSME in type I diabetic patients over a 4-year period was 3.4%. The 4-year incidence of CSME in type I and type II insulin-treated diabetic patients was found to be 4.3 and 5.1%, while type II noninsulin-treated patients had a 1.3% incidence (Williams et al., 2004)[10].

Diagnosis

Macular edema is clinically defined as retinal thickening of the macula as seen on biomicroscopy. When moderate, the thickening may be difficult to diagnose, and contact lenses with good stereoscopy, such as Centralis Direct® (Volk), or noncontact lenses of 60, 78, or 90 dpt could be used.

The biomicroscopic assessment of the retinal thickness is subjective, and the clinical examination can only quantify thicknesses at above 1.6 times the normal rate (Brown et al., 2004)[12]. Today, the OCT evaluation for retinal thickness is objective.

Ancillary Tests

Fluorescein Angiography

Fluorescein angiography visualizes leakage from incompetent vessels that have lost their ability to prevent the egress of dye into the retinal tissue. Additionally, in the early phase of the angiogram, capillary dilatation may be seen in the perifoveal region. Late pooling of the dye may be evident assuming a petaloid pattern when accumulation of dye involves the perifoveal region, or it may show a honeycomb appearance when occurring outside the perifoveal area.

Fluorescein angiography shows the cause of leakage from microaneurysms or macular capillaries. It may also enable assessment as to the extent of macular nonperfusion, which has a significant prognostic value. Fluorescein leakage is not, however, sufficient to diagnose macular edema; a simple diffusion of fluorescein without retinal thickening is not included as part of the definition of macular edema.

Optical Coherence Tomography

OCT imaging helps in immediately estimating intraretinal modifications, pinpointing the eventual existence of infraclinical foveolar detachment, assessing the vitreoretinal juncture, and precisely measuring the thickened retina (Massin et al., 2006)[13]. In the case of DME, OCT demonstrates increased retinal thickness with areas of low intraretinal reflectivity prevailing in the outer retinal layers and the loss of foveal depression. Spectral domain OCT (SD-OCT) can show small cysts, sometimes in the inner retina, even when retinal thickening is moderate (fig. 6, 7). Hard exudates are detected as spots of high reflectivity with low reflective areas behind them and are found primarily in the outer retinal layers. Two

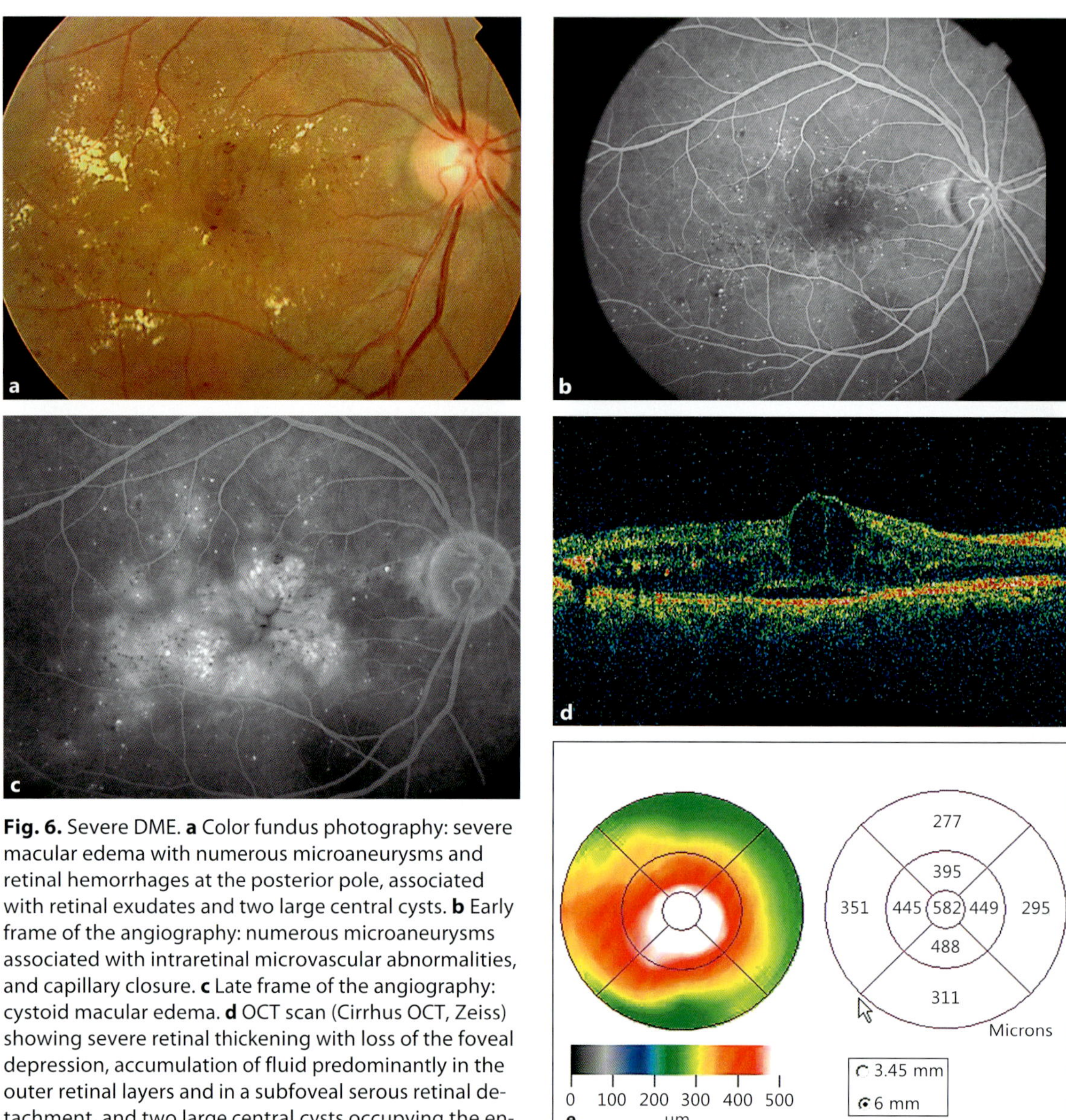

Fig. 6. Severe DME. **a** Color fundus photography: severe macular edema with numerous microaneurysms and retinal hemorrhages at the posterior pole, associated with retinal exudates and two large central cysts. **b** Early frame of the angiography: numerous microaneurysms associated with intraretinal microvascular abnormalities, and capillary closure. **c** Late frame of the angiography: cystoid macular edema. **d** OCT scan (Cirrhus OCT, Zeiss) showing severe retinal thickening with loss of the foveal depression, accumulation of fluid predominantly in the outer retinal layers and in a subfoveal serous retinal detachment, and two large central cysts occupying the entire thickness of the retina. **e** Corresponding OCT mapping.

distinct features (Otani et al., 1999)[14] can be observed: cystoid spaces, which appear as small round hyporeflective lacunae with high-signal elements bridging the retinal layers, and outer retinal swelling, characterized by an ill-defined, widespread hyporeflective area of thickening. It is distinguished from serous retinal detachment by the absence of the highly anterior reflective boundary. Small spots with high reflectivity may be seen with SD-OCT, which may be due to protein or lipid deposits secondary to an early breakdown of the BRB (fig. 7) (Bolz et al., 2009)[15]. OCT

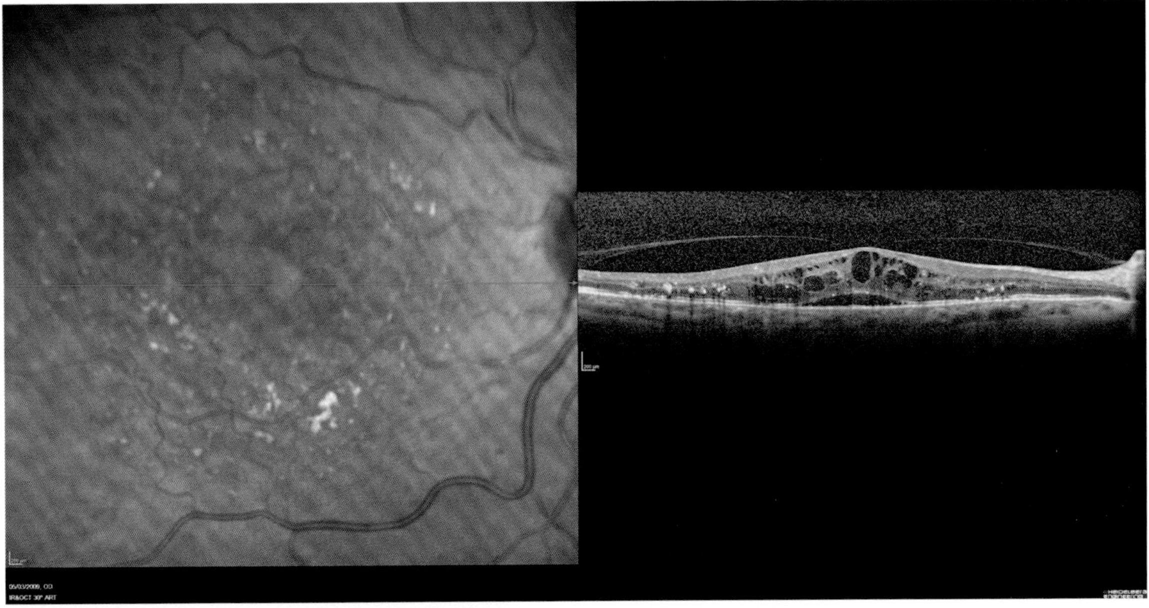

Fig. 7. Severe DME on Spectralis OCT (Heidelberg). Left: Fundus photography with OCT scan. Right: Severe retinal thickening with serous retinal detachment. Several intraretinal cysts are visible, prevailing in the outer retinal layers, but small cysts are located in the inner layers as well. Retinal exudates appear as spots of high reflectivity with low reflective areas behind them, and small spots with high reflectivity are also seen with SD-OCT, which may be due to protein or lipid deposits. In addition, a perifoveolar detachment of the posterior hyaloid is well visible. The line of the photoreceptors is relatively well preserved.

is particularly useful in detecting a feature combined with macular edema not easily seen on biomicroscopy, i.e., *serous retinal detachment* (fig. 7) (Ozdemir et al., 2005, Catier et al., 2005)[16, 17].

Serous retinal detachment, seen in 15% of eyes with DME, appears as a shallow elevation of the retina, with an optically clear space between the retina and the RPE, and a distinct outer border of the detached retina. The pathogenesis and the functional consequences of serous retinal detachment associated with cystoid macular edema are still unknown. However, in a series of 78 eyes with macular edema examined on OCT, the presence of serous retinal detachment was not correlated with poorer visual acuity (Catier et al., 2005)[17]. It has been shown that a serous retinal detachment could be present combined with moderate retinal thickening and

disappear when DME worsens (Gaucher et al., 2008)[18]. It may be a sign of early dysfunction of the outer BRB.

OCT seems particularly relevant to analyze the *vitreomacular relationship*. Indeed OCT is much more accurate than biomicroscopy in determining the status of a posterior hyaloid when it is only slightly detached from the macular surface (Gaucher et al., 2005)[19]. In some cases of DME, the posterior hyaloid on OCT is thick and hyperreflective. It is partially detached from the posterior pole and taut over it, but remains attached to the disk and to the top of the raised macular surface, on which it exerts obvious vitreomacular traction (fig. 8). In these cases, vitrectomy is beneficial (Lewis et al., 1992; Massin et al., 2003; Thomas et al., 2005; Pendergast et al., 2000)[5, 20–22]. In other cases, the posterior hyaloid

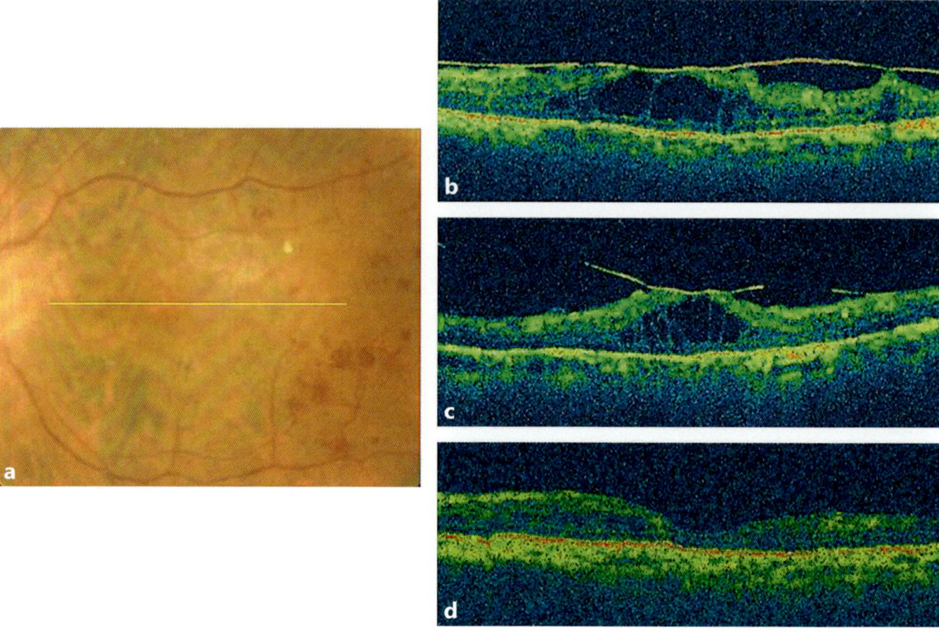

Fig. 8. DME associated with traction. **a** Fundus photography before vitrectomy. **b, c** Retinal thickening is combined with a thickened epiretinal membrane. **d** After vitrectomy, retinal thickness had decreased, with a normal foveal depression.

appears slightly reflective, detached from the retinal surface in the perifoveolar area, and attached at the foveolar center. This aspect is quite common and corresponds to early posterior vitreous detachment (fig. 7) (Gaucher et al., 2005; Uchino et al., 2001)[19, 23].

One major advantage of OCT is that it allows *measurement of retinal thickness* from the tomograms by means of computer image-processing techniques (Hee et al., 1995, 1998)[24, 25]. OCT allows retinal thickness to be calculated as the distance between the anterior and posterior highly reflective boundaries of the retina, which are located by a thresholding algorithm. The anterior boundary corresponds to the internal limiting membrane (ILM) and is well defined because of the contrast between the nonreflective vitreous and the backscattering of the retina. In SD-OCT, the posterior boundary is located as the hyperreflective band visible just

above the RPE band, which is thought to correspond to the signal of the photoreceptor and especially to the junction between the inner and outer photoreceptor segments. Finally, on SD-OCT, the posterior boundary is located differently according to the various devices. Since the commercialization of OCT systems, several types of software have become available to quantify macular thickening. Hee et al. (1998)[25] and associates have developed a standardized mapping OCT protocol, which consists of 6 radial tomograms 6 mm long in a spoke pattern centered on the fovea, which has the advantage of concentrating measurements in the central fovea. The retinal thickness is computed for a total of 600 macular locations along these 6 intersecting lines.

Retinal thickness is typically displayed in two different manners: first as a 2-dimensional color-coded map of retinal thickness in the posterior pole, with brighter colors indicating areas of increased retinal thickness and, for quantitative evaluation, retinal thickness is reported as a numeric average of the 9 ETDRS-type areas.

Regarding SD-OCT, a new type of macular mapping is utilized: macular mapping in a 3-dimensional cube, a system for scanning multiple parallel lines, which provides a more homogenous distribution of measured points within the macular region and is also a real source of 3-dimensional image reconstruction. A number of studies have demonstrated good reproducibility of OCT measurements of single scans and retinal mapping in normal eyes and in eyes with DME (Massin et al., 2001; Polito et al., 2005)[26, 27]. Excellent reproducibility of retinal thickness measurements with the SD-OCT has been reported as well, especially with Spectralis OCT (Wolf-Schnurrbusch et al., 2009; Menke et al., 2009)[28, 29]. The Diabetic Retinopathy Clinical Research Network (DRCR. net) has calculated that for the Stratus OCT, an 11% change or more of macular thickness can be considered as clinically significant (Diabetic Retinopathy Clinical Research Network et al., 2007)[30]. Finally, OCT may allow detection of early thickening of the macular area, which may be calculated as follows: when the mean retinal thickness of an area is greater than the mean thickness +2 SD in the corresponding area in healthy subjects (Strom et al., 2002)[31].

A novel OCT-based imaging technique is gaining popularity in the medical retina community. OCT angiography uses decorrelation between resampled images to detect flow to construct images of blood flow. OCT angiography is able to identify FAZ enlargement and irregularity, and capillary drop out. However, this noninvasive, dyeless imaging technique has some limitations: the field of view is still small when compared to the 20–30° standard photographic field, the identification of microaneurysms is difficult due to the slow blood flow, and vascular leakage is not detectable.

Medical Care

Systemic Control

Solid evidence has been provided regarding the principle that the control of systemic risk factors is strictly related to the course of macular edema secondary to DR. The attention of researchers has been especially focused on the effect of hyperglycemia, and many single studies, together with several multicenter clinical trials, have clearly demonstrated that persistent hyperglycemia is strongly associated with the incidence and progression of macular edema (Klein et al., 1989; Klein et al., 1995; Klein et al., 1998; Vitale et al., 1995; Diabetes Control and Complications Trial Research Group, 1997; Diabetes Control and Complications Trial Research Group, 2000; Aroca et al., 2004; Roy and Affouf, 2006; White et al., 2008; UK Prospective Diabetes Study Group, 1998; UK Prospective Diabetes Study Group, 1998; Matthews et al., 2004; Kohner et al., 2001; Kohner, 2008; Adler et al., 2000)[32–46].

Lower levels of glycosylated hemoglobin, in particular, have turned out to be associated with a lower incidence of macular edema, independent of the duration of diabetes mellitus. An increase of 1% in the glycosylated hemoglobin value between baseline and subsequent follow-up was associated with a 22% increase in the 21-year cumulative incidence of macular edema (Klein et al., 2009)[47]. These data are similar to those obtained by the Diabetes Control and Complications Trial, which found that intensive glycemic control was associated with a 46% reduction in the incidence of macular edema at the end of the trial, and with a 58% reduction 4 years later in the patients undergoing intensive treatment (3 or more daily insulin injections or a continuous subcutaneous insulin infusion), in comparison to those in the conventional group (with 1 or 2 daily injections of insulin) (Diabetes Control and Complications Trial Research Group, 2000)[37].

Exenatide is a novel glucagon-like peptide-1 receptor agonist that is administered subcutaneously and has been reported to improve DR and macular edema (Sarao et al., 2014; Varadhan et al., 2014)[48, 49]. However, when a too-fast amelioration of glycemic control is obtained, an initial and transient progression of DR may be possible. A possible consequence of strict metabolic control is represented by the potential development of severe hypoglycemic episodes (Diabetes Control and Complications Trial Research Group, 1997; Davis et al., 2007)[36, 50]. A rapid worsening of the macular edema can occur following improvement of glycemic control that is too fast, and a gradual metabolic balance is generally advisable.

Systolic blood pressure was found to be associated with the incidence of macular edema by several studies (Klein et al., 1989; Klein et al., 1995; Klein et al., 1998; Vitale et al., 1995; Aroca et al., 2004; Roy and Affouf, 2006; Klein et al., 2009; Jaross et al., 2005)[32–35, 38, 39, 47, 51]. Rigid control of hypertension is also mandatory in an effort to reduce the progression of microvascular damage typical of DR, including macular edema (Matthews et al., 2004; Funatsu and Yamashita, 2003)[43, 52]. In particular, the level of blood pressure, rather than the type of drug used, is critical in an attempt to limit the course of macular edema, as shown by the UK Prospective Diabetes Study (Matthews et al., 2004)[43]. Moreover, some investigators have indicated that, among the blood pressure-controlling drugs, special consideration should be given to angiotensin II-converting enzyme inhibitors (Sjolie, 2007)[53].

A number of investigations have also described an association between the prevalence of diabetic nephropathy, as manifest by microalbuminuria or gross proteinuria, and the incidence and progression of macular edema (West et al., 1980; Knuiman et al., 1986; Jerneld, 1988; Kostraba et al., 1991; Cruickshanks et al., 1993; Klein et al., 1993; Romero et al., 2007)[54–60].

Smoking has inconsistently been found to be associated with the prevalence and incidence of macular edema (Klein et al., 1983; Moss et al., 1996)[61, 62]. Smoking might influence the course of macular edema due to its effect on coagulation and the inflammatory response to the disease. Regardless of its association, smoking should be avoided because of its relation to increased risk of death and other systemic complications.

Lastly, hyperlipidemia has been linked to the occurrence of retinal hard exudates and macular edema in patients with DR (Sjolie, 2007; Chew et al., 1996)[53, 63]. The control of serum lipid level through pharmacologic therapies, including simvastatin, can retard the progression of macular edema and can lead to the reduction of hard deposition and microaneurysm formation (Sen et al., 2002; Rechtman et al., 2007)[64, 65]. In essence, a number of investigations have clearly pointed out that good systemic control can effectively slow the natural evolution of macular edema secondary to DR. Objectives of systemic therapy must address several aspects, including the attainment of good glycemic control, both by achieving the target glycosylated hemoglobin and minimizing the variability in the serum glucose levels and by obtaining blood pressure stabilization.

Special attention must be paid to make the risk of severe hypoglycemia occurrence as minimal as possible. On the basis of these data, the ophthalmologist must recommend that the patients comply with the suggested therapy, have their glycemia, glycosylated hemoglobin, and blood pressure frequently checked, and have regular physical examinations with their general practitioner and retina specialist, in any attempt to steer clear of the ocular complications of diabetes mellitus.

Ocular Pharmacotherapy

Corticosteroids
Photocoagulation has been the standard of care for DME for decades. However, a substantial group of patients are unresponsive to laser therapy and fail to improve after photocoagulation. It

has been reported that 3 years after initial grid treatment, visual acuity improved in 14.5% of patients with DME, did not change in 60.9%, and decreased in 24.6% (Lee and Olk, 1991)[66]. Thus, other treatment modalities for DME have been investigated.

In recent years, the *intravitreal administration of steroids* has provided promising results for the treatment of DME (Sarao et al., 2014)[67]. The anti-inflammatory, angiostatic, and antipermeability properties of these compounds have gained interest in chronic retinal conditions such as DME. A complete understanding of the mechanism of action of corticosteroids has not been fully clarified. However, corticosteroids have been shown to interfere with many regulatory components of gene expression inhibiting the expression of vascular endothelial growth factor (VEGF) and key proinflammatory genes (tumor necrosis factor α and other inflammatory chemokines), while inducing gene functioning as anti-inflammatory factors [pigment epithelium-derived growth factor (PEDF)] (Tsaprouni et al., 2002; Juergens et al., 2004; Tong et al., 2006; Kim et al., 2007; Zhang et al., 2006)[68–72]. The anti-inflammatory activity of steroids is also related to the inhibition of the phospholipase A_2 pathway, to the lower release of inflammatory cell mediators, and to the reduced leukocyte chemotaxis (Abelson and Butrus, 1994)[73]. Additionally, triamcinolone acetonide (TA) seems to reduce the expression of matrix metalloproteinases (MMPs) and downregulates intercellular adhesion molecule 1 on choroidal endothelial cells (Mizuno et al., 2007)[74].

Intravitreal Triamcinolone Acetonide
Injection of intravitreal TA has been used for treatment of DME in a number of randomized clinical trials and has demonstrated improvements in morphological and functional outcomes (Audren et al., 2006; Jonas et al., 2006; Gillies et al., 2006)[75–77]. A carefully designed prospective, randomized trial conducted by the DRCR.net investigated the efficacy and safety of 1- and 4-mg doses of preservative-free intravitreal TA in comparison with focal or grid laser photocoagulation (Diabetic Retinopathy Clinical Research Network, 2008)[78]. In this study, photocoagulation was shown to be more effective over time and had fewer side effects than TA.

More recently, a new, large, randomized, DRCR.net study investigated the efficacy of intravitreal TA in combination with laser photocoagulation in comparison with intravitreal ranibizumab with prompt or deferred laser photocoagulation or laser photocoagulation alone. At the 2-year visit, compared with the sham + prompt laser arm, the difference in mean change in visual acuity from baseline was +3.7 letters in the ranibizumab + prompt laser group (p = 0.03), +5.8 letters in the ranibizumab + deferred laser group (p < 0.01), and 1.5 letters in the TA + prompt laser group (p = 0.35). A worsening of visual acuity of 3 or more lines occurred in 10, 4, 2, and 13% of eyes, respectively, and an improvement in visual acuity by 3 or more lines occurred in 18, 29, 28, and 22% of eyes, respectively. The mean change (µm ± SD) in central retinal thickness from baseline was –141 in the ranibizumab + prompt laser group, –150 in ranibizumab + deferred laser group, –107 in the TA + prompt laser group, and –138 in the sham + prompt laser group. The development of cataract in the steroid-treated eyes may have significantly influenced the results. Among the eyes that were pseudophakic at baseline, the mean change (± SD) in the visual acuity letter score from baseline was +5 in the ranibizumab + prompt laser group, +9 in ranibizumab + deferred laser group, +8 in the TA + prompt laser group, and +5 in the sham + prompt laser group (Diabetic Retinopathy Clinical Research Network et al., 2010)[79].

Intravitreal TA injections carry some risks, including acute infectious endophthalmitis, pseudoendophthalmitis, and iatrogenic retinal breaks. One review reported an estimated incidence rate of endophthalmitis after intravitreal administration of TA of 1.4% per injection (24/1,739) (Jager et al., 2004)[80]. In both the 2008 and 2010 DRCR. net (Protocol B and Protocol I) studies, no cases of endophthalmitis or inflammatory pseudoendophthalmitis were reported. An intraocular pressure (IOP)-lowering medication was required in 5% of eyes in the sham + prompt laser and ranibizumab + prompt laser groups, in 3% of eyes in the ranibizumab + deferred laser group, and in 28% of patients of the TA + laser group.

It must be pointed out that different commercially available TA formulations have been used in the different trials, and this may influence the results. An in vitro study demonstrated that differences in formulation (more specifically the dimension and distribution in size of TA crystals) have an impact on drug efficacy (Veritti et al., 2011)[81]. This aspect needs to be further investigated.

Peribulbar Triamcinolone Acetonide Injection
Evidence has shown the efficacy of the transscleral pathway in delivering drugs to the macular retina (Geroski and Edelhauser, 2001; Olsen et al., 1995; Kato et al., 2004)[82–84]. Transscleral delivery of TA is routinely used for the treatment of various inflammatory eye diseases and has been proposed for the treatment of DME. Some studies report that intravitreal injection of TA may be more effective than posterior juxtascleral infusion for the treatment of refractory DME (Bonini-Filho et al., 2005; Cardillo et al., 2005; Ozdek et al., 2006)[85–87]. A modified formulation of TA injected via juxtascleral infusion was proposed (Veritti et al., 2009)[88], which proved a sustained effect of 6 months.

Corticosteroid Implants
Several intravitreal steroid-releasing implants have been designed in an attempt to provide long-term drug delivery to the macular region. These include nonbiodegradable and biodegradable dexamethasone, fluocinolone acetonide (FA), and TA implants. Dexamethasone is synthetic glucocorticoid, which is relatively small, water-soluble, and has a pharmacokinetic half-life of about 3 h and a biological half-life of 36–45 h (Graham and Peyman, 1974; Hardman et al., 2001)[89, 90]. Consequently, a sustained-release formulation is attractive to prolong its efficacy in the target tissue. Ozurdex™ (Allergan Inc., Irvine, Calif., USA) is a biodegradable extended-release form of dexamethasone. The polymer matrix composed of polylactide-co-glycolide copolymer releases dexamethasone over approximately 1 month with a potential therapeutic effect for about 4–6 months (Fialho et al., 2008)[91]. It is injected via the pars plana with a 22-gauge device. Ozurdex™ has been approved for the treatment of macular edema secondary to retinal vein occlusion (RVO), DME, and noninfectious uveitis.

The efficacy and safety of Ozurdex™ in DME was investigated in the large, randomized, phase III MEAD trial. In the MEAD study, 1,048 eyes with DME, visual acuity between 34 and 68 ETDRS letters, and central retinal thickness ≥300 µm were randomly assigned to treatment with dexamethasone implant 0.7 mg, dexamethasone implant 0.35 mg, or sham procedure.

Patients who met retreatment eligibility criteria could be retreated no earlier than 6 months after previous treatment. The primary endpoint was improvement of ≥15 letters in best-corrected visual acuity (BCVA) from baseline to the 3-year study visit. There were 22.2% of eyes with ≥15-letter improvement in the 0.7-mg group, 18.4% in the 0.35-mg group, and 12% in the sham group (p ≤ 0.018). Mean average reduction in central retinal thickness from baseline during the study was greater with dexamethasone implant 0.7 mg (–112 µm) and with dexamethasone implant 0.35 mg (–108 µm) than with sham (–42 µm) (p < 0.001). Cataract development in phakic eyes was detected in 68, 64, and 20% in the dexamethasone implant 0.7 mg, dexamethasone implant 0.35 mg, and sham groups, respectively (Boyer et al., 2014)[92].

IOP-lowering medication was required during the study by 41.5, 37.6, and 9.1% of patients in the dexamethasone implant 0.7-mg, dexamethasone implant 0.35-mg, and sham groups, respectively. The initial IOP increase typically occurred after the first or second injection. Mean IOP peaked at 1.5 or 3 months after each injection; IOP returned to within the normal range by 6 months after injection. One (0.3%) eye treated with dexamethasone implant 0.7-mg and 1 eye (0.3%) treated with dexamethasone implant 0.35-mg underwent glaucoma incisional surgery to manage steroid-induced increased IOP (Boyer et al., 2014)[92].

FA is a synthetic steroid with a solubility of 1/24 in aqueous solution of dexamethasone and a short systemic half-life. FA can be released in a linear manner in vivo over an extended period of time by nonerodible drug delivery devices (Ashton et al., 1994; Jaffe et al., 2000)[93, 94].

Iluvien® (Alimera Sciences, Alpharetta, Ga., USA) is a nonerodable injectable fluocinolone intravitreal implant, which delivers a low dose of drug for up to either 18 or 36 months and either 0.2 or 0.5 µg of drug per day. It is designed to be injected with a 25-gauge needle through the pars plana. The FAME study program consisted of two identical 36-month, phase III clinical trials that evaluated the efficacy and the safety of two doses of FA implant in patients with DME (Campochiaro et al., 2011; Campochiaro et al., 2012)[95, 96]. In this study, 956 eyes were randomized to receive a high-dose implant (0.5 µg/day), a low-dose implant (0.2 µg/day), or a sham procedure. After 36 months, an improvement in visual acuity by 3 or more lines occurred in 28.7, 27.8, and 18.9% of eyes, respectively. Mean (± SD) reductions in central macular thickness were 185 ± 174 µm in the high-dose FA group, 180 ± 160 µm in the low-dose FA group, and 142 ± 152 µm in the sham group. Among patients with a duration of DME of more than 3 years, the proportion of eyes showing a gain of 15 letters or more was 13.4% of patients in the sham group compared with 34% in the low-dose FA group (p < 0.001) and 28.8% in the high-dose FA group (p = 0.002). An improvement of 3 or more lines in patients with DME for less than 3 years occurred in 27.8% of the eyes in the sham group, 22.3% of the eyes in the low-dose FA group, and 26.4% of the eyes in high-dose FA group. The mean change in BCVA letter score between baseline and month 36 in long-duration DME subjects was 1.8 in the sham group compared with 7.6 in low-dose FA group (p < 0.004) and 6.2 in high-dose FA group (p < 0.024). The most common adverse event was cataract. Among phakic eyes, 81.7% of the low-dose group, 88.7% of the high-dose group, and 50.7% of the sham group experienced development of cataract. IOP-lowering medications were needed in 47.3% of the high-dose group, 38.4% of the low-dose group, and 14.1% of the sham group. Incisional IOP-lowering surgery was performed in 8.1% of the high-dose group, 4.8% of the low-dose group, and 0.5% of the sham group. The US Food and Drug Administration (FDA) approved Iluvien® for the treatment of DME for patients treated with a course of corticosteroids and did not have a significant rise in IOP, and it has received marketing authorization in 17 EU countries for use in the treatment of vision impairment associated with chronic DME considered insufficiently responsive to other available therapies.

Verisome® (Icon Bioscience Inc., Sunnyvale, Calif., USA) is a biodegradable implant designed to be injected intravitreously, and can be used to release a broad range of pharmaceutical agents, including small molecules, peptides, proteins, and monoclonal antibodies. When loaded with TA, preclinical studies have demonstrated sustained levels of the drug in the vitreous for up to 6 months (6.9-mg formulation) and 12 months (13.8-mg formulation). This implant appears to be well tolerated in rabbit eyes (Hu et al., 2008)[97]. In a phase II study, Lim et al. treated 10 patients with macular edema secondary to RVO with a single injection of either 6.9 mg (25 µl) or 13.8 mg (50 µl) triamcinolone and then followed them for 1 year. Five patients who received 13.8 mg (50 µl) experienced a significant and sustained reduction in mean central subfield OCT thickness from 518 μm at baseline to 289 μm at day 30, 207 μm at day 180, and 278 μm at day 360. Three patients in the study had elevated IOP, of which 2 cases were due to neovascular glaucoma (Lim JI et al., 2011)[98].

Vascular Endothelial Growth Factor Inhibitors
In the pathophysiologic sequence of events leading to DME, chronic hyperglycemia induces oxidative damage to endothelial cells and an inflammatory response (Gardner et al., 2002)[99]. The subsequent overexpression of a number of growth factors, including VEGF, insulin-like growth factor 1, angiopoietin 1 and 2, stromal-derived factor 1, fibroblast growth factor 2, and tumor necrosis factor α, leads to BRB breakdown in the ischemic retina (Grant et al., 2004)[100]. Thus, anti-VEGF agents, interfering with a critical stimulus for the development of BRB breakdown, have been investigated in the treatment of DME.

Ranibizumab
Ranibizumab (Lucentis, Genentech) is a humanized antigen-binding fragment directed against VEGF. It is currently labeled by the FDA for the treatment of wet AMD, macular edema following RVO, DME, and DR in patients with DME. It is approved by the European Medicines Agency (EMA) for the therapy of wet AMD, DME, macular edema following RVO, and choroidal neovascularization due to pathologic myopia. In the US, ranibizumab is given at a dosage of 0.3 mg for the treatment of DME, while its use is recommended at a dosage of 0.5 mg in Europe.

In the phase III RISE study, 377 patients were randomized to receive monthly injections of 0.3-mg ranibizumab, 0.5-mg ranibizumab or sham injections. In the parallel RIDE study, 382 patients were randomized to receive the same treatment options. After 3 months, macular laser photocoagulation was available to all patients as rescue treatment, if necessary. After 2 years, patients in the sham group were eligible to receive monthly injections of 0.5-mg ranibizumab. At 24 months, 18% of patients in the sham arm gained at least 15 letters, compared to 45% of 0.3-mg (p < 0.0001) and 39% of 0.5-mg ranibizumab-treated eyes (p < 0.001). In RIDE, significantly more patients in the ranibizumab arms gained 15 letters or more: 34% of 0.3-mg patients (p < 0.0001) and 46% of 0.5-mg ranibizumab patients (p < 0.0001), compared to 12% of sham patients (Nguyen et al., 2012)[101].

The 36-month extension of RISE-RIDE showed that the strong VA gains and improvement in retinal anatomy achieved with ranibizumab at month 24 were sustained through month 36. Delayed treatment in patients randomized initially to sham treatment did not seem to result in the same extent of VA improvement observed in patients originally randomized to ranibizumab (Brown et al., 2013)[102].

In the RESTORE study, 0.5-mg ranibizumab monotherapy or ranibizumab combined with laser was compared to laser alone in 345 patients. Patients received 3 initial monthly ranibizumab injections or sham procedures. Retreatments were performed if needed. Laser or sham was performed at baseline and during the follow-up if needed. Ranibizumab alone and combined with laser was superior to laser alone in improving mean average change in the BCVA letter score from baseline to month 1 through 12 (+6.1 and +5.9 vs. +0.8; both p < 0.0001). At month 12, a significantly greater proportion of patients had a BCVA letter score ≥15 and BCVA letter score level >73 (20/40 Snellen equivalent) with ranibizumab (22.6 and 53%, respectively) and ranibizumab + laser (22.9 and 44.9%) versus laser (8.2 and 23.6%). Moreover, health-related quality of life, assessed by the National Eye Institute Visual Function Questionnaire (NEI VFQ-25), improved significantly from baseline with ranibizumab alone and combined with laser (p < 0.05 for composite score and vision-related subscales) versus laser alone. Patients received ~7 (mean) ranibizumab/sham injections over 12 months (Mitchell et al., 2011)[103]. Consecutive individualized ranibizumab treatment during the 36-month extension study led to an overall maintenance of BCVA and central retinal subfield thickness. Moreover, at month 36, 14.8% of patients in the prior ranibizumab group, 28.3% of patients in the prior ranibizumab + laser group, and 16.0% of patients in the prior laser group had an improvement in ETDRS severity score (≥3 steps) from baseline, whereas 1.6, 7.5, and 4.0% of patients, respectively, had a worsening of ETDRS score (≥3 steps) from baseline to month 36 (Schmidt-Erfurth et al., 2014)[104]. Ranibizumab treatment in both the RESTORE trial and RISE-RIDE trial program showed an excellent systemic and ocular safety profile.

The DRCR.net protocol S trial was conducted to evaluate the efficacy of intravitreal ranibizumab in the treatment of proliferative DR compared to the gold standard panretinal photocoagulation. The study showed that mean peripheral visual field sensitivity loss was worse (p < 0.001), vitrectomy was more frequent (9% difference; p < 0.001), and DME development was more frequent (19% difference; p < 0.001) in the PRP group versus the ranibizumab group, respectively. Eyes without active or regressed neovascularization at 2 years were not significantly different (35% in the ranibizumab group vs. 30% in the PRP group). In the ranibizumab group, eyes without DME at baseline received a median of 7 injections through 1 year and 10 injections through 2 years. Eyes with DME at baseline received a median of 9 injections through 1 year and 14 injections through 2 years (Writing Committee for the Diabetic Retinopathy Clinical Research Network et al., 2015)[105].

Aflibercept

Aflibercept is a recombinant fusion protein composed of portions from the extracellular domains of human VEGF receptors 1 and 2 fused to the Fc portion of human IgG1. It is characterized by a high binding affinity to VEGF-A. It is approved by EMA and FDA for the use in patients with wet AMD, DME, macular edema secondary to RVO, and myopic choroidal neovascularization. The FDA registered intravitreal aflibercept for wet AMD, macular edema secondary to RVO, DME, and DR in patients with DME. The safety and efficacy of aflibercept were assessed in two randomized, multicenter, double-masked, controlled studies in 862 patients with DME: VIVID and VISTA.

In each study, patients were randomly assigned in a 1:1:1 ratio to 1 of 3 dosing regimens: (1) aflibercept administered 2 mg every 8 weeks following 5 initial monthly injections (2Q8); (2) aflibercept administered 2 mg every 4 weeks (2Q4), and (3) macular laser photocoagulation (at baseline and then as needed). Beginning at week 24, patients meeting a prespecified threshold of vision loss were eligible to receive additional treatment: patients in the aflibercept groups could receive laser and patients in the laser group could receive aflibercept. In both studies, the primary efficacy endpoint was the mean change from baseline in BCVA at week 52 as measured by the ETDRS letter score. Efficacy of both the aflibercept 2Q8 and aflibercept 2Q4 groups was statistically superior to the control group. This statistically superior improvement in BCVA was maintained at week 100 in both studies. Mean BCVA changes from baseline in the 2Q4, 2Q8, and laser groups were +10.7, +10.5, and +1.2 letters at week 52 and +11.4, +9.4, and 0.7 letters at week 100, respectively, in VIVID. Corresponding improvements in BCVA in VISTA were +12.5, +10.7, and +0.2 letters at week 52 and +11.5, +11.1, and 0.9 letters at week 100.

In the VIVID and VISTA studies, an efficacy outcome was the change in the (ETDRS) Diabetic Retinopathy Severity Scale (ETDRS-DRSS).

At week 100, approximately 30–38% of patients in the aflibercept arms improved by 2 steps or more, compared to 7–16% in the laser group (Korobelnik et al., 2014)[106].

Bevacizumab

Bevacizumab (Avastin; Genentech) is a full-length humanized antibody against VEGF. It is widely used off-label in the treatment of retinal conditions characterized by excessive VEGF. It is approved for the treatment of metastatic cancer and a randomized, phase II DRCR.net trial evaluated the short-term effects of intravitreal bevacizumab and demonstrated a beneficial action in DME (Scott et al., 2007)[105].

A randomized, placebo-controlled clinical trial compared the efficacy of 3 intravitreal injections of bevacizumab alone or combined with intravitreal triamcinolone in the first injection versus sham injection. A total of 115 eyes were randomly assigned to 1 of 3 groups (bevacizumab alone, bevacizumab combined with intravitreal triamcinolone, or sham injection). Central macular thickness was reduced significantly in both treatment groups. At week 24, retinal thickness reduction was 95.7 μm in the bevacizumab group and 92.1 μm in the combination group, compared with a mean increase of 34.9 μm in the control group. Significant gains in visual acuity were noted compared with the sham group (monotherapy: p = 0.01; combination therapy: p = 0.006). The addition of a steroidal drug in this study had no significant effect on retinal thickness, but did result in a trend toward earlier visual improvements (Ahmadieh et al., 2008)[108]. Similar overall results were also found in another randomized study (Soheilian et al., 2009)[109].

The Intravitreal Triamcinolone Acetonide versus Intravitreal Bevacizumab for Refractory Diabetic Macular Edema (IBEME) study was a trial comparing morphological and functional outcomes in 28 patients treated with a single injection of either bevacizumab or TA in DME. Central macular thickness was significantly reduced in the triamcinolone group compared with the bevacizumab group at weeks 4, 8, 12, and 24. Visual acuity was significantly higher in the triamcinolone group at weeks 8 and 12. A significant increase in intraocular pressure was seen only in the triamcinolone group at week 4 (Paccola et al., 2008)[110].

Recently, DRCR.net designed and conducted a randomized trial comparing the three anti-VEGF drugs: ranibizumab, aflibercept and bevacizumab. Eighty-nine clinical sites enrolled 660 participants with center-involving DME. Patients were randomized to receive injections of 2-mg aflibercept, 1.25-mg bevacizumab, or 0.3-mg ranibizumab. The anti-VEGF agents were administered every 4 weeks. At the 24-week visit, injection was withheld if there was no improvement or worsening after two consecutive injections. Treatment was resumed if visual acuity or retinal thickness worsened. After 1 year of treatment, aflibercept produced overall better visual acuity outcomes, with the mean BCVA improving by 13.3 letters, versus 9.7 letters with bevacizumab, and 11.2 letters with ranibizumab. However, the investigators judged these differences to be not clinically meaningful. At 1 year, central retinal thickness decreased on average by 169 μm (aflibercept), 147 μm (ranibizumab), and 101 μm (bevacizumab). When the initial visual acuity letter score was between 20/32 and 20/40, mean improvement was similar between the drugs. When baseline visual acuity was 20/50 or worse, mean improvement was 18.9 with aflibercept, 11.8 with bevacizumab, and 14.2 with ranibizumab. This difference was statistically significant (Diabetic Retinopathy Clinical Research Network et al., 2015)[111].

The Protocol T two-year data provide longer-term evidence that anti-VEGF therapy is efficacious in treating DME. The main difference between year 1 and year 2 results was that at 2 years, the superior visual results of aflibercept over ranibizumab in the lower vision group were no longer present. At year 2, bevacizumab-treated eyes, with a baseline BCVA of 20/50 or worse, still showed less vision improvement compared to the other agents. No significant differences were noted in the number of intravitreal injections required in the three groups: approximately 10 in the first year and 5 in the second year. The incidence of adverse events in all three groups of Protocol T was consistent with previous trials (Wells et al., 2016)[112].

Other Drugs

Novel prophylactic and therapeutic interventions in DR are being investigated in either systemic or ocular delivery. Ocular pharmacologic therapies include MMP inhibitors and PEDF inducers as an alternative to growth factor modulators and steroids. ALG-001 is a synthetic anti-integrin oligopeptide. It mediates integrin subunits implicated in the angiogenic cascade ($\alpha_5\beta_1$, $\alpha v\beta_3$, $\alpha v\beta_5$), as well as integrin subunits implicated in posterior vitreous detachment and vitreous liquefaction ($\alpha_3\beta_1$). It has a dual activity for turning off the angiogenic cascade and for causing vitreolysis. Moreover, its activity may persist for at least 90 days after injection. In a phase I DME study, ALG-001 has been shown to improve vision by approximately 9 letters in 15 patients with advanced DME during a follow-up of 5 months. A phase II study (DEL MAR) is currently underway.

VAP-1 is expressed in retinal capillaries and acts as an amine oxidase and as an endothelial adhesion molecule for leukocytes. In a preclinical study performed in a streptozocin-induced diabetic rat model, treatment with ASP-8232 improved retinal hyperpermeability and inhibited plasma VAP-1 activity; combination treatment with an anti-VEGF antibody was associated with greater benefit than that achieved with either agent alone.

VAP-1 Inhibition in Diabetes (VIDI), an ongoing phase II study, is a controlled study being conducted at 15 centers across the United States.

Abicipar pegol is a DARPin that binds soluble isoforms of VEGF-A. DARPins are small protein therapies derived from natural ankyrin repeat proteins, one of the most common binding proteins in nature. They are responsible for diverse functions, such as cell signaling and receptor binding. They are characterized by small size, high potency, high stability, high affinity (strong binding), and flexible architecture. Abicipar has shown promising results in wet AMD trials and is currently being evaluated in DME patients in a phase II study.

AKB-9778 is a Tie2 activator and inhibits human protein tyrosine phosphatase β (HPTPβ) that activates the Tie2 pathway to promote vascular stability, preventing abnormal blood vessel growth and vascular leakage. In a phase Ib/II dose-escalation study (TIME-1), this investigational product showed good tolerability when administered subcutaneously for 28 days as monotherapy in patients with DME. After treatment at doses of 15 mg or greater, 7 out of 18 patients demonstrated a reduction in central subfield thickness in the study eye of greater than 50 μm, and 13 out of 18 patients gained 5 or more letters of visual acuity.

Encapsulated cell technology is a treatment modality developed by Neurotech (Lincoln, R.I., USA), which involves the implantation of a semipermeable polymer capsule in the vitreous cavity. The small capsule contains cells that have been genetically modified to produce desired proteins or peptides. The structure of the hollow-fiber membrane is designed to allow influx of oxygen and nutrients while guaranteeing immune privilege. Encapsulated cell technology can also be engineered to secrete antiangiogenic and anti-inflammatory factors. Encapsulated cell technology has been investigated in phase II clinical trials including subjects with geographic atrophy and retinitis pigmentosa.

Surgical Care

Photocoagulation

Many studies have demonstrated a beneficial effect of laser photocoagulation on DME. The ETDRS, which identified macular edema as a study objective, provided the most comprehensive directives for the management of affected patients and the strongest support for the therapeutic benefit of photocoagulation. In the ETDRS, focal/grid laser photocoagulation of eyes with edema involving or threatening the fovea reduced the

3-year risk of moderate visual loss (defined as a loss of ≥15 letters) by approximately 50%, from 24% in the control group, to 12% in the laser group (Early Treatment Diabetic Retinopathy Study Research Group, 1985)[3].

As a result, the clinical and therapeutic approach to DME is largely based on the findings and conclusions of the ETDRS. Laser photocoagulation leads to visual improvement in a minority of patients. For the majority of cases, the goal of laser treatment is to stabilize visual acuity, and patients should be informed of this when laser photocoagulation is planned. Furthermore, the visual and functional prognosis in the subgroup of patients with diffuse DME is poor, and in those cases, macular edema is often refractory to multiple treatments. With the advent of new imaging modalities, it has come into question whether the presence of CSME on fundus biomicroscopy is still to be considered as the best indicator to apply laser. In the ETDRS, the diagnosis of macular edema was based on clinical examination, regardless of visual acuity, and fluorescein angiography was used to help direct laser treatment. In recent years, the use of OCT has gained increasing popularity as an objective tool to measure retinal thickness and other aspects associated with DME. Standard OCT assessment of macular edema has been adopted in multicenter trials in patients with DME and has been demonstrated to correlate well with fundus biomicroscopy (Strom, 2002)[31].

Some studies have demonstrated a good correlation between OCT and fluorescein angiography in patients with CSME, with a greater sensitivity of OCT to detect earlier stages of macular edema (Kang, 2004; Jittpoonkuson et al., 2010)[7, 113]. Combined fluorescein angiography and OCT data could be helpful to disclose the pathogenesis of the edema, to diagnose and optimize early treatment, when necessary, thereby reducing visual loss. It remains to be evaluated with longitudinal studies if earlier treatment decisions based on fluorescein angiographic and tomographic features reflect a more favorable visual prognosis.

Mechanism of Action of Laser Photocoagulation
The specific mechanisms of action of laser photocoagulation in DME are still unclear. Pigments involved in the process of light absorption during laser photocoagulation are xanthophylls (outer and inner plexiform layers), melanin (RPE cells, choroidal melanocytes), and hemoglobin (retinal and choroidal vessels).

The primary effect of laser treatment is thermal damage, mainly induced at the level of the RPE. However, concurrent damage to the adjacent choriocapillary and outer retinal layers, such as the photoreceptors, usually occurs as a consequence of heat transmission. Two different mechanisms of action can be hypothesized: direct and indirect.

The effectiveness of focal laser photocoagulation could be due, at least partially, to direct thrombosis caused by absorption of light by hemoglobin with consequent closure of leaky microaneurysms. Several hypotheses suggesting an indirect effect of laser photocoagulation have been proposed, and these seem to be supported by the efficacy of grid treatment alone (without focal, direct treatment of microaneurysms), light photocoagulation, and micropulse techniques (Bandello et al., 2005)[114]. One possible explanation is that the laser-induced destruction and consequent reduction of retinal, RPE, and choriocapillaris tissue following treatment could lead to direct oxygen diffusion from the choriocapillaris to the inner retina, through the laser scars, ultimately relieving retinal hypoxia (Stefansson, 2001)[115].

Furthermore, laser photocoagulation could reduce the oxygen demand by destroying the outer retinal layers, allowing an increased oxygen supply to the inner retina. Contrasting evidence exists on this point: some authors demonstrated increased preretinal oxygen partial pressure in photocoagulated areas, while others revealed choriocapillaris loss and reduction of retinal capillaries in areas of laser photocoagulation (Wolbarsht and Landers, 1980; Molnar et al., 1985)[116, 117].

However, both conventional continuous-wave laser and micropulse laser have been shown to induce reduction of outer retinal oxygen consumption and increased oxygen level within the retina in animal models (Stefansson et al., 1981)[118]. The latter finding supports the hypothesis that loss of retinal capillary after laser photocoagulation would result in the reduction of abnormal leaking vessels and consequent improvement of macular edema (Yu et al., 2005)[119].

Another theory proposes that laser treatment may stimulate improvement of retinal oxygenation and induce autoregulatory vasoconstriction of macular arterioles and venules, thus reducing retinal blood flow and consequently macular edema (Wilson et al., 1988)[120]. Some investigators have hypothesized that laser injury to the RPE induces both anatomic remodeling and functional restoration. Laser photocoagulation may restore the RPE barrier, leading to cell proliferation, resurfacing, and inducing the production of cytokines that antagonize the permeabilizing effect of VEGF (Guyer et al., 1992; Han et al., 1992; Gottfredsdottir et al., 1993; Xiao et al., 1999; Ogata et al., 2001)[121–125].

Despite theoretical advantages of some wavelengths over others, several studies have shown a similar efficacy for all the wavelengths (yellow, green, red, infrared) commonly used for the treatment of DME.

Timing of Laser Photocoagulation
An indispensable requirement for successful laser treatment is the presence of prevalently retinovascular DME. There is no proven indication for laser treatment when the cause of macular edema is tractional (epiretinal membrane, taut, attached posterior hyaloid), and often in such cases laser photocoagulation is even contraindicated since treatment could worsen the tractional component.

Analysis of early- and late-frame fluorescein angiography provides information about the nature of the edema and its possible causal mechanisms. Prevalently retinovascular DME is typically characterized by an exact correspondence between microvascular abnormalities, well defined in the early phases, and dye leakage evident in the late frames. On the contrary, biomicroscopic examination, however carefully performed, allows an evaluation of the presence of retinal thickening, but only occasionally (especially for focal edema where there are circinate lipid exudates in which leaking lesions are often obvious within the lipid ring) consents to disclose the exact cause of macular edema.

Fluorescein angiography is currently the most reliable diagnostic technique to identify retinovascular DME and should be mandatory for early and adequate laser treatment. Furthermore, fluorescein angiography identifies the presence and severity of macular ischemia that, if extensive, contraindicates laser photocoagulation.

Laser treatment is most effective when initiated before visual acuity declines, therefore treatment should be initiated as soon as CSME is detected (Early Treatment Diabetic Retinopathy Study Research Group, 1985; Early Treatment Diabetic Retinopathy Study Research Group, 1995)[3, 126]. When treatment is planned, risks and benefits of laser photocoagulation should be discussed with the patient. Patients should be informed that the treatment aim is to stabilize vision and prevent further visual loss, and that visual improvement, although possible, is uncommon. In asymptomatic patients with excellent visual acuity (20/20), it is possible to consider deferring focal laser treatment and scheduling close follow-up appointments (every 2–4 months). In such cases, assessment of the proximity of exudates to the fovea, status of the fellow eye, scheduled cataract surgery, and presence of retinopathy approaching high-risk characteristics should guide treatment decision. In patients with optimal visual acuity, treatment can be deferred in the presence of macular edema without central involvement.

If careful, serial examinations and documentation (fundus stereophotography is a valuable tool to document clinical findings and to allow compari-

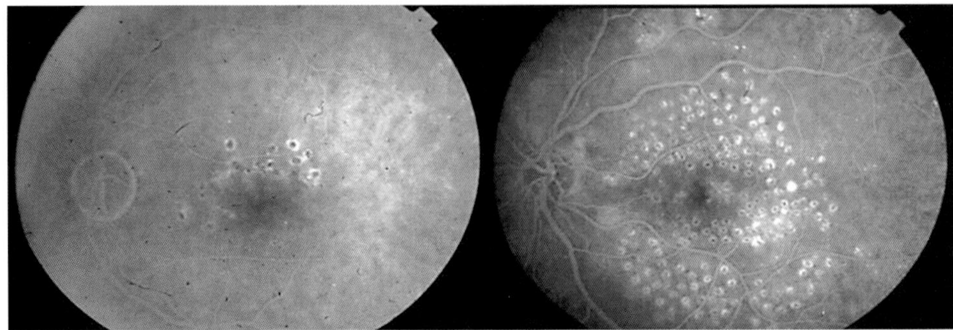

Fig. 9. Examples of laser treatment techniques. Left: focal. Right: grid.

son) reveal progression of the edema toward the center. Patients should be considered for laser treatment especially if treatable lesions are located 500 μm outside of the macular center. When panretinal photocoagulation is needed for severe NPDR or non-high-risk PDR in eyes with macular edema, it is preferable to perform focal photocoagulation before panretinal photocoagulation, starting treatment in the nasal and inferior sectors, since there is evidence that panretinal photocoagulation as used in the ETDRS may exacerbate macular edema. However, panretinal and focal laser photocoagulation should be concomitantly performed in the presence of CSME and high-risk PDR (if retinal or disk neovascularization is extensive or vitreous/preretinal hemorrhage has occurred recently).

A follow-up examination for individuals with CSME should be scheduled within 3–4 months of laser treatment. Retreatment of up to 300 μm (unless there is perifoveal capillary dropout) or including the FAZ should be considered if macular edema persists or recurs. Close monitoring, at least every 3–4 months, should be planned and retreatment deferred if visual acuity has improved and an objective reduction of retinal thickness is observed.

Treatment Procedures
Even though the principles of macular laser therapy were established more than 20 years ago, the ETDRS recommendations still constitute the basis of the current treatment guidelines.

Laser photocoagulation techniques for DME can traditionally be classified as focal or grid (fig. 9). The ETDRS treatment strategy involves treating discrete areas of leaking microaneurysms considered to produce retinal thickening or hard exudates with focal photocoagulation.

The grid technique was applied to treat areas of diffuse leakage, including microaneurysms, intraretinal microvascular abnormalities, leaking capillary segments, and areas of nonperfusion. Both techniques are usually performed after pupil dilation and under topical anesthesia, with the application of a contact lens.

Focal Treatment
The ETDRS protocol requires the direct treatment of all focal points of leakage located between 500 and 3,000 μm from the center of the macula. At the initial session, lesions located between 300 and 500 μm from the macular center could be optionally treated if visual acuity is 20/40 or worse, and if treatment would not destroy the remaining perifoveal capillary network.

Initial treatment requires a whitening of microaneurysms with 50- to 100-μm spots for a duration of 0.1 s. Repeat focal burns are applied, if needed, to obtain the desired effect, especially for microaneurysms larger than 40 μm. Retreatment is required if macular edema persists and the abovementioned criteria are not met. Clusters of microaneurysms could be treated with larger and

Bandello · Battaglia Parodi · Lanzetta · Loewenstein · Massin · Menchini · Veritti confluent spots (200–500 μm) if the lesions are not located within 750 μm from the center of the macula. Additional treatment is recommended if residual CSME with treatable lesions is seen on examination 4 months after the initial treatment. Intervals between laser sessions need to be at least 4 months.

Focal Treatment: Practical Guidelines
Laser strategy for macular edema has changed and evolved over the years in order to maintain the same results and reduce potential complications.

There is a trend toward larger spot sizes, longer exposure times, and lower energy levels. Most retinal specialists do not directly treat microaneurysms, as performed in the ETDRS, since 'whitening' or 'darkening' of the aneurysms is not necessary and requires higher energy. Light, small-sized (100–200 μm in diameter) burns to leaking microaneurysms in the macula (500–3,000 μm from the center of the macula, but not within 500 μm of the disk), with a relatively long exposure time of 0.1–0.3 s, are preferable if patients provide adequate compliance and immobility (table 3).

The initial power setting varies according to media opacities, degree of fundus pigmentation, and type of wavelength employed. Laser wavelengths with great affinity for hemoglobin are preferred (yellow, green). Red and infrared laser wavelengths can be useful in the presence of cataract; blue and blue-green wavelengths should not be employed due to their potential to damage the ILM and their absorption by macular xanthophylls. When using krypton red or diode infrared lasers, it is recommended to employ low energy and longer exposure time. If an infrared diode laser is chosen, retinal whitening should be barely visible, otherwise there is a high risk of provoking tears of the Bruch's membrane. Independent of the wavelength selected, the power should be gradually increased, by 10–20 mW, until the desired effect is reached. Whitening of microaneurysms is not required, but at least a mild gray-

white burn should be evident beneath all microaneurysms. Exposure time should be as long as possible to obtain the desired effect, unless the target area is paracentral: in such cases, shorter exposure times are preferred. It is advisable to avoid overtreating, which causes almost inevitably large chorioretinal atrophy and scotomata.

As established by the ETDRS, initial focal treatment should not be applied to focal lesions located within 300–500 μm from the center of the FAZ: treatment can be applied within 500 μm if retinal thickening persists at the 4-month follow-up, and if such treatment does not destroy the perifoveal capillary network and visual acuity is worse than 20/40. In the presence of numerous microaneurysms that would require the destruction of extensive retinal areas and the risk of progressive confluence of the laser scars, it is advisable to perform grid treatment.

Grid Treatment
In the ETDRS, the grid strategy for diffuse macular edema consisted of burns of 50–200 μm in size, a duration of 0.1 s, and of lighter intensity than that required for panretinal photocoagulation, placed one burn width apart. Laser spots can be placed in the papillomacular bundle but not within 500 μm from the margin of the optic disk and the center of the macula. Retreatment criteria are the same as for focal laser: further treatment is advisable if residual CSME is present on examination at 4-month intervals.

Table 3. Parameters for focal photocoagulation

Spot size	100–200 μm
Exposure time	0.1–0.3 s
Change in microaneurysm color	Whitening/darkening of microaneurysms is not required, but at least a mild gray-white burn beneath all microaneurysms

Table 4. Parameters for grid photocoagulation

Spot size	100–200 µm
Exposure time	0.1–0.3 s
Burn intensity	Light whitening (barely visible burns)
Power increase	10–20 mW
Spot spacing	At least 1 spot width apart

Grid Photocoagulation: Practical Guidelines
In the grid technique, a grid or pattern of nonconfluent spots (100–200 µm spot size, with 1 burn width spacing) is placed to the entire leaking area and/or segments of capillary nonperfusion, producing a light-gray burn (table 4). Three to 4 concentric rows of spots with a ring-like pattern are usually applied. The grid is centered on the FAZ and extended up to 2 papillary diameters or to the margin of a preexisting panphotocoagulative treatment, including the interpapillomacular bundle (but not within 500 µm from the disk).

Laser power is lower compared to that used for focal treatment since the target of grid photocoagulation should be to obtain a barely visible whitening at the level of the retina and RPE. Since the severity of retinal thickening and the degree of fundus pigmentation may vary in the course of diffuse edema, photocoagulative parameters must be modified many times during each session, requiring higher power in more edematous areas. Therefore, it is sensible to start laser treatment in areas scarcely thickened and then proceed to treat more thickened zones, gradually increasing the power by 10 mW. Special care should be taken in treating large intraretinal hemorrhages, particularly if green and yellow wavelengths are used since their absorption by the innermost retinal layers can damage the ILM and the nerve fiber layer. In such cases, red or infrared wavelengths must be used.

In some patients, due to extensive retinal thickness, it can be difficult to ascertain the exact localization of the edge of the FAZ. In these cases, it is rational to begin with a conservative treatment. Following initial laser photocoagulation, the leakage and edema are likely to decrease, permitting an easier recognition of the FAZ and consenting to bring the treatment up to the edge of the FAZ. In case of bilateral grid treatment, it is advisable to spare the median raphe in order to avoid paracentral scotomata.

Modified Grid Photocoagulation
In clinical practice, it is common to encounter mixed forms of DME, where focal and diffuse leakage are combined and clearly visible on fluorescein angiography. In such cases, the use of a modified grid technique that has been shown to have comparable efficacy to the ETDRS grid is advisable. Modified grid photocoagulation was introduced more than 15 years ago (Lee and Olk, 1991; Early Treatment Diabetic Retinopathy Study Research Group, 1987; Ferris and Davis, 1999)[66, 127, 128].

This technique primarily consists of a grid treatment to areas of diffuse leakage, with occasional focal treatment of localized leakage situated either within or outside areas of diffuse edema. Grid treatment leads to visual improvement in 14.5% of treated eyes, stabilization in 60.9%, and worsening in 24.6% of eyes. Modified grid photocoagulation is applied to edematous perifoveal retina, including the edge of the FAZ, using 2–3 rows of 100-µm spots, placed 100 µm apart. The remaining areas of retinal thickening and/or capillary nonperfusion are then treated with 150- to 200-µm spots, placed 200 µm apart. The end point of laser treatment is to obtain a barely visible light-intensity burn at the level of the retina and RPE. Associated focal leakage is treated with 100- to 150-µm spots to achieve a slightly darker burn. Additional treatment is usually applied after 3–4 months if residual retinal thickening involving the center of the FAZ is noted. An alternative ap-

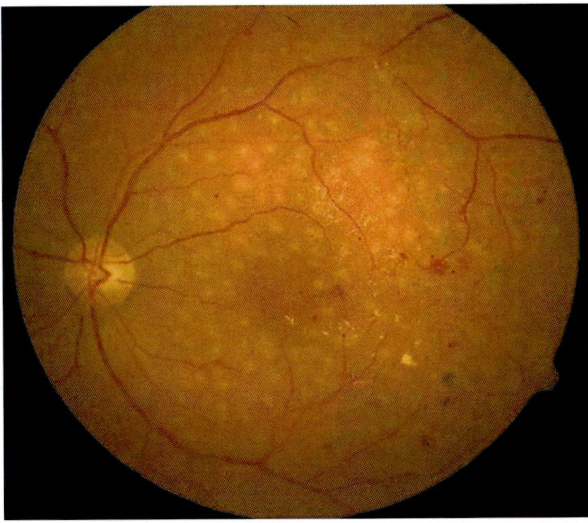

Fig. 10. Mild macular grid.

proach is the mild macular grid (fig. 10). With this technique, mild, widely spaced, 50-μm burns are applied to the entire area considered for grid treatment, including unthickened retina and avoiding the foveal region. A total of 200–300 evenly distributed, light burns are usually performed. However, the mild macular grid technique appears to be less effective than the modified ETDRS laser, leading to a slightly worse visual acuity outcome and slightly smaller reduction in retinal thickening compared to the latter one (Olk, 1986)[129].

Complications of Photocoagulation

Although effective, the ETDRS technique involves placing burns close to the center of the macula, with potential complications. Complications of laser treatment can occur, although most side effects are transient and resolve spontaneously, and therefore the possible adverse effects should be discussed with the patient. Iris stromal burns caused by inappropriate focusing of the laser beam on the retina are much more common following panretinal photocoagulation and are rarely observed after macular treatment.

Perception of symptomatic paracentral scotomata is often the result of confluence of adjacent spots placed close to the fovea. This complication is more common when the blue-green wavelength is used in macular treatment, due to the absorption of this particular wavelength by the nerve fiber layer. One of the most serious complications of focal and grid techniques associated with permanent visual loss is inadvertent foveolar burn. This can be avoided by careful observation of the macular topography, possibly with the aid of a recent fluorescein angiography, which helps in finding foveal landmarks. If the edema is massive and the exact localization of the macula is difficult, selecting the cobalt blue filter of the slit lamp can be useful: the fovea can be located through the selective absorption of the blue light by the macular xanthophylls. Alternatively, the operator may ask the patient to fixate on the laser beam; however, in the course of edema, the fixation point may not correspond to the anatomical fovea. A nonexperienced operator can be misled by the use of inverting fundus lenses; therefore, it is always useful to locate the macula before and during treatment. If the patient is uncooperative, moves, or is unable to understand the operator's instructions during treatment, short exposure times or peribulbar anesthesia may be indicated. It is important to avoid excessively intense and/or short-duration burns, especially for focal laser photocoagulation since there is the risk of rupture of the Bruch's membrane and consequent iatrogenic choroidal neovascularization (fig. 11). In this case, an immediate hemorrhage may herald the Bruch's membrane tear, but a clinically visible break is not always observable.

Choroidal neovascularization arising from areas where Bruch's membrane was ruptured can develop 2 weeks to 5 months after treatment (Olk, 1990)[130]. Iatrogenic choroidal neovascularization, usually type II and subretinal, can be successfully treated with anti-VEGF drugs or with photodynamic therapy. To reduce the risk of this complication, it is recommended to use the low-

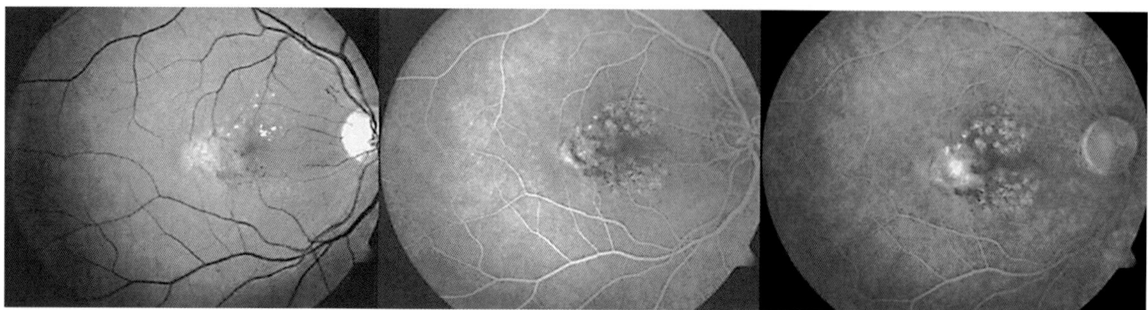

Fig. 11. Iatrogenic choroidal neovascularization. Red-free photograph (left) and early (center) and late (right) fluorescein angiography reveal the presence of a classic choroidal neovascularization which arose from a laser burn following grid photocoagulation for DME.

est intensity needed to obtain a light-gray burn, a spot size greater than 50 μm, and avoid repeated burns over a single microaneurysm.

Epiretinal fibrosis is an uncommon complication of macular laser treatment, usually secondary to intense treatment and direct treatment of intraretinal hemorrhage. Another serious complication, usually associated with poor visual prognosis, is the development of subretinal fibrosis (Guyer et al., 1992; Han et al., 1992; Writing Committee for the Diabetic Retinopathy Clinical Research Network, 2007)[121, 122, 131]. Only 8% of cases of subretinal fibrosis are directly related to focal laser photocoagulation. In these cases, strands of subretinal fibrosis originating from laser scars are noted, suggesting that a rupture of the Bruch's membrane secondary to high-intensity burns is the causal mechanism. Most of the cases are correlated with the presence of extensive hard exudates, especially following the reabsorption of macular edema. In these cases, subretinal fibrosis results from fibrous metaplasia of the RPE stimulated by the presence of the exudates. The most important predictive factors for the development of subretinal fibrosis include the presence of severe exudation in the macula, usually seen as plaque of hard exudates, and elevated serum lipids prior to laser photocoagulation (Writing Committee for the Diabetic Retinopathy Clinical Research Network, 2007)[131]. The ETDRS reported the presence of subretinal fibrosis in 31% of patients with intense exudation versus 0.05% of eyes without hard exudates.

Scar enlargement over time is a complication described following grid treatment for diffuse DME in about 5% of treated eyes (Lewis et al., 1990)[132]. The causal mechanism is usually intense treatment, which may lead to RPE hyperplastic changes and atrophy. If small-sized intense burns are applied close to the fovea, scar enlargement may lead to significant visual loss. The occurrence of this complication following macular treatment for DME is much less than that seen in eyes treated with photocoagulation for choroidal neovascularization, and the progressive trend toward lower energy and larger spot sizes has reduced its frequency (fig. 12) (Schatz et al., 1991; Fong et al., 1997)[133, 134].

Advancements in Laser Photocoagulation

Light and Subthreshold Laser Photocoagulation
Laser photocoagulation is a photothermal process in which heat is produced by the absorption of laser energy in targeted tissues. This treatment modality is the standard of care for a number of retinal and choroidal diseases. The current end point of laser photocoagulation is ophthalmoscopically visible retinal whitening, the sign that the retina itself has been thermally damaged. This

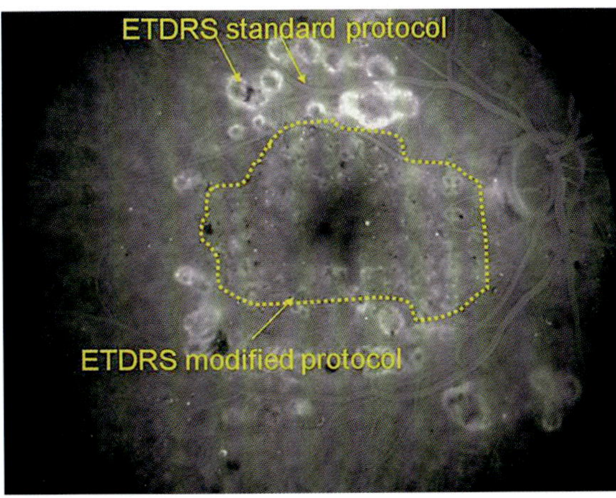

Fig. 12. ETDRS-modified protocol versus standard ETDRS photocoagulation: difference in laser burns. Laser burns applied superiorly to the macula and performed using the standard ETDRS parameters are larger and confluent compared to the spots placed in a grid pattern using a smaller spot diameter and lower intensity.

thermal tissue injury is the origin of many potential complications of laser photocoagulation including preretinal and subretinal fibrosis, choroidal neovascularization, and progressive expansion of laser scans. Light, minimally invasive laser treatment for clinically significant DME has been compared to conventional photocoagulation in a prospective, randomized clinical trial (Bandello et al., 2005)[114]. Low levels of energy were employed to produce barely visible burns at the level of the RPE. This 29-eye study suggested that light photocoagulation is as effective as conventional laser treatment in the reduction of foveal retinal thickness and improvement of visual acuity. Recently, subthreshold nonvisible retinal laser irradiation has been proposed as a less invasive treatment modality, associated with less side effects and maintained efficacy (Lanzetta et al., 2001)[135].

Micropulse Retinal Photocoagulation
Subthreshold nonvisible photocoagulation with repetitively pulsed (micropulse) photocoagulators has been proposed to avoid or minimize un-necessary retinal damage. In micropulse irradiation, laser pulses (pulse envelopes) contain a series (pulse train) of very brief micropulses. The pulse train of micropulses has a characteristic frequency (repetition rate in hertz) and duty cycle (percentage of time that the laser is on during the pulse envelope).

Typically, a train of repetitive, short- and low-energy laser pulses is used to confine laser damage to the minimum level that is sufficient to evoke a biological response, leaving the surrounding tissue unaffected. Each pulse induces a temperature rise that decays quickly in the interpulse time, so the thermal gradient in adjacent structures stays below the threshold to obtain visible damage. Such laser treatment does not leave a visible sign of laser exposure on the retina tissue and is therefore not ophthalmoscopically detectable (Dorin, 2003)[136]. However, OCT may be used to detect early changes in retinal reflectivity during subclinical and retinal sparing photocoagulation (Lanzetta et al., 2008; Veritti et al., 2012)[137, 138]. The OcuLight SLx laser system (Iridex Corporation, Mountain View, Calif., USA) is an infrared (810 nm) diode laser, which can be used either for continuous-wave conventional photocoagulation or for subthreshold micropulse photocoagulation. A typical micropulse treatment modality employs a 200-ms exposure enveloping 100 micropulses of 0.3 ms (500 Hz, 15% duty cycle). Repetitively pulsed laser irradiation seems to localize the thermal effect to the RPE layer. The very short micropulses offer little time for heat conduction from the RPE cells to the surrounding tissue. Recently, a meta-analysis of randomized and controlled trials comparing micropulse laser to conventional laser photocoagulation in DME was conducted. A total 398 eyes (203 eyes in the subthreshold micropulse diode laser group and 195 eyes in the conventional laser group) were considered for the analysis. The authors concluded that subthreshold micropulse laser was superior to conventional laser in terms of mean change of logMAR BCVA at 3, 9, and 12 months after treatment (p = 0.02, p = 0.04, and p = 0.03, respectively), and it showed a similar trend at 6 months (p = 0.05). The two types of treatment seem to have similar anatomical outcome (Chen et al., 2016)[139].

Selective Retina Therapy
Selective retina therapy is a laser modality regime that can be used for retinal diseases associated with a degeneration of the RPE. The goal of treatment is to selectively harm RPE cells without damaging the photoreceptors (and thus avoiding scotomata), the neural retina, and the choroid (Brinkmann et al., 2006)[140]. Typically, heat diffuses from the absorbing RPE at a speed of approximately 1 μm/s. Thus, traditional laser expositions of 100 ms and more lead to significant heat conduction. Selective retina treatment involves the delivery of 30 light pulses of 1.7 μs at a repetition rate of 100 Hz using a 527-nm frequency doubled Q-switched Nd:YLF laser. Repeated irradiation with those very-short-duration pulses seems to confine energy to the RPE while sparing the photoreceptors.

Whereas after standard argon laser photocoagulation a grayish white spot is ophthalmoscopically perceivable, lesions produced with selective retina treatment are not visible but are detectable by fluorescein angiography. This differs from micropulse retinal photocoagulation in which laser spots are not visible with ophthalmoscopy and fluorescein angiography. Possibly, submillisecond and submicrosecond repetitive pulse laser treatment are dissimilar in the localization of laser irradiance effects to RPE cells or their melanin granules.

The effects of selective retina treatment Q-switched laser pulses of only 8 ns have been investigated in a rabbit model with a double-frequency Nd:YAG laser (532 nm) (Framme et al., 2008)[141]. Ophthalmoscopic and angiographic damage thresholds were determined to be 266 and 72 mJ/cm^2, respectively, for a repetition of 10 pulses. Histologic examination of lesions revealed damaged RPE with an intact Bruch's membrane. However, selective damage of the RPE without affecting the photoreceptors can only rarely be achieved due to the small safety range.

Recently, selective retina treatment has been evaluated in 19 patients with various macular disorders (including DME) with 200-ns and 1.7-μs laser pulses. Ophthalmic and angiographic threshold irradiances were recorded. Among the 200-ns treatments, nearly all could be individuated angiographically (angiographic threshold: 115 μJ) but could not be visualized ophthalmoscopically. ED_{50} cell damage threshold energies were 99.6 μJ for 200-ns laser pulses and 196.3 μJ for 1.7-μs pulses (Framme et al., 2008)[142]. Recently, in a prospective nonrandomized study, selective retina therapy has been shown to improve BCVA by 1–2 ETDRS lines in 41% of eyes and by more than 2 ETDRS lines in 29% of cases (Park et al., 2016)[143].

Retinal Regeneration Therapy
Retinal regeneration therapy (Ellex Medical, Adelaide, S.A., Australia) has been proposed as a laser treatment modality that uses extremely short pulses to stimulate the RPE to produce a renewal process, with a reduction in retinal disease progression. The goal of retinal regeneration therapy is to cause RPE cell migration in a sort of biostimulation, releasing MMPs. The Ellex retinal regeneration therapy laser system uses a Q-switched double-frequency Nd:YAG laser to produce a single 3-ns pulse at 532 nm.

A preliminary report on 29 eyes with DME treated with retinal regeneration therapy has been presented (Hamilton, 2007)[144]. Central macular thickness at 3 months decreased by more than 5 in 55% of eyes, remained stable in 24% of cases, and increased in 20% of eyes. A majority of patients manifested an improvement in visual acuity, while no evidence of laser damage to the photoreceptor cells was demonstrated by microperimetry.

Semiautomated Patterned Scanning Laser Photocoagulation

The Pattern Scan Laser (Pascal, Optimedica Corporation, Santa Clara, Calif., USA) is a double-frequency Nd:YAG diode-pumped solid-state laser, which produces laser beams with a wavelength of 532 nm and can deliver multiple spots in predetermined patterns. It is based on a galvanometric scanner system (Blumenkranz et al., 2006)[145]. Two output channels send x-axis and y-axis coordinates to an x-y galvanometer, which changes the mirror angle for the laser pulse delivery. The Pascal photocoagulator was the first system to deliver a series of different pattern arrays. Nowadays, a number of models with pattern-scan technology are available.

The operator can select the pattern, the number of spots, and spacing between them. Predetermined patterns include single-spot, square arrays, octants, quadrants, full and modified macular grid, triple arcs, and single-line arcs. To allow the system to apply multiple spots, pulse durations are reduced to 10–20 ms. Shorter pulse durations are also associated with reduced pulse energy requirements and with decreased heat conduction to the surrounding tissues. Theoretically, the decreased anterior diffusion would lead to less damage to the inner retina and nerve fiber layer and the lower posterior diffusion would be associated with less discomfort to the patient. This leaves space for less invasive treatment modalities and less time-consuming procedures (Sheth et al., 2011)[146].

Typically, the pattern scan laser photocoagulator allows uniform whitening with less scar expansion. The feasibility of a rapid application of a precise array of spots allows the physician to deliver adequate-spaced treatment in the absence of an ophthalmoscopically visible end point. This can be particularly suitable for subthreshold laser irradiation, permitting a more accurate placement of subthreshold lesions in a predetermined pattern.

Conclusion

In recent years, advances in laser therapy for retinal disease have been directed toward reducing the unnecessary disruptive effect that laser photocoagulation causes to retinal tissues. To obtain such treatment, pulse duration should be lowered to reduce thermal conduction and spare the neural retina. However, short exposition times may reduce the safety power range between a threshold photocoagulation burn and photo-disruptive phenomena. Therefore, an appropriate treatment window should be prudently individuated. Furthermore, the physician needs to know when an appropriate laser dose has been delivered in the absence of a visible end point with a dedicated on-line detection system.

Vitrectomy

Lewis et al. (1992)[5] and Van Effenterre et al. (1993)[147] were the first to provide results on surgery for tractional DME. This intervention consists of a vitrectomy with a posterior vitreous cortex peeling. Pendergast and colleagues (Pendergast et al., 2000)[22] later confirmed the beneficial results observed in the first studies in a retrospective study of 55 eyes with an average of 23 months of follow-up. Following the vitrectomy, 27 eyes (49%) regained at least 2 lines of visual acuity, 23 eyes (42%) had stable visual acuity, and 5 eyes (9%) had a loss of at least 2 lines. The authors described a decrease in clinical features of cystoid macular edema for 52 patients (95%), and the complete disappearance for 45 patients (92%).

Other studies have confirmed a beneficial result of vitrectomy for tractional DME (table 5) (Harbour et al., 1996; Massin et al., 2003; Gandorfer et al., 2000)[6, 20, 148]. The functional prognosis is even better when vitrectomy is performed at an early stage.

Authors have also reported their experience of vitrectomy for macular edema, without any vit-

Table 5. Vitrectomy results on eyes with diffuse macular edema combined with taut and thickened posterior hyaloid

Studies	Eyes	Improvement in VA of ≥2 lines	Anatomical improvement	Follow-up, months
(Lewis et al., 1992)[5]	10	6 (60%)	10 (100%)	16
(Van Effenterre et al., 1993)[147]	22	22 (100%)	19 (86%)	14
(Harbour et al., 1996)[6]	7	4 (57%)	6 (86%)	12
(Pendergast et al., 2000)[22]	55	27 (49%)	52 (95%)	23
(Gandorfer et al., 2000)[148]	10	10 (100%)	10 (100%)	16
(Massin et al., 2003)[20]	7	5 (70%)	7 (100%)	18

VA = Visual acuity.

Table 6. Results of randomized studies on vitrectomy for eyes with diffuse macular edema syndrome without vitreomacular traction

Studies	Eyes	Type of intervention	Improvement in VA of ≥2 lines	Mean decrease of retinal thickening on OCT, µm
(Stolba et al., 2005)[155]	56	PPV + ILM vs. spontaneous evolution	52% 13%	63 null
(Thomas et al., 2005)[21]	40	PPV + ILM vs. laser	NS	73 29
(Yanyali et al., 2005)[157]	24	PPV + ILM vs. laser	50% 25%	219 29
(Patel et al., 2006)[154]	15	PPV vs. laser	NS	27 (NS) 107
(Kumar et al., 2007)[153]	12	PPV + ILM vs. laser	6 (50%), NS 3 (25%)	300 106

NS = Not significant; PPV = pars plana vitrectomy.

reomacular traction syndrome. The results are more controversial, as they are retrospective and have not yet been confirmed (Ikeda et al., 1999; Ikeda et al., 2000; Otani and Kishi, 2000; Yamamoto et al., 2001)[149–152].

The results of 5 randomized studies have recently been published (table 6) (Kumar et al., 2007; Patel et al., 2006; Stolba et al., 2005; Thomas et al., 2005; Yanyali et al., 2005)[153–157]. These studies compare the outcome of vitrectomy, including the peeling of the ILM in 3 studies, to laser treatment in 4 studies, and to the spontaneous evolution of macular edema in 1 study (Stolba et al., 2005)[155]. The studies, however, have a small patient base and the results are contradictory. Only Yanyali and colleagues have shown beneficial results of vitrectomy in a study comprising 24 eyes, both in terms of visual acuity and in reduction of the macular thickening, but the follow-up was short. In addition, the patients from the 'laser' group have only received one photocoagulation session. Stolba and colleagues demonstrated significant improvement of visual acuity but had a less successful result related to macular thickening. Thomas and colleagues as well as Patel and colleagues did not demonstrate any significant difference between the two treatments, although Patel and colleagues showed a slight preference for laser treatment. Kumar and colleagues did not obtain a significant difference in improved visual acuity between groups. Thus, the randomized studies have currently not demonstrated any advantage for recommending a vitrectromy for DME without associated traction.

Follow-Up and Prognosis

The evolution of DME is slow. It may wax and wane, probably under the effect of systemic factors, such as high blood pressure and glycemia (Massin-Korobelnik et al., 1994; Polito et al., 2006)[158, 159]. In the control group of the ETDRS trial, only 15% of patients with CSME had significant visual loss after a 3-year follow-up (Early Treatment Diabetic Retinopathy Study Research Group, 1985)[3]. The long-term prognosis of DME, however, is poor in eyes with persistent macular edema in the absence of treatment. Factors of poor visual prognosis include long duration of edema, severe macular nonperfusion, subfoveal plaque exudates, and subfoveal fibrosis.

Conclusion

DME remains among the first causes of visual loss in the working-age population, and its frequency will increase due to significant development of diabetes mellitus incidence throughout the world.

Laser treatment was the gold standard of therapy for reducing visual loss from DME. Attempts have been made in recent years to make laser treatment less invasive and with fewer associated complications. In some clinical trials, light and subthreshold laser approaches have appeared as effective as the classic technique. Although there is still a lack of strong supporting evidence, a less destructive technique using a reduced amount of energy is currently favored by many ophthalmologists in their daily practice.

Significant improvement in diagnostic tools has greatly changed the management of DME. The advent of OCT and its pervasive clinical use has been particularly important in determining a correct interpretation of pathogenic mechanisms involved in the appearance of macular edema, particularly when an anomalous adherence of posterior hyaloid makes pars plana vitrectomy a more rational approach than laser photocoagulation.

OCT is also needed when quantification of edema is the basis for determining efficacy of different treatment modalities, both in multicenter clinical trials and in daily practice.

The advent of the intravitreal approach for treatment of posterior segment disease by using different compounds is one of the most important innovations in the field of macular edema of the last few years. Steroids and anti-VEGF drugs can be injected inside the eye, reaching high concentrations with few or no systemic side effects. Multicenter clinical trials have already been completed showing an excellent efficacy of these compounds; moreover, in the next few years, new drugs will become available making treatment of DME even more effective. Considering the complexity of DME pathogenesis, it is also possible that a combination of different therapeutic approaches will soon become the standard of care for this disease.

References

1 King H, Aubert RE, Herman WH: Global burden of diabetes, 1995–2025: prevalence, numerical estimates, and projections. Diabetes Care 1998;21:1414–1431.
2 Antonetti DA, Lieth E, Barber AJ, Gardner TW: Molecular mechanisms of vascular permeability in diabetic retinopathy. Semin Ophthalmol 1999;14:240–248.
3 Early Treatment Diabetic Retinopathy Study Research Group: Photocoagulation for diabetic macular edema. Early Treatment Diabetic Retinopathy Study report number 1. Arch Ophthalmol 1985;103:1796–1806.
4 Weinberger D, Fink-Cohen S, Gaton D, Priel E, Yassur Y: Non-retinovascular leakage in diabetic maculopathy. Br J Ophthalmol 1995;79:728–731.
5 Lewis H, Abrams GW, Blumenkranz MS, Campo RV: Vitrectomy for diabetic macular traction and edema associated with posterior hyaloidal traction. Ophthalmology 1992;99:753–759.
6 Harbour JW, Smiddy WE, Flynn HWJ, Rubsamen PE: Vitrectomy for diabetic macular edema associated with a thickened and taut posterior hyaloid membrane. Am J Ophthalmol 1996;121:405–413.
7 Kang SW, Park CY, Ham DI: The correlation between fluorescein angiographic and optical coherence tomographic features in clinically significant diabetic macular edema. Am J Ophthalmol 2004;137:313–322.
8 Wilkinson CP, Ferris FL, Klein RE, Lee PP, Agardh CD, Davis M, Dills D, Kampik A, Pararajasegaran R, Verdaguer JT, Global Diabetic Retinopathy Project Group: Proposed international clinical diabetic retinopathy and diabetic macular edema disease severity scales. Ophthalmology 2003;110:1677–1682.
9 Girach A, Lund-Andersen H: Diabetic macular oedema: a clinical overview. Int J Clin Pract 2007;61:88–97.
10 Williams R, Airey M, Baxter H, Forrester J, Kennedy-Martin T, Girach A: Epidemiology of diabetic retinopathy and macular oedema: a systemic review. Eye 2004;18:963–983.
11 Varma R, Torres M, Peña F, Klein R, Azen S; Los Angeles Latino Eye Study Group: Prevalence of diabetic retinopathy in adult Latinos. Ophthalmology 2004;111:1298–1306.

12 Brown JC, Solomon SD, Bressler SB, et al: Detection of diabetic foveal edema. Contact lens biomicroscopy compared with optical coherence tomography. Arch Opthalmol 2004;122:330–335.
13 Massin P, Girach A, Erginay A, Gaudric A: Optical coherence tomography: a key to the future management of patients with diabetic macular oedema. Acta Ophthalmol Scand 2006;84:466–474.
14 Otani T, Kishi S, Maruyama Y: Patterns of diabetic macular edema with optical coherence tomography. Am J Ophthalmol 1999;127:688–693.
15 Bolz M, Schmidt-Erfurth U, Deak G, Mylonas G, Kriechbaum K, Scholda C: Optical coherence tomographic hyperreflective foci: a morphologic sign of lipid extravasation in diabetic macular edema. Ophthalmology 2009;116:914–920.
16 Ozdemir H, Karacorlu M, Karacorlu S: Serous macular detachment in diabetic cystoid macular oedema. Acta Ophthalmol Scand 2005;83:63–66.
17 Catier A, Tadayoni R, Paques M, et al: Optical coherence tomography characterization of macular edema according to various etiology. Am J Ophthalmol 2005;140:200–206.
18 Gaucher D, Sebah C, Erginay A, et al: Optical coherence tomography features during the evolution of serous retinal detachment in patients with diabetic macular edema. Am J Ophthalmol 2008;145:289–296.
19 Gaucher D, Tadayoni R, Erginay A, et al: Optical coherence tomography assessment of the vitreorelationship in diabetic macular edema. Am J Ophthalmol 2005;139:807–813.
20 Massin P, Duguid G, Erginay A, et al: Optical coherence tomography for evaluating diabetic macular edema before and after vitrectomy. Am J Ophthalmol 2003;135:169–177.
21 Thomas D, Bunce C, Moorman C, Laidlaw AH: Frequency and associations of a taut thickened posterior hyaloid, partial vitreomacular separation, and subretinal fluid in patients with diabetic macular edema. Retina 2005;25:883–888.
22 Pendergast SD, Hassan TS, Williams GA, et al: Vitrectomy for diffuse diabetic macular edema associated with a taut premacular posterior hyaloid. Am J Ophthalmol 2000;130:178–186.

23 Uchino E, Uemura A, Ohba N: Initial stages of posterior vitreous detachment in healthy eyes of older persons evaluated by optical coherence tomography. Arch Ophthalmol 2001;119:1475–1479.
24 Hee MR, Puliafito CA, Wong C, Duker JS, Reichel E, Rutledge B, et al: Quantitative assessment of macular edema with optical coherence tomography. Arch Ophthalmol 1995;113:1019–1029.
25 Hee MR, Puliafito CA, Duker JS, Reichel, E, Coker JG, Wilkins JR, et al: Topography of diabetic macular edema with optical coherence tomography. Ophthalmology 1998;105:360–370.
26 Massin P, Haouchine B, Gaudric A: Macular traction detachment and diabetic edema associated with posterior hyaloidal traction. Am J Ophthalmol 2001;132:599–600.
27 Polito A, Del Borrello M, Isola M, et al: Repeatability and reproducibility of fast macular thickness mapping using stratus optical coherence tomography. Arch Ophthalmol 2005;123:1330–1337.
28 Wolf-Schnurrbusch UE, Ceklic L, Brinkmann CK, et al: Macular thickness measurements in healthy eyes using six different optical coherence tomography instruments. Invest Ophthalmol Vis Sci 2009;50:3432–3437.
29 Menke MN, Dabov S, Knecht P, Sturm V: Reproducibility of retinal thickness measurements in healthy subjects using spectralis optical coherence tomography. Am J Ophthalmol 2009;147:467–472.
30 Diabetic Retinopathy Clinical Research Network, Krzystolik MG, Strauber SF, Aiello LP, et al: Reproducibility of macular thickness and volume using Zeiss optical coherence tomography in patients with diabetic macular edema. Ophthalmology 2007;114:1520–1525.
31 Strom C, Sander B, Larsen N, et al: Diabetic macular edema assessed with optical coherence tomography and stereo fundus photography. Invest Ophthalmol Vis Sci 2002;43:241–245.
32 Klein R, Moss SE, Klein BE, et al: The Wisconsin Epidemiologic Study of Diabetic Retinopathy. XI. The incidence of macular edema. Ophthalmology 1989;96:1501–1510.

33 Klein R, Klein BE, Moss SE, Cruickshanks KJ: The Wisconsin Epidemiologic Study of Diabetic Retinopathy. XV. The long-term incidence of macular edema. Ophthalmology 1995;102:7–16.

34 Klein R, Klein BE, Moss SE, Cruickshanks KJ: The Wisconsin Epidemiologic Study of Diabetic Retinopathy: XVII. The 14-year incidence and progression of diabetic retinopathy and associated risk factors in type 1 diabetes. Ophthalmology 1998;105:1801–1815.

35 Vitale S, Maguire MG, Murphy RP, et al: Clinically significant macular edema in type I diabetes: incidence and risk factors. Ophthalmology 1995;102:1170–1176.

36 Diabetes Control and Complications Trial Research Group: Hypoglycemia in the Diabetes Control and Complications Trial. Diabetes 1997;46:271–286.

37 Diabetes Control and Complications Trial/Epidemiology of Diabetes Interventions and Complications Research Group: Retinopathy and nephropathy in patients with type 1 diabetes four years after a trial of intensive therapy. N Engl J Med 2000;342:381–389.

38 Aroca PR, Salvat M, Fernandez J, Mendez I: Risk factors for diffuse and focal macular edema. J Diabetes Complications 2004;18:211–215.

39 Roy MS, Affouf M: Six-year progression of retinopathy and associated risk factors in African American patients with type 1 diabetes mellitus: the New Jersey 725. Arch Ophthalmol 2006;124:1297–1306.

40 White NH, Sun W, Cleary PA, Danis RP, Davis MD, Hainsworth DP, Hubbard LD, Lachin JM, Nathan DM: Prolonged effect of intensive therapy on the risk of retinopathy complications in patients with type 1 diabetes mellitus: 10 years after the Diabetes Control and Complications Trial. Arch Ophthalmol 2008;126:1707–1715.

41 UK Prospective Diabetes Study (UKPDS) Group: Intensive blood glucose control with sulphonylureas or insulin compared with conventional treatment and risk of complications in patients with type 2 diabetes (UKPDS 33). Lancet 1998;352:837–853.

42 UK Prospective Diabetes Study Group: Tight blood pressure control and risk of macrovascular and microvascular complications in type 2 diabetes: UKPDS 38. BMJ 1998;317:708–713.

43 Matthews DR, Stratton IM, Aldington SJ, et al: Risk of progression of retinopathy and visual loss related to tight control of blood pressure in type 2 diabetes mellitus (UKPDS 69). Arch Ophthalmol 2004;122:1631–1640.

44 Kohner EM, Stratton IM, Aldington SJ, Holman RR, Matthews DR; UK Prospective Diabetes Study (UKPDS) Group: Relationship between the severity of retinopathy and progression to photocoagulation in patients with type 2 diabetes mellitus in the UKPDS (UKPDS 52). Diabet Med 2001;18:178–184.

45 Kohner EM: Microvascular disease: what does the UKPDS tell us about diabetic retinopathy? Diabet Med 2008;25:20–24.

46 Adler AI, Stratton IM, Neil HA, et al: Association of systolic blood pressure with macrovascular and microvascular complications of type 2 diabetes (UKPDS 36): prospective observational study. BMJ 2000;321:412–419.

47 Klein R, Knudtson MD, Lee KE, et al: The Wisconsin Epidemiologic Study of Diabetic Retinopathy XXIII. The twenty-five-year incidence of macular edema in persons with type 1 diabetes. Ophthalmology 2009;116:497–503.

48 Sarao V, Veritti D, Lanzetta P: Regression of diabetic macular edema after subcutaneous exenatide. Acta Diabetol 2014;51:505–508.

49 Varadhan L, Humphreys T, Walker AB, Varughese GI: The impact of improved glycemic control with GLP-1 receptor agonist therapy on diabetic retinopathy. Diabetes Res Clin Pract 2014;103:e37–e39.

50 Davis MD, Beck RW, Home PD, Sandow J, Ferris FL: Early retinopathy progression in four randomized trials comparing insulin glargine and NPH (corrected) insulin. Exp Clin Endocrinol Diabetes 2007;115:240–243.

51 Jaross N, Ryan P, Newland H: Incidence and progression of diabetic retinopathy in an Aboriginal Australian population: results from the Katherine Region Diabetic Retinopathy Study (KRDRS). Report No. 2. Clin Exp Ophthalmol 2005;33:26–33.

52 Funatsu H, Yamashita H: Pathogenesis of diabetic retinopathy and the renin-angiotensin system. Ophthalmic Physiol Opt 2003;23;495–501.

53 Sjolie AK: Prospects for angiotensin receptor blockers in diabetic retinopathy. Diabetes Res Clin Pract 2007;76:S31–S39.

54 West KM, Erdreich LJ, Stober JA: A detailed study of risk factors for retinopathy and nephropathy in diabetes. Diabetes 1980;29:501–508.

55 Knuiman MW, Welborn TA, McCann VJ, et al: Prevalence of diabetic complications in relation to risk factors. Diabetes 1986;35:1332–1339.

56 Jerneld B: Prevalence of diabetic retinopathy: a population study from the Swedish island of Gotland. Acta Ophthalmol 1988;188:3–32.

57 Kostraba JN, Klein R, Dorman JS, et al: The Epidemiology of Diabetes Complications Study. IV. Correlates of diabetic background and proliferative retinopathy. Am J Epidemiol 1991;133:381–391.

58 Cruickshanks KJ, Ritter LL, Klein R, Moss SE: The association of microalbuminuria with diabetic retinopathy: the Wisconsin Epidemiologic Study of Diabetic Retinopathy. Ophthalmology 1993;100:862–867.

59 Klein R, Moss SE, Klein BE: Is gross proteinuria a risk factor for the incidence of proliferative diabetic retinopathy? Ophthalmology 1993;100:1140–1146.

60 Romero P, Baget M, Mendez I, et al: Diabetic macular edema and its relationship to renal microangiopathy: a sample of type I diabetes mellitus patients in a 15-year follow-up study. J Diabetes Complications 2007;21:172–180.

61 Klein R, Klein BE, Davis MD: Is cigarette smoking associated with diabetic retinopathy? Am J Epidemiol 1983;118:228–238.

62 Moss SE, Klein R, Klein BE: Cigarette smoking and ten-year progression of diabetic retinopathy. Ophthalmology 1996;103:1438–1442.

63 Chew EY, Klein ML, Ferris FL III, et al: Association of elevated serum lipid levels with retinal hard exudate in diabetic retinopathy. Early Treatment Diabetic Retinopathy Study (ETDRS) Report 22. Arch Ophthalmol 1996;114:1079–1084.

64 Sen K, Misra A, Kumar A, Pandey RM: Simvastatin retards progression of retinopathy in diabetic patients with hypercholesterolemia. Diabetes Res Clin Pract 2002;56:1–11.

65 Rechtman E, Harris A, Garzozi HJ, Ciulla TA: Pharmacologic therapies for diabetic retinopathy and diabetic macular edema. Clin Ophthalmol 2007;1:383–391.

66 Lee CM, Olk RJ: Modified grid laser photocoagulation for diffuse diabetic macular edema. Long-term visual results. Ophthalmology 1991;98:1594–1602.

67 Sarao V, Veritti D, Boscia F, Lanzetta P: Intravitreal steroids for the treatment of retinal diseases. ScientificWorldJournal 2014;2014:989501.

68 Tsaprouni LG, Ito K, Punchard N, Adcock IM: Triamcinolone acetonide and dexamethasome suppress TNF-alpha-induced histone H4 acetylation on lysine residues 8 and 12 in mononuclear cells. Ann NY Acad Sci 2002;973:481–483.

69 Juergens UR, Jager F, Darlath W, Stober M, Vetter H, Gillissen A: Comparison of in vitro activity of commonly used topical glucocorticoids on cytokine- and phospholipase inhibition. Eur J Med Res 2004;9:383–390.

70 Tong JP, Lam DS, Chan WM, Choy KW, Chan KP, Pang CP: Effects of triamcinolone on the expression of VEGF and PEDF in human retinal pigment epithelial and human umbilical vein endothelial cells. Mol Vis 2006;12:1490–1495.

71 Kim YH, Choi MY, Kim YS, et al: Triamcinolone acetonide protects the rat retina from STZ-induced acute inflammation and early vascular leakage. Life Sci 2007;81:1167–1173.

72 Zhang SX, Wang JJ, Gao G, Shao C, Mott R, Ma JX: Pigment epithelium-derived factor (PEDF) is an endogenous antiinflammatory factor. FASEB J 2006;20:323–325.

73 Abelson MB, Butrus S: Corticosteroids in ophthalmic practice; in Abelson MB, Neufeld AH, Topping TM (eds): Principles and Practice of Ophthalmology. Philadelphia, WB Saunders, 1994, p 1014.

74 Mizuno S, Nishiwaki A, Morita H, Miyake T, Ogura Y: Effects of periocular administration of triamcinolone acetonide on leukocyte-endothelium interactions in the ischemic retina. Invest Ophthalmol Vis Sci 2007;48:2831–2836.

75 Audren F, Erginay A, Haouchine B, et al: Intravitreal triamcinolone acetonide for diffuse macular oedema: 6-month results of a prospective controlled trial. Acta Ophthalmol Scand 2006;84:624–630.

76 Jonas JB, Kamppeter BA, Harder B, Vossmerbaeumer U, Sauder G, Spandau UH: Intravitreal triamcinolone acetonide for diabetic macular edema: a prospective, randomized study. J Ocul Pharmacol Ther 2006;22:200–207.

77 Gillies MC, Sutter FK, Simpson JM, Larsson J, Ali H, Zhu M: Intravitreal triamcinolone for refractory diabetic macular edema: two-year results of a double masked, placebo-controlled, randomized clinical trial. Ophthalmology 2006;113:1533–1538.

78 Diabetic Retinopathy Clinical Research Network: A randomized trial comparing intravitreal triamcinolone acetonide and focal/grid photocoagulation for diabetic macular edema. Ophthalmology 2008;115:1447–1449, 1449.e1–e10.

79 Diabetic Retinopathy Clinical Research Network, Elman MJ, Aiello LP, et al: Randomized trial evaluating ranibizumab plus prompt or deferred laser or triamcinolone plus prompt laser for diabetic macular edema. Ophthalmology 2010;117:1064–1077.e35.

80 Jager RD, Aiello LP, Patel SC, Cunningham ET Jr: Risks of intravitreous injection: a comprehensive review. Retina 2004;24:676–698.

81 Veritti D, Perissin L, Zorzet S, Lanzetta P: The effect of triamcinolone acetonide, sodium hyaluronate, and chondroitin sulfate on human endothelial cells: an in vitro study. Eur J Ophthalmol 2011;21(suppl 6):S75–S79.

82 Geroski DH, Edelhauser HF: Transscleral drug delivery for posterior segment disease. Adv Drug Deliv Rev 2001;52:37–48.

83 Olsen TW, Edelhauser HF, Lim JI, Geroski DH: Human scleral permeability. Effects of age, cryotherapy, transscleral diode laser, and surgical thinning. Invest Ophthalmol Vis Sci 1995;36:1893–1903.

84 Kato A, Kimura H, Okabe K, Okabe J, Kunou N, Ogura Y: Feasibility of drug delivery to the posterior pole of the rabbit eye with an episcleral implant. Invest Ophthalmol Vis Sci 2004;45:238–244.

85 Bonini-Filho MA, Jorge R, Barbosa JC, Calucci D, Cardillo JA, Costa RA: Intravitreal injection versus sub-Tenon's infusion of triamcinolone acetonide for refractory diabetic macular edema: a randomized clinical trial. Invest Ophthalmol Vis Sci 2005;46:3845–3849.

86 Cardillo JA, Melo LA Jr, Costa RA, et al: Comparison of intravitreal versus posterior sub-Tenon's capsule injection of triamcinolone acetonide for diffuse diabetic macular edema. Ophthalmology 2005;112:1557–1563.

87 Ozdek S, Bahceci UA, Gurelik G, Hasanreisoglu B: Posterior subtenon and intravitreal triamcinolone acetonide for diabetic macular edema. J Diabetes Complications 2006;20:246–251.

88 Veritti D, Lanzetta P, Perissin L, Bandello F: Posterior juxtascleral infusion of modified triamcinolone acetonide formulation for refractory diabetic macular edema: one-year follow-up. Invest Ophthalmol Vis Sci 2009;50:2391–2397.

89 Graham RO, Peyman GA: Intravitreal injection of dexamethasone. Treatment of experimentally induced endophthalmitis. Arch Ophthalmol 1974;92:149–154.

90 Hardman JG, Limbird LE, Molinoff PB: Goodman & Gilman's The Pharmacological Basis of Therapeutics, ed 9. New York, McGraw Hill, 2001.

91 Fialho SL, Behar-Cohen F, Silva-Cunha A: Dexamethasone-loaded poly(epsiloncaprolactone) intravitreal implants: a pilot study. Eur J Pharm Biopharm 2008;68:637–646.

92 Boyer DS, et al: Three-year randomized, sham-controlled trial of dexamethasone intravitreal implant in patients with diabetic macular edema. Ophthalmology 2014;121:1904–1914.

93 Ashton P, Blandford DL, Pearson PA, Jaffe GJ, Martin DF, Nussenblatt RB: Review: implants. J Ocul Pharmacol 1994;10:691–701.

94 Jaffe GJ, Yang CH, Guo H, Denny JP, Lima C, Ashton P: Safety and pharmacokinetics of an intraocular fluocinolone acetonide sustained delivery device. Invest Ophthalmol Vis Sci 2000;41:3569–3575.

95 Campochiaro PA, et al: Long-term benefit of sustained-delivery fluocinolone acetonide vitreous inserts for diabetic macular edema. Ophthalmology 2011;118:626–635.e2.

96 Campochiaro PA, et al: Sustained delivery fluocinolone vitreous inserts provide benefit for at least 3 years in patients with diabetic macular edema. Ophthalmology 2012;119:2125–2132.

97 Hu M, Huang G, Karasina F, Wong VG: Verisome, a novel injectable, sustained release, biodegradable, intraocular drug delivery system and triamcinolone acetonide. Annu Meet Assoc Res Vis Ophthalmol, Ft Lauderdale, 2008.

98 Lim JI, et al: Sustained-release intravitreal liquid drug delivery using triamcinolone acetonide for cystoid macular edema in retinal vein occlusion. Ophthalmology 2011;118:1416–1422.

99 Gardner TW, Antonetti DA, Barber AJ, LaNoue KF, Levison SW: Diabetic retinopathy: more than meets the eye. Surv Ophthalmol 2002;47(suppl 2):S253–S262.

100 Grant MB, Afzal A, Spoerri P, Pan H, Shaw LC, Mames RN: The role of growth factors in the pathogenesis of diabetic retinopathy. Expert Opin Investig Drugs 2004;13:1275–1293.

101 Nguyen QD, et al: Ranibizumab for diabetic macular edema: results from 2 phase III randomized trials: RISE and RIDE. Ophthalmology: 2012;119:789–801.

102 Brown DM, et al: Long-term outcomes of ranibizumab therapy for diabetic macular edema: the 36-month results from two phase III trials: RISE and RIDE. Ophthalmology 2013;120:2013–2022.

103 Mitchell P, et al: The RESTORE study: ranibizumab monotherapy or combined with laser versus laser monotherapy for diabetic macular edema. Ophthalmology 2011;118:615–625.

104 Schmidt-Erfurth U, et al: Three-year outcomes of individualized ranibizumab treatment in patients with diabetic macular edema: the RESTORE extension study. Ophthalmology 2014;121:1045–1053.

105 Writing Committee for the Diabetic Retinopathy Clinical Research Network, Gross JG, et al: Panretinal photocoagulation vs intravitreous ranibizumab for proliferative diabetic retinopathy: a randomized trial. JAMA 2015;314:2137–2146.

106 Korobelnik JF, et al: Intravitreal aflibercept for diabetic macular edema. Ophthalmology 2014;121:2247–2254.

107 Scott IU, Edwards AR, Beck RW, et al: A phase II randomized clinical trial of intravitreal bevacizumab for diabetic macular edema. Ophthalmology 2007;114:1860–1867.

108 Ahmadieh H, Ramezani A, Shoeibi N, et al: Intravitreal bevacizumab with or without triamcinolone for refractory macular edema: a placebo-controlled, randomized clinical trial. Graefes Arch Clin Exp Ophthalmol 2008;246:483–489.

109 Soheilian M, Ramezani A, Obudi A, et al: Randomized trial of intravitreal bevacizumab alone or combined with triamcinolone versus macular photocoagulation in diabetic macular edema. Ophthalmology 2009;116:1142–1150.

110 Paccola L, Costa RA, Folgosa MS, Barbosa JC, Scott IU, Jorge R: Intravitreal triamcinolone versus bevacizumab for treatment of refractory diabetic macular oedema (IBEME study). Br J Ophthalmol 2008;92:76–80.

111 Diabetic Retinopathy Clinical Research Network, Wells JA, et al: Aflibercept, bevacizumab, or ranibizumab for diabetic macular edema. N Engl J Med 2015;372:1193–1203.

112 Wells JA, et al: Aflibercept, bevacizumab, or ranibizumab for diabetic macular edema: two-year results from a comparative effectiveness randomized clinical trial. Ophthalmology 2016;123:1351–1359.

113 Jittpoonkuson T, Garcia P, Rosen RB: Correlation between fluorescein angiography and spectral domain optical coherence tomography in the diagnosis of cystoid macular edema. Br J Ophthalmol 2010;94:1197–1200.

114 Bandello F, Polito A, Del Borrello M, Zemella N, Isola M: 'Light' versus 'classic' laser treatment for clinically significant diabetic macular oedema. Br J Ophthalmol 2005;89:864–870.

115 Stefansson E: The therapeutic effects of retinal laser treatment and vitrectomy. A theory based on oxygen and vascular physiology. Acta Ophthalmol Scand 2001;79:435–440.

116 Wolbarsht ML, Landers MB 3rd: The rationale of photocoagulation therapy for proliferative diabetic retinopathy: a review and a model. Ophthalmic Surg 1980;11:235–245.

117 Molnar I, Poitry S, Tsacopoulos M, et al: Effect of laser photocoagulation on oxygenation of the retina in miniature pigs. Invest Ophthalmol Vis Sci 1985;26:1410–1414.

118 Stefansson E, Landers MB 3rd, Wolbarsht ML: Increased retinal oxygen supply following pan-retinal photocoagulation and vitrectomy and lensectomy. Trans Am Acad Ophthalmol Soc 1981;79:307–334.

119 Yu D, Cringle S, Su E, Yu PK, Humayun MS, Dorin G: Laser-induced changes in intraretinal oxygen distribution in pigmented rabbits. Invest Ophthalmol Vis Sci 2005;46:988–999.

120 Wilson DJ, Finkelstein D, Quigley HA, Green WR: Macular grid photocoagulation. An experimental study on the primate retina. Arch Ophthalmol 1988;106:100–105.

121 Guyer DR, D'Amico DJ, Smith CW: Subretinal fibrosis after laser photocoagulation for diabetic macular edema. Am J Ophthalmol 1992;113:652–656.

122 Han DP, Mieler WF, Burton TC: Submacular fibrosis after photocoagulation for diabetic macular edema. Am J Ophthalmol 1992;113:513–521.

123 Gottfredsdottir MS, Stefansson E, Jonasson F, Gislason I: Retinal vasoconstriction after laser treatment for diabetic macular edema. Am J Ophthalmol 1993;115:64–67.

124 Xiao M, McLeod D, Cranley J, Williams G, Boulton M: Growth factor staining patterns in the pig retina following retinal laser photocoagulation. Br J Ophthalmol 1999;83:728–736.

125 Ogata N, Ando A, Uyama M, Matsumura M: Expression of cytokines and transcription factors in photocoagulated human retinal pigment epithelial cells. Graefes Arch Clin Exp Ophthalmol 2001;239:87–95.

126 Early Treatment Diabetic Retinopathy Study Research Group: Focal photocoagulation treatment of diabetic macular edema. Relationship of treatment effect to fluorescein angiographic and other retinal characteristics at baseline. ETDRS report number 19. Arch Ophthalmol 1995;113:1144–1155.

127 Early Treatment Diabetic Retinopathy Study Research Group: Treatment techniques and clinical guidelines for photocoagulation of diabetic macular edema. Early Treatment Diabetic Retinopathy Study report number 2. Ophthalmology 1987;94:761–774.

128 Ferris FL III, Davis MD: Treating 20/20 eyes with diabetic macular edema. Arch Ophthalmol 1999;117:675–676.

129 Olk RJ: Modified grid argon (blue-green) laser photocoagulation for diffuse diabetic macular edema. Ophthalmology 1986;93:938–950.

130 Olk RJ: Argon green (514 nm) versus krypton red (647 nm) modified grid laser photocoagulation for diffuse diabetic macular edema. Ophthalmology 1990;97:1101–1113.

131 Writing Committee for the Diabetic Retinopathy Clinical Research Network: Comparison of modified early treatment diabetic retinopathy study and mild macular grid laser photocoagulation strategies for diabetic macular edema. Arch Ophthalmol 2007;125: 469–480.

132 Lewis H, Schachat AP, Haimann MH, et al: Choroidal neovascularization after laser photocoagulation for diabetic macular edema. Ophthalmology 1990;97:503–511.

133 Schatz H, Madeira D, McDonald R: Progressive enlargement of laser scars following grid laser photocoagulation for diffuse diabetic macular edema. Arch Ophthalmol 1991;109:1549–1551.

134 Fong DS, Segal PP, Myers F, et al: Subretinal fibrosis in diabetic macular edema. ETDRS report 23. Early Treatment Diabetic Retinopathy Study Research Group. Arch Ophthalmol 1997; 115:873–877.

135 Lanzetta P, Dorin G, Pirracchio A, Bandello F: Theoretical bases of non-ophthalmoscopically visible endpoint photocoagulation. Semin Ophthalmol 2001;16:8–11.

136 Dorin G: Subthreshold and micropulse diode laser photocoagulation. Semin Ophthalmol 2003;18:147–153.

137 Lanzetta P, Polito A, Veritti D: Subthreshold laser. Ophthalmology 2008; 115:216–216.e1.

138 Veritti D, et al: Online optical coherence tomography during subthreshold laser irradiation. Eur J Ophthalmol 2012;22:575–579.

139 Chen G, Tzekov R, Li W, Jiang F, Mao S, Tong Y: Subthreshold micropulse diode laser versus conventional laser photocoagulation for diabetic macular edema: a meta-analysis of randomized controlled trials. Retina 2016;36:2059–2065.

140 Brinkmann R, Roider J, Birngruber R: Selective retina therapy (SRT): a review on methods, techniques, preclinical and first clinical results. Bull Soc Belge Ophtalmol 2006;302:51–69.

141 Framme C, Schuele G, Kobuch K, Flucke B, Birngruber R, Brinkmann R: Investigation of selective retina treatment (SRT) by means of 8 ns laser pulses in a rabbit model. Lasers Surg Med 2008;40:20–27.

142 Framme C, Walter A, Prahs P, Theisen-Kunde D, Brinkmann R: Comparison of threshold irradiances and online dosimetry for selective retina treatment (SRT) in patients treated with 200 nanoseconds and 1.7 microseconds laser pulses. Lasers Surg Med 2008;40:616–624.

143 Park YG, Kim JR, Kang S, Seifert E, Theisen-Kunde D, Brinkmann R, Roh YJ: Safety and efficacy of selective retina therapy (SRT) for the treatment of diabetic macular edema in Korean patients. Graefes Arch Clin Exp Ophthalmol 2016;254:1703–1713.

144 Hamilton P: Selective laser retinal pigment epithelium treatment for diabetic macular edema. Retina Subspecialty Day AAO Annu Meet, New Orleans, 2007.

145 Blumenkranz MS, Yellachich D, Andersen DE, et al: Semiautomated patterned scanning laser for retinal photocoagulation. Retina 2006;26: 370–376.

146 Sheth S, Lanzetta P, Veritti D, Zucchiatti I, Savorgnani C, Bandello F: Experience with the Pascal® photocoagulator: an analysis of over 1,200 laser procedures with regard to parameter refinement. Indian J Ophthalmol 2011; 59:87–91.

147 Van Effenterre G, et al: Macular edema caused by contraction of the posterior hyaloids in diabetic retinopathy. Surgical treatment of a series of 22 cases (in French). J Fr Ophtalmol 1993;16: 602–610.

148 Gandorfer A, Messmer EM, Ulbig MW, Kampik A: Resolution of diabetic macular edema after surgical removal of the posterior hyaloid and the inner limiting membrane. Retina 2000;20: 126–133.

149 Ikeda T, Sato K, Katano T, Hayashi Y: Vitrectomy for cystoid macular oedema with attached posterior hyaloid membrane in patients with diabetes. Br J Ophthalmol 1999;83:12–14.

150 Ikeda T, Sato K, Katano T, Hayashi Y: Improved visual acuity following pars plana vitrectomy for diabetic cystoid macular edema and detached posterior hyaloid. Retina 2000;20:220–222.

151 Otani T, Kishi S: Tomographic assessment of vitreous surgery for diabetic macular edema. Am J Ophthalmol 2000;129:487–494.

152 Yamamoto T, Akabane N, Takeuchi S: Vitrectomy for diabetic macular edema: the role of posterior vitreous detachment and epimacular membrane. Am J Ophthalmol 2001;132:369–377.

153 Kumar A, Sinha S, Azad R, Sharma YR, Vohra R: Comparative evaluation of vitrectomy and dye-enhanced ILM peel with grid laser in diffuse diabetic macular edema. Graefes Arch Clin Exp Ophthalmol 2007;245:360–368.

154 Patel JI, Hykin PG, Schadt M, et al: Diabetic macular oedema: pilot randomised trial of pars plana vitrectomy vs macular argon photocoagulation. Eye (Lond) 2006;20:873–881.

155 Stolba U, Binder S, Gruber D, Krebs I, Aggermann T, Neumaier B: Vitrectomy for persistent diffuse diabetic macular edema. Am J Ophthalmol 2005; 140:295–301.

156 Thomas D, Bunce C, Moorman C, Laidlaw DA: A randomized controlled feasibility trial of vitrectomy versus laser for diabetic macular oedema. Br J Ophthalmol 2005;89:81–86.

157 Yanyali A, Nohutcu AF, Horozoglu F, Celik E: Modified grid laser photocoagulation versus pars plana vitrectomy with internal limiting membrane removal in diabetic macular edema. Am J Ophthalmol 2005;139:795–801.

158 Massin-Korobelnik P, Gaudric A, Coscas G: Spontaneous evolution and treatment of diabetic cystoid macular edema. Graefes Arch Ophthalmol 1994;232:279–289.

159 Polito A, Borello M, Polini G, et al: Diurnal variation in clinically significant diabetic macular edema measured by the Stratus OCT. Retina 2006;26:14–20.

Prof. Francesco Bandello
Department of Ophthalmology, University Vita-Salute, Scientific Institute San Raffaele
Via Olgettina 60
IT–20132 Milano (Italy)
E-Mail bandello.francesco@hsr.it

Coscas G (ed): Macular Edema. 2nd, revised and extended edition.
Dev Ophthalmol. Basel, Karger, 2017, vol 58, pp 139–167 (DOI: 10.1159/000455278)

Retinal Vein Occlusions

Jost B. Jonas[a] · Jordi Monés[b] · Agnès Glacet-Bernard[c] · Gabriel Coscas[c]

[a]Department of Ophthalmology, Medical Faculty Mannheim, University of Heidelberg, Mannheim, Germany; [b]Institut de la Màcula i de la Retina, Barcelona, Spain; [c]Service Universitaire d'Ophtalmologie, Hôpital Intercommunal de Créteil, Créteil, France

Abstract

Retinal vein occlusions (RVOs) have been defined as retinal vascular disorders characterized by dilatation of retinal veins with retinal and subretinal hemorrhages, macular edema, and a varying degree of retinal ischemia. Retinal angiography, either as fluorescein and indocyanine green (ICG) angiography or in the form of optical coherence tomography (OCT)-based angiography, is essential for the diagnosis and assessment of the prognosis of RVOs. It allows the differentiation of diverse types of RVOs, such as perfused or nonperfused, as well as the detection of different modalities in the natural history of RVOs. OCT angiographic imaging in combination with dye angiography (fluorescein or ICG) is the most effective method to assess the amount and location of cystoid macular edema and the persistence, regression, and degree of ischemia. OCT can additionally display the presence and integrity of the outer limiting membrane and of the inner and outer segments of the photoreceptors as useful biomarkers for the prognosis and as a guide for the treatment of RVO. Due to the relatively often benign and self-limiting course of nonischemic RVOs, therapy may initially be delayed. If macular edema extends into the foveolar region and persists, intravitreal medical therapy including steroids (triamcinolone; fluocinolone or dexamethasone in slow-release devices) and/or anti-VEGF (vascular endothelial growth factor) drugs (bevacizumab, ranibizumab, aflibercept) may be intravitreally administered, avoiding the irreversibly destructive effect of laser coagulation, which previously was applied in a 'grid' pattern over the extrafoveolar leaking area. The side effects of intraocularly applied steroids in relatively young patients including cataract formation and ocular hypertension have to be considered. © 2017 S. Karger AG, Basel

Retinal vein occlusions (RVOs) have been defined as retinal vascular disorders characterized by engorgement and dilatation of the retinal veins due to increased retinal venous blood pressure, with secondary (mostly) intraretinal hemorrhages; (mostly) intraretinal (and partially subretinal) edema which can also include the foveal region and which can lead to hard retinal exudates as deposits of lipids; and a varying degree of retinal ischemia including cotton wool spots as signs of it (Hayreh, 1964; Hayreh, 1965; Coscas et al., 1978; Hayreh, 1983; The Central Vein Occlusion Study, 1993; The Central Vein Occlusion Study Group M report, 1995; The Central Vein Occlusion Study Group N report, 1995; Hayreh et al., 1990; Coscas et al., 1984)[1–9].

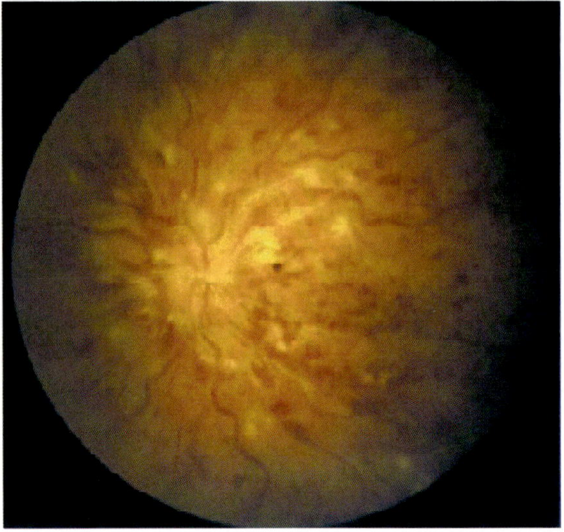

Fig. 1. Fundus photograph showing a CRVO.

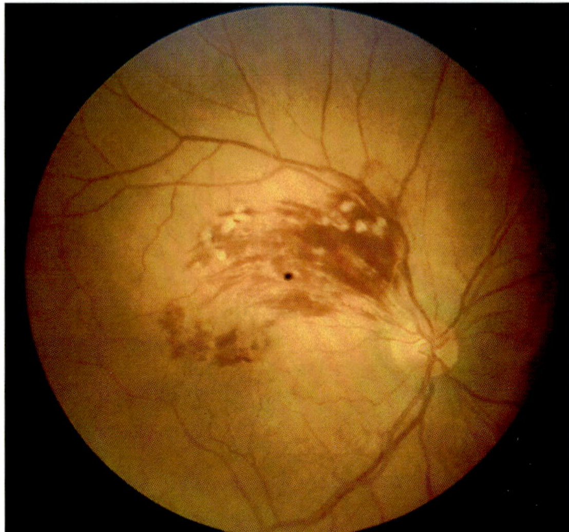

Fig. 2. Fundus photograph showing a superior temporal BRVO.

As soon as the foveal region is involved in macular edema, central visual acuity drops.

RVOs are differentiated into:

- *Central retinal vein occlusion* (CRVO), if the whole retinal venous retinal system is involved, and if the presumed site of an increased venous outflow resistance is located in the lamina cribrosa and/or posterior to it[a] (fig. 1)
- *Branch retinal vein occlusion* (BRVO), if the venous engorgement involves only branches of the whole retinal venous system; depending on the site where the engorgement starts, one can further subdivide into BRVOs which originate in the optic disc and BRVOs which originate at an arteriovenous crossing (fig. 2)

Based on the seminal works by Hayreh, the degree of ischemia has been used to further classify the RVOs into ischemic and nonischemic types (Hayreh, 1964; Hayreh, 1965; Coscas et al., 1978)[1-3]. In ischemic RVO, there are well-established stigmata of inner retinal ischemia, including marked retinal capillary nonperfusion, cotton wool spots mainly in the acute phase, visual acuity of counting fingers or less, perimetric defects so that only the Goldmann target V4e can be detected, a relative afferent pupillary defect of more than 1.2 logarithmic units, and later, intraocular neovascularization. In nonischemic (or perfused) RVO, there is essentially a relative stasis of retinal venous blood flow and macular edema associated with leakage from the altered retinal capillary bed.

Epidemiology

RVOs are one of the most common causes of a retinal vascular abnormality and a frequent cause of visual loss. Being recognized at least as early as

---

[a] If the superior or the inferior hemisphere of the fundus is involved, the presumed site of the occlusion is one of the two trunks of the intraneural central retinal vein where this congenital abnormality exists. This entity (hemicentral RVO) is considered a variant of CRVO.

1855 (Liebreich, 1855)[10], RVOs have been the subject of more than 3,000 publications so far. Current estimates of the prevalence of RVOs are derived from major population-based studies, such as the Blue Mountains Eye Study, the Beaver Dam Eye Study, and a combined analysis of the Atherosclerosis Risk in Communities and Cardiovascular Health Studies (Klein et al., 2000; Mitchell et al., 1996; Wong et al., 2005)[11–13].

More recent data have been published from other *ethnic groups*: the Beijing Eye Study (Liu et al., 2007; Zhou et al., 2013)[14, 15], the Multiethnic Study of Atherosclerosis (Cheung et al., 2008)[16], the Singapore Malay Eye Study (Lim et al., 2008)[17], and the Central India Eye and Medical Study (Jonas et al., 2013)[18]. The reported *prevalence of RVOs* varied widely across these studies, ranging from 0.3% (Mitchell et al., 1996)[12] to 1.6%. The variability between the prevalence rates among the various studies is likely related to the relatively small number of RVO patients in any single study, differences in the study methodologies (e.g., retinal photography), and possible ethnic differences in the distribution of RVO risk factors. As a result of these limitations, estimations of RVO prevalence are relatively imprecise.

Furthermore, most single studies rarely report on the *prevalence of different RVO subtypes,* namely CRVO and BRVO, which are important to distinguish as they differ in their risk factors (Hayreh et al., 2001; O'Mahoney et al., 2008)[19, 20], prognosis, and treatment (Hayreh, 2005; McIntosh et al., 2006; Mohamed et al., 2006)[21–23].

A recent multicenter study pooled individual level data of more than 70,000 adults in 15 studies around the world (Rogers et al., 2009)[24]. The prevalence rates per 1,000 persons were 4.42 for BRVO and 0.80 for CRVO, with these prevalence rates being age- and gender-standardized to the 2008 world population aged 30 years and older. The prevalence of RVOs was similar between men and women, and increased with age. Overall, the prevalence of BRVO was highest in Asians and Hispanics and lowest in whites, although the overlapping confidence intervals suggested that ethnic differences were not statistically significant. In the Multiethnic Study of Atherosclerosis (Cheung et al., 2008)[16], the only study with four ethnic groups examined in one investigation, the crude prevalence of any RVO was similar across whites, blacks, Chinese, and Hispanics.

It is worth noting that in the Multiethnic Study of Atherosclerosis, sample sizes of each ethnic group were relatively small, particularly the Chinese subgroup (n = 724), and that all participants were United States residents who were free from clinical cardiovascular disease (i.e., generally healthier study participants). Therefore, the Multiethnic Study of Atherosclerosis might not be sufficiently powered to detect meaningful ethnic difference in RVO prevalence, and should not be expected to represent different ethnic groups outside the US. Other studies of multiple ethnic samples as a single study also did not have sufficient numbers of RVO cases to examine ethnic differences by RVO subtypes. The higher prevalence of BRVO in some ethnic groups may reflect different population distributions of RVO risk factors. For example, the prevalence of arterial hypertension and uncontrolled hypertension has been reported to be higher in Asians (Leenen et al., 2008)[25] and Hispanics (Read et al., 2007)[26] than in whites (Giles et al., 2007; Ostchega et al., 2008)[27, 28].

Summarizing all available data on the prevalence rates of RVOs worldwide, one may estimate that 14–19 million adults are affected by the disease worldwide. The prevalence of both BRVO and CRVO increases significantly with age, but does not differ by gender. Possible ethnic differences in the prevalence of RVO may reflect differences in the prevalence of vascular risk factors, particularly arterial hypertension; ethnic-related differences in the prevalence of glaucomatous optic neuropathy as the major ocular risk factor; or other unknown factors. Although population-based investigations revealed a significantly higher prevalence of BRVOs than of CRVOs, CRVOs cause considerably more visual burden. Differences between the results of population-based studies and the findings obtained in hospital-based investigations may be due to the fact that population-based studies count any RVO including those RVOs located outside of the fovea and without drop in visual acuity, while patients with extrafoveal RVOs usually do not go to a hospital and are thus not included in the hospital-based investigations.

Factors Associated with RVOs
In probably the largest study on associations between RVOs and other factors, Hayreh et al. (2001)[19] prospectively investigated 1,090 consecutive patients with RVOs, almost all of whom were Caucasians. They found that there was a significantly higher prevalence of arterial hypertension in BRVO compared with CRVO and hemicentral RVO. BRVO also had a significantly higher prevalence of peripheral vascular disease, venous disease, peptic ulcer, and other gastrointestinal disease compared with CRVO.

The proportion of patients with BRVO with cerebrovascular disease was also significantly greater than that of the combined group of patients with CRVO and patients with hemicentral RVO. There was no significant difference in the prevalence of any systemic disease between CRVO and hemicentral RVO. A significantly greater prevalence of arterial hypertension and diabetes mellitus was present in the ischemic CRVO group compared with the nonischemic CRVO group. Similarly, arterial hypertension and ischemic heart disease were more prevalent in major BRVO than in macular BRVO.

Relative to the US white control population, the combined group of patients with CRVO and patients with hemicentral RVO had a higher prevalence of arterial hypertension, peptic ulcer, diabetes mellitus (in the ischemic type only), and thyroid disorder. The patients with BRVO showed a greater prevalence of arterial hypertension, cerebrovascular disease, chronic obstructive pulmonary disease, peptic ulcer, diabetes (in young

patients only), and thyroid disorder compared with the US white control population.

A variety of systemic disorders may be present in association with different types of RVO and in different age groups, and their relative prevalence differs significantly, so that the common practice of generalizing about these disorders for an entire group of patients with RVO can be misleading. Apart from a routine medical evaluation, an extensive and expensive workup for systemic diseases seems unwarranted in the vast majority of patients with RVO (Hayreh et al., 2001)[19].

In a second study, the same authors investigated hematological abnormalities associated with the various types of RVO (Hayreh et al., 2002)[29]. A variety of hematological abnormalities may be seen in association with different types of RVOs, but the routine inexpensive hematological evaluation may usually be sufficient for RVO patients. Based on their findings in the study and on a literature review, Hayreh and colleagues additionally suggested that treatment with anticoagulants or platelet antiaggregating agents may adversely influence the visual outcome, without any evidence of a protective or beneficial effect. Similar findings were reported from other hospital-based studies (The Eye Disease Case-Control Study Group, 1993)[30], which underlined that CRVO patients display a cardiovascular risk profile. A decreased risk was observed with increasing levels of physical activity, increasing levels of alcohol consumption, and in women using postmenopausal estrogens.

Evidence gathered in population-based studies on associations between RVO and ocular and systemic factors confirms that RVOs are significantly associated with glaucomatous optic neuropathy and arterial hypertension, as shown in the Blue Mountains Eye Study, the Beaver Dam Eye Study, and the Beijing Eye Study, to name only a few (Klein et al., 2000; Mitchell et al., 1996; Liu et al., 2007)[11, 12, 14]. Corresponding with the association with arterial hypertension, the studies also suggested increased mortality for patients with RVOs and an age of less than 70 years (Cugati et al., 2007; Xu et al., 2007)[31, 32].

Familial clustering of RVOs has been observed, yet the role of gene mutation in RVO remains uncertain (Girmens et al., 2008)[33]. It has remained unclear whether RVOs are associated with abnormalities of the blood clotting system, such as factor V Leiden, factor XII deficiency, glucose-6-phosphate dehydrogenase deficiency, decreased plasma homocysteine level, presence of antiphospholipid antibodies, or intake of warfarin and aspirin (The Central Vein Occlusion Study Group, 1997; Glacet-Bernard et al., 1994; Arsène et al., 2005; Kuhli et al., 2002; Kuhli et al., 2004; Pinna et al., 2007)[34–39]. In a recent pilot project, higher estimated cerebrospinal fluid pressure was associated with a higher incidence of RVOs originating at the optic nerve head (i.e., CRVOs, hemicentral RVOs, and BRVOs originating at the optic nerve head) in a 10-year follow-up examination of the Beijing Eye Study (Jonas et al., 2015)[40]. From a pathogenic point of view, this association may explain the association between the incidence of RVOs and arterial hypertension since arterial blood pressure is correlated with cerebrospinal fluid pressure (Berdahl et al., 2012; Ren et al., 2013)[41, 42]. The association may also fit with the observation that RVOs are usually noticed by the patients in the morning after sleeping. During sleeping, cerebrospinal fluid pressure is increased due to hydrostatic reasons. The association also agrees with the finding that wider retinal vein diameters are associated with higher estimated cerebrospinal fluid pressure (Jonas et al., 2014)[43]. Interestingly, obstructive sleep apnea syndrome (OSAS) has recently been shown to be associated with RVOs and also to be an independent risk factor of RVO (Glacet-Bernard et al. 2010; Chou et al., 2012)[44, 45]. The local and systemic effects of OSAS could contribute to the development of RVOs: nocturnal hypoxemia and hypercapnia, respiratory efforts, increased intrathoracic, intracranial and cerebral spinal fluid pressure, elevated arterial pressure during arousal from sleep, oxidative stress, and a hypercoagulable state. The prevalence of OSAS is particularly high in obese patients. The authors concluded that OSAS is largely underdiagnosed and that it may account for the occurrence RVOs in many patients, particularly since RVOs may develop predominantly during sleeping. In clinical practice, it appears to be important to take into account the strong potential association between OSAS and RVOs since the treatment of OSAS has been demonstrated to reduce the risk of cardiovascular and cerebrovascular disorders.

Interestingly, the amount of macular edema in patients with RVOs shows diurnal changes. Paques et al. (2005)[46] and Gupta et al. (2009)[47] examined patients with macular edema due to CRVO and observed a significantly thicker macular edema at 7:00 am than at 7:00 pm, parallel to changes in visual acuity. In a parallel manner, the choroid is slightly thicker in the morning than in the afternoon (Usui et al., 2012; Tan et al., 2012)[48, 49]. Since both the central retinal vein and the vortex veins with the choroidal blood drain via the superior orbital vein into the brain, the findings of diurnal changes in macular edema in patients with RVO and in choroidal thickness point to a potential role the cerebrospinal fluid pressure may play for RVOs and potentially other conditions: due to hydrostatic reasons, the cerebrospinal fluid pressure is higher at night and in the early morning than during daytime (Jonas et al., 2016)[50]. Correspondingly, also for choroidal thickness, a positive association with estimated cerebrospinal fluid pressure has been found (Jonas et al., 2014)[51]. Interestingly, chronic RVOs were not significantly associated with choroidal thickness (Du et al., 2013)[52], while a study by Tsuiki et al. (Tsuiki et al., 2013)[53] on patients with unilateral CRVO revealed an abnormally thick subfoveal choroid. Tsuiki et al. additionally detected that after treatment with intravitreal bevacizumab, subfoveal choroidal thickness significantly decreased to normal values. Central corneal thickness was not related with the prevalence of RVOs (Xu et al., 2010)[54], nor was the size of the optic nerve head (Xu et al., 2012)[55].

Clinical Course

The natural history and prognosis of RVOs have been examined in only a few prospective studies (Koizumi et al., 2007)[56]. The natural history of CRVO has been assessed in the Central Retinal Vein Occlusion Study (The Central Vein Occlusion Study Group, 1997)[32], a prospective cohort study with randomized clinical trials of specific subgroups of patients. It included 725 patients with CRVO who were observed for a 3-year follow-up every 4 months. Visual acuity outcome was largely dependent on initial acuity:

- Sixty-five percent of patients with initially good visual acuity (20/40 or better) maintained visual acuity in the same range at the end of the study.
- Patients with intermediate initial acuity (20/50 to 20/200) showed a variable outcome: 19% improved to better than 20/50, 44% stayed in the intermediate group, and 37% had final visual acuity worse than 20/200.
- Patients who had poor visual acuity at the first visit (<20/200) had an 80% chance of having a visual acuity less than 20/200 at the final visit, whether perfused or nonperfused initially.

In the first 4 months of follow-up, 81 (15%) of the 547 eyes with good perfusion developed ischemia. During the next 32 months of follow-up, an additional 19% of eyes were found to have developed ischemia, yielding a total of 34% after 3 years. The development of nonperfusion or ischemia was most rapid in the first 4 months and progressed continuously throughout the entire duration of follow-up. When iris or angle neovascularization occurred, it was treated promptly with panretinal photocoagulation. The strongest predictors of iris or angle neovas-

cularization were low visual acuity and a high amount of nonperfusion seen by fluorescein angiography (FA). Of eyes initially categorized as nonperfused or indeterminate, 35% (61/176) developed iris or angle neovascularization, compared with 10% (56/538) of eyes initially categorized as perfused. Other risk factors were venous tortuosity, extensive retinal hemorrhage, and duration of less than 1 month. Neovascular glaucoma that was unsuccessfully managed with medical treatment developed in only 10 eyes. No eye was enucleated. Thus, visual acuity at baseline is a strong predictor of visual acuity at 3 years for eyes with good baseline vision and eyes with poor baseline vision, but a poor predictor for intermediate acuities. Visual acuity is also a strong predictor for the development of iris and angle neovascularization, as is nonperfusion. During the course of follow-up, one third of the eyes with perfusion became ischemic. Some systemic factors have also been demonstrated to be associated with retinal ischemia, such as an elevated hematocrit level, elevated fibrinogen, older age, and male gender (Glacet-Bernard et al., 1996)[57]. Some patients may present with pronounced perivenular whitening and abrupt visual loss. While the fundus shows minimal signs of venous obstruction, careful examination can reveal areas of retinal opacification in a perivenous pattern (fig. 3). These patients usually recover, even in cases with severe visual loss at presentation, often with residual microscotomas (Browning, 2002; Paques et al., 2003)[58, 59]. In these patients the prognostic value of visual acuity at the initial examination may be questionable. Another important aspect is duration of the disease. In some reports on the natural course, 26% of patients had transient macular edema with spontaneous resolution (Gutman, 1977)[60]. This finding may explain the relatively good results even in the control groups of some studies such as GENEVA, BRAVO, and CRUISE, in which patients with recent-onset macular edema due to RVO were included (Thach et al., 2014;

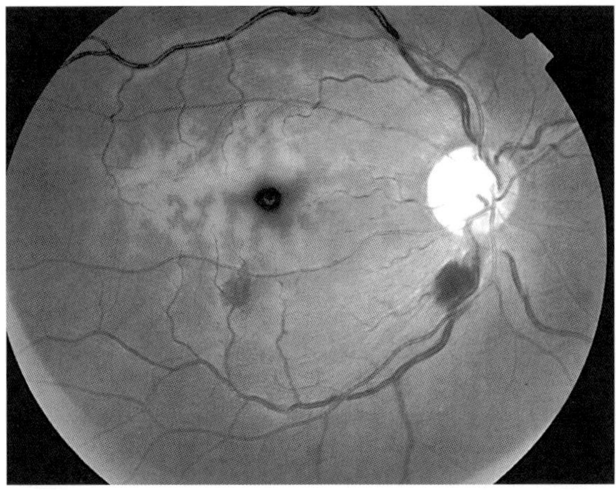

Fig. 3. Blue reflectance photograph of a patient with CRVO and perivenular whitening.

Campochiaro et al., 2010; Haller et al., 2010; Haller et al., 2011)[61–64]. In contrast, chronic macular edema is associated with poor visual prognosis and needs to be treated.

Diagnosis: Imaging and Functional Testing, Stages, and Classifications

Clinical Signs

Patients with an RVO usually notice a painless loss in vision, which may affect parts of the whole visual field, depending on whether it is a BRVO or CRVO. If the drop in vision is experienced shortly after its development, the majority of the patients report they noticed the visual impairment in the morning (Hayreh et al., 1980)[65]. This may imply that the RVO occurred at night during sleep.

Increasing pain is rarely the first symptom noticed by the patient. It can occur if a previously unnoticed ischemic RVO led to the development of iris neovascularization and neovascular glaucoma.

The ophthalmologic diagnosis of RVO is made primarily by conventional ophthalmoscopy.

Recent RVOs are characterized by the presence of retinal edema, optic disk hyperemia or edema, scattered superficial or deep hemorrhages, cotton wool spots, and venous dilatation. Old RVOs are characterized by (occluded and) sheathed retinal veins, venous-venous collaterals, and intraretinal hard exudates.

The ophthalmoscopic examination allows the differentiation into CRVO and BRVO, and the subclassification into BRVO originating in the optic nerve head and BRVO originating at arteriovenous crossings or limited to macular venules (fig. 1, 2). In addition, the differentiation into ischemic RVOs (with large deep hemorrhage) and nonischemic RVOs (with mainly flame hemorrhage) is of high clinical importance, particularly with respect to the prognosis of the disease.

Slit lamp biomicroscopy of the anterior segment is mandatory for all patients with RVOs to detect *iris neovascularization* as early as possible. A vascular congestion of iris vessels may be considered as an early evidence of the presence of vasodilator factors released from the retina that precede in many patients the actual onset of iris neovascularization (Hayreh et al., 2005; Paques et al., 2004)[21, 66].

Fluorescein Angiography

Besides the recently developed OCT-based angiography FA is the only examination which directly visualizes not only large retinal vessels but also the retinal macular capillary bed (Casselholmde Salles et al., 2016; Coscas et al., 2016; Abri Aghdam et al., 2016; Kashani et al., 2015; Suzuki et al., 2016)[67–71]. FA both confirms the slow-down of retinal blood circulation and evaluates the effects of the vein obstruction on the capillary bed. FA is therefore the 'clue tool' for the diagnosis and prognosis of RVO, permitting the differentiation between the nonischemic type and the ischemic form (Hayreh, 1965; Coscas et al., 1978; Hayreh et al., 1990; Glacet-Bernard et al., 1996; Laatikainen et al., 1976)[1, 3, 8, 57, 72]. FA is essential in diagnosing RVO and before choosing the therapeutic option (fig. 4).

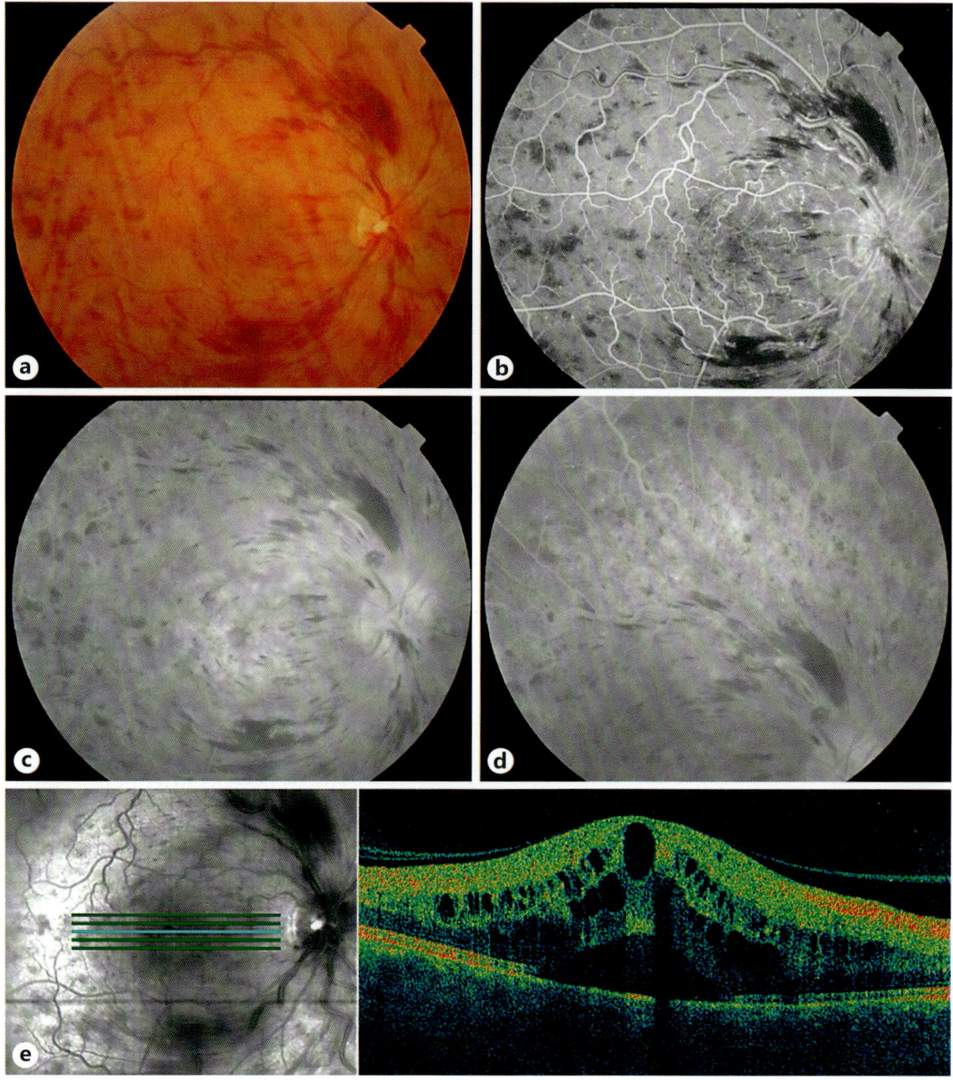

Fig. 4. Nonischemic CRVO with persistent macular edema (courtesy of Agnes Glacet-Bernard). **a** Color photography: well-perfused CRVO with flame-shaped hemorrhages. **b** FA displaying the slowdown of retinal blood circulation and dilation of the capillary bed, visible in the macular area. **c** On the late frame, fluorescein leakage is collected in pseudocystic cavities. **d** Peripheral retinal quadrants remained well-perfused. **e** SD-OCT: macular thickness was increased to 755 µm.

The confirmation of the RVO diagnosis is mainly related to the increase in the length of the retinal transit time, defined as the time between the first fluorescein appearance in the main retinal arteries and its appearance as a laminar flow in the main posterior veins. A transit time of less than 2–3 s is regarded as 'normal' and a longer time (more than 5 s) is considered 'delayed'. Nevertheless, the quantification of retinal transit time by FA is not significantly accurate because it depends on the rapidity of the antecubital intravenous injection and on the frequency of the frames.

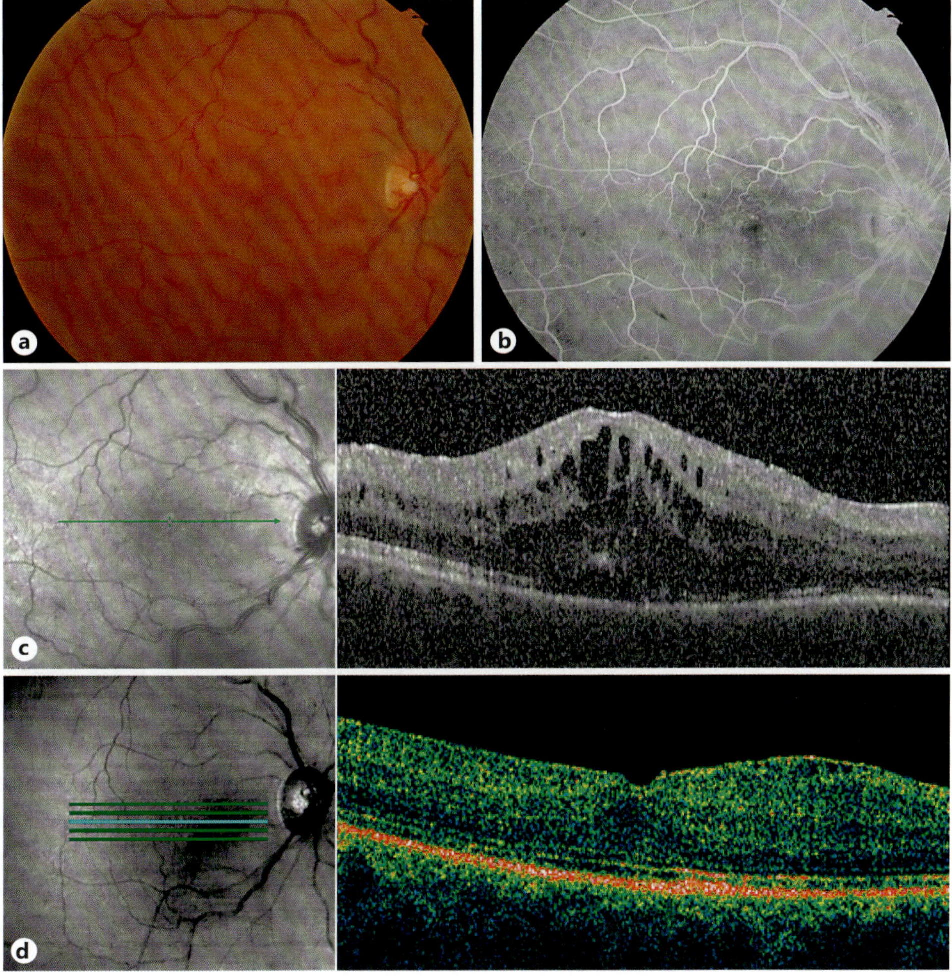

Fig. 5. Nonischemic CRVO with persistent macular edema (courtesy of Agnes Glacet-Bernard). **a** One year after the onset, fundus aspect returned grossly to normal. **b** FA showing persistent dilation of the capillary bed in the macular area. **c** SD-OCT (Spectralis): central macular thickness was 601 μm. **d** SD-OCT (Cirrus): 1 month after bevacizumab injection, macular edema completely disappeared.

However, video angiography using a scanning laser ophthalmoscope showed an improvement in the evaluation and the measurement of retinal circulation times, which is particularly important for the diagnosis of combined retinal occlusion, such as RVO associated with cilioretinal artery occlusion or combined retinal artery and vein occlusion.

FA also permits the localization and the qualitative evaluation of retinal capillary bed changes that includes hyperpermeability and/or nonperfusion.

Dilatation of retinal veins and capillaries, observed on the early frames of FA, is generally seen in all forms of RVO, with late leakage in the macular area and late staining at the level of the wall of the main posterior veins. Hyperpermeability can be more marked showing early and intense leakage from the macular capillary bed and collection of the dye on the late frames of FA in radially oriented pseudocystic cavities forming the typical cystoid macular edema with a 'petaloid pattern' (fig. 4, 5).

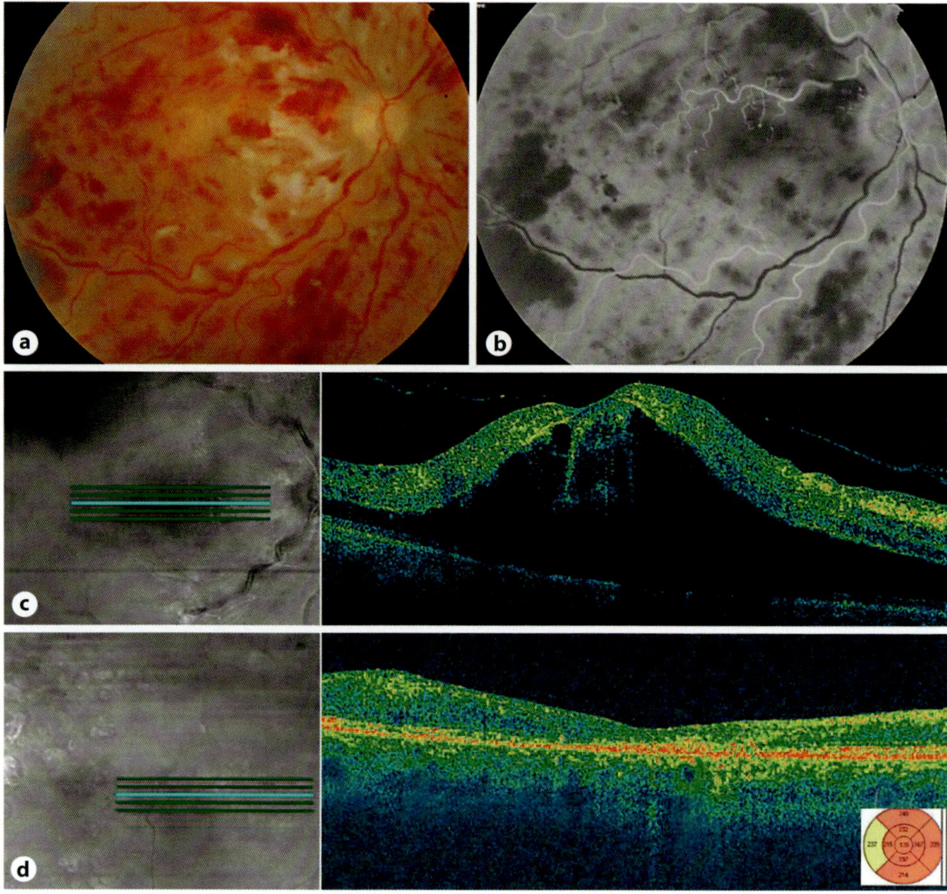

Fig. 6. Ischemic CRVO (courtesy of Agnes Glacet-Bernard). **a** Color photography of a CRVO with numerous cotton wool spots and deep hemorrhages. **b** FA displaying the slowdown of retinal blood circulation and widespread capillary nonperfusion. **c** OCT: macular thickness was dramatically increased up to more than 1,000 μm; a foveal detachment is visible. **d** Final OCT (16 months after the onset of the CRVO and after panretinal photocoagulation): macular atrophy. The photoreceptor layer is no longer visible. Central retinal thickness was 139 μm.

Capillary nonperfusion is most analyzable on the early frames of FA, at the arteriovenous time, before leakage. Macular nonperfusion is correlated with a bad visual prognosis and its diagnosis must be done in the pretherapeutic evaluation of a macular edema. Peripheral nonperfusion characterizes the ischemic forms, which are prone to ocular neovascularization (fig. 6). Sudden interruption of the blood flow can be observed giving the aspect of a dead tree, with late staining and/or leakage at the level of the wall of the vessels crossing over the ischemic area (Coscas et al., 1978)[3].

When retinal hemorrhages are numerous and deep, it can be impossible to assess the integrity of the retinal capillary bed. Extensive hemorrhagic RVO usually corresponds to ischemic RVO. The diagnosis of ischemic RVO is confirmed by clinical data such as severe and sudden loss in visual acuity, the presence of absolute central scotomas, and the iris and angle aspect.

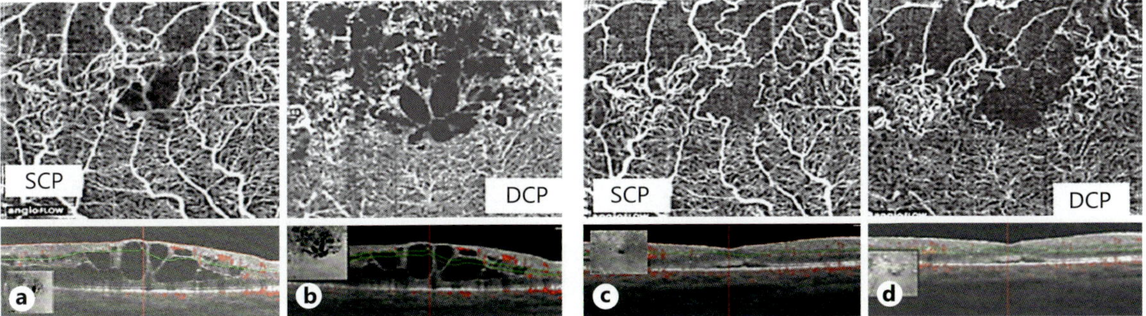

Fig. 7. BRVO with cystoid macular edema: comprehensive assessment on OCT angiography (top images: C-Scan – bottom images: B-Scan), including multiple, large, cystoid spaces, deeply 'black', without any signal in the superior temporal quadrant (**a, b**) and the regression of the cysts after 3 anti-VEGF injections, leaving the area as nonperfused and no change in the retinal capillaries: disorganization with dilation and disruption (**c, d**).

FA is a relatively easy method to recognize the diverse types of RVO, both perfused and nonperfused (and mixed types), as well as to detect the different modalities in natural history [regression of the macular edema or progression to ischemic type (acutely or slowly)].

FA is an effective method to determine the presence (or absence) of macular cystoid edema, its extension, persistence, or regression. Moreover, in BRVO, FA examination makes it easy to differentiate the cases threatening the macula and evaluate the extension of nonperfused capillary bed areas.

Optical Coherence Tomography
Optical coherence tomography (OCT) examination is widely used to detect changes in the retinal architecture of eyes affected by various macular diseases and to quantitatively measure retinal thickness (Catier et al., 2005)[73].

In RVO, OCT can display intraretinal cystoid spaces responsible for the increase in retinal thickness often associated with serous detachment of the neurosensory retina. The retinal cystoid spaces can be numerous and confluent, forming a large central cystoid space. Associated findings can be observed such as vitreous macular adherence, epiretinal membrane, hyperreflexivity

of the posterior layer corresponding to atrophy or fibrosis of the retinal pigment epithelium, subretinal accumulation of material (fibrosis), lamellar macular hole, intraretinal lipid exudates, and intraretinal hemorrhage (fig. 4–6).

Recent studies have suggested that in BRVOs, visual function and recovery of vision is correlated with thickness of the central macula, and that is correlated with the integrity of the inner and outer segments of the photoreceptors in the fovea (Ota et al., 2008)[74].

Spectral domain OCT (SD-OCT) helps to quantify the amount of cystoid macular edema and supplies additional information, such as whether the accumulated fluid is located mostly within the retinal layers or additionally in the subretinal space (Shroff et al., 2008)[75]. Thanks to a better definition of the scans, SD-OCT can display the presence and integrity of the outer limiting membrane and of the inner and outer segments of the photoreceptors, which provides useful information for prognosis (fig. 4–6).

OCT-Based Angiography
OCT-based angiography, which has recently been introduced into clinical practice, is a very promising technique to visualize the vascular

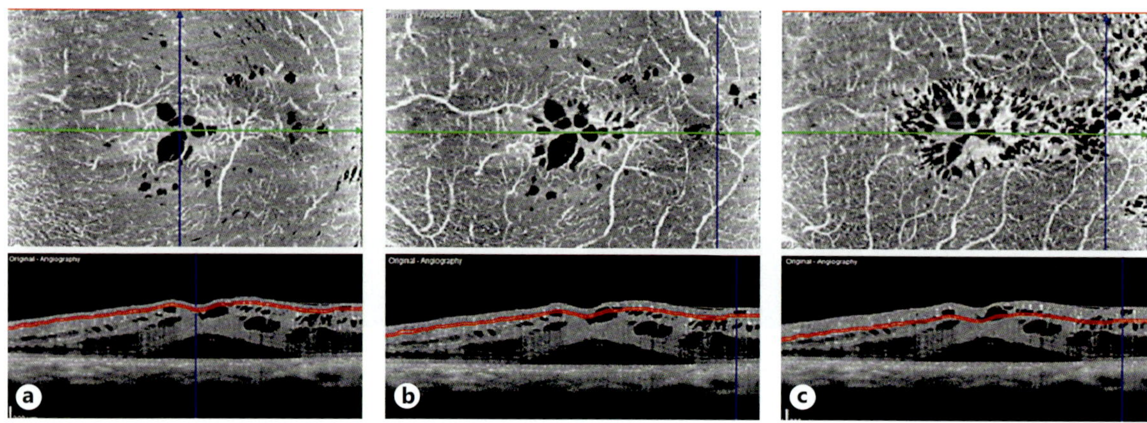

Fig. 8. RVO with cystoid macular edema: comprehensive assessment on OCT angiography, including a C-scan section taken at the level of the ganglion cell layer (superficial capillary plexus) (**a**), another one taken at the inner nuclear layer (deep capillary plexus) (**b**), and the corresponding B-scan passing through the foveal depression (**c**). The cystoid spaces are deeply 'black', without any signal. Note the capillary network disorganization with scarcity, dilation, and disruption. Slides obtained with manual segmentation.

system of the retina and choriocapillaris in different layers in a noninvasive manner (Wei et al., 2013; Wang et al., 2014; Jia et al., 2014; Jia et al., 2015; Yu et al. 2015; Pechauer et al., 2015; Glacet-Bernard et al., 2016; Sellam et al., 2016)[76–83]. Its disadvantage as compared to FA is that OCT angiography does not show leakage and pooling of fluid, so that a conventional SD-OCT is necessary to detect macular swelling and edema. The advantages of OCT angiography are that it is not invasive and that it allows the visualization of the different vascular systems of the retina, optic nerve head, and choriocapillaris separately in the different layers of the retina and optic nerve head. There is also a need to enlarge the field of examination so that the whole macular region and the fundus periphery can be explored (as it is actually possible upon FA). Some preliminary investigations have suggested that OCT angiography may in some clinical situations become a substitute for FA in the clinical assessment of macular edema in RVOs. OCT angiography allows the specific analysis of both macular edema and the macular capillary bed architecture with more contrast (as compared to FA), more specific seg-

mentation, and no risk of an allergy. OCT angiography also allows the distinction between the superficial capillary plexus and deep capillary plexus. OCT angiography may soon be automatically quantified for a specific analysis of follow-up (fig. 7, 8).

OCT angiography is a fast noninvasive exam that allows the imaging of both plexuses in vein retinal occlusion. The deep capillary plexus is predominantly affected. Recent studies have demonstrated correlations between vascular densities, superficial foveal avascular zone, visual acuity, and FA peripheral ischemia.

The follow-up of macular edema and hypoperfusion and also of peripheral ischemia will become more efficient with OCT angiography, which is undergoing continuous development.

Additional Examinations

Additional diagnostic clues may be obtained by a modified type of ophthalmodynamometry (Hitchings et al., 1976; Jonas, 2003; Jonas, 2003; Jonas, 2003; Jonas, 2004)[84–88]. The Goldmann contact lens-associated ophthalmodynamometric device provides a direct visualization of the optic disk when manually asserting pressure onto the globe, and it allows an assessment of the blood pressure in the central retinal artery and central retinal vein (Harder et al., 2007; Jonas et al., 2007)[89, 90]. In particular, ophthalmodynamometry is helpful in the differentiation between the ischemic type of CRVO versus the nonischemic type. The central retinal vein pressure was usually higher than the diastolic arterial blood pressure in eyes with ischemic CRVO, and it was usually lower than the diastolic arterial blood pressure in eyes with a nonischemic CRVO (Jonas et al., 2007)[90]. Future studies may examine whether an increased central retinal vein pressure in asymptomatic eyes may indicate an increased risk for the eventual development of RVOs.

Management

Treatment of Associated Conditions
Since the population-based studies mentioned above and multicenter prospective studies such as the Central Retinal Vein Occlusion Study have shown associations between RVOs, glaucoma, and arterial hypertension (Klein et al., 2000; Mitchell et al., 1996; Wong et al., 2005)[11–13], glaucoma and arterial hypertension should be excluded in patients with RVOs. It has remained unclear so far whether lowering of the intraocular pressure in glaucoma patients or a better control of blood pressure in patients with arterial hypertension is beneficial for the final visual outcome after RVOs.

Laser Photocoagulation
Central Retinal Vein Occlusion
In 1990, a prospective study of argon laser panretinal photocoagulation performed over a 10-year period in 123 eyes with ischemic CRVO was reported (Hayreh et al., 1990)[91]. Eyes treated by laser coagulation as compared with untreated eyes did not differ significantly in the incidence of anterior chamber angle neovascularization, neovascular glaucoma, retinal and/or optic disk neovascularization, vitreous hemorrhage, or visual acuity. The study revealed, however, a statistically significant difference in the incidence of iris neovascularization between the two groups. Consequently, the Central Retinal Vein Occlusion Study was conducted in the year 1997 (The Central Vein Occlusion Study Group, 1997)[34]. According to the results of the study, attention to visual acuity is a crucial element of the initial examination because it is an important indicator of final visual prognosis and neovascularization risk. A visual acuity worse than 20/200 is highly correlated with the presence and development of retinal ischemia and neovascularization. The study suggested that at the patient's initial visit it would be important to perform a careful slit lamp examination and gonioscopy to evaluate any iris or anterior chamber angle neovascularization. If true neovascularization is already present, a panretinal laser photocoagulation should be considered. (In the rare clinical situation of simultaneous bilateral CRVOs, the possibility of hyperviscosity should be considered and diagnostically excluded.) A follow-up schedule should be established depending on the duration and severity of the occlusion and the patient's circumstances.

- Patients with initial visual acuity less than 20/200 may be examined every month for the initial 6 months.
- Prognosis is mixed for patients with visual acuity between 20/50 and 20/200; either monthly or bimonthly follow-ups may be instituted initially (and possibly revised) depending on exactly where on the scale the patient's visual acuity falls, whether the CRVO is progressing or improving, and other factors.
- If visual acuity decreases at any time during follow-up to less than 20/200, it is likely that extensive nonperfusion has developed in the eye.
- If visual acuity is 20/40 or better, the patient may be asked to return every 1–2 months for 6

months, with precise examination of the macular area using FA and OCT.

A decrease in visual acuity may also be frequently associated with macular edema, persistent or recurrent, easily recognized with the help of FA and quantified in OCT examinations, during follow-up. In 1995, The Central Retinal Vein Occlusion Study evaluated the efficacy of grid laser treatment on macular edema compared to a control group (The Central Retinal Vein Occlusion Study Group, 1995)[6]. Grid laser treatment clearly reduced the angiographic evidence of macular edema compared to controls but visual acuity was not statistically improved in the treated group: after a 3-year follow-up, visual acuity improved spontaneously in 24% of the control group versus 27% after grid laser treatment. Nevertheless, grid laser treatment could be offered to young patients, even if no positive result but only a trend is shown in patients less than 60 years of age.

In conclusion, the first essential step in the management of CRVO is to determine the type of CRVO since the prognosis, complications, visual outcome, and management of nonischemic and ischemic CRVO are different. Ocular neovascularization is a complication of ischemic RVO only. (It is important to remember that the conventional prevalent use of a 10-disk area of retinal capillary obliteration is not a valid parameter to differentiate ischemic from non-ischemic RVO, or to predict ocular neovascularization.) The natural history of the disease with the possibility of a spontaneous improvement particularly in the nonischemic group, with macular edema, should not be mistaken for a beneficial effect of treatment in studies without a control group.

Branch Retinal Vein Occlusion
The Branch Vein Occlusion Study's multicenter randomized controlled clinical trial was designed to address questions regarding the management of complications of branch vein occlusion (The Branch Vein Occlusion Study Group, 1984; The Branch Vein Occlusion Study Group, 1986)[92, 93]. With respect to the question whether grid argon laser photocoagulation was useful in improving visual acuity in eyes with BRVO and macular edema and vision reduced to 20/40 or worse, the study included 139 eyes, which were randomly assigned to either a treated group or an untreated control group with a mean follow-up of 3.1 years for all study eyes. The gain in visual acuity from baseline maintained for 2 consecutive visits was significantly greater in the treated eyes (at least 2 Snellen lines). Grid laser photocoagulation was, therefore, recommended for patients with macular edema associated with BRVO who met the eligibility criteria of this study (visual acuity of 20/40 or less, persistent macular edema lasting for 4 months or longer, resorption of macular hemorrhages).

In 1993, another prospective study was reported on 271 eyes with major BRVO and ischemic hemicentral RVO, which either underwent scatter argon laser photocoagulation to the involved sector (n = 61 eyes) or remained untreated (n = 210 eyes) (Hayreh et al., 1993)[94]. This study concluded that argon laser photocoagulation treatment should be given only when neovascularization was seen and not otherwise, because in the latter case, the detrimental effects of laser coagulation might outweigh its beneficial effects. In the assessment of published studies on the effect of laser treatment on visual outcome of patients with RVO, every laser coagulation spot in the macular region led to a scotoma in the pericentral visual field.

Several other investigations were focused on the laser treatment of RVO (Arnarsson et al., 2000; Maár et al., 2004; Ohashi et al., 2004; Esrick et al., 2005; Parodi et al., 2006; Hayreh, 2003)[95–100]. Laser photocoagulation in a 'grid' pattern over the area, demonstrated as leaking by FA, remains to be one of the 'reference treatments for macular edema' due to BRVO. The Pascal® laser is useful for the comfort and safety of the patient, as it avoids overdosed or confluent impacts.

Ophthalmic: Surgical Treatment
Besides retinal laser coagulation, surgical treatment modalities have been reported for RVOs. For BRVO originating at arteriovenous crossings, a *sheathotomy* has been suggested to liberalize the retinal venule and the retinal arteriole from their surrounding adventitious tissue at the crossing site (Opremcak et al., 1999; Shah et al., 2000; Le Rouic et al., 2001; Cahill et al., 2003; Fujii et al., 2003; Mason et al., 2004; Charbonnel et al., 2004; Yamaji et al., 2004; Yamamoto et al., 2004)[101–109]. Randomized trials with an untreated control group and a clear differentiation between the ischemic type of BRVO and the nonischemic type of BRVO have been scarce. It may be questionable, therefore, whether sheathotomy is a recommended therapy for BRVOs originating at the arteriovenous crossing site. In most clinical sites, this surgical technique was not introduced or has been abandoned.

Radial neurotomy has been suggested as therapy for CRVO (Opremcak et al., 2001; García-Arumí et al., 2003; Weizer et al., 2003; Spaide et al., 2004; Arevalo et al., 2008)[110–114]. However, randomized prospective trials have not yet shown beneficial effects of radial neurotomy for the treatment of CRVO, so it is unclear whether the technique should be recommended (Hayreh, 2002)[115]. Again, in most clinical sites, this surgical technique was not introduced or has been abandoned.

Another surgical technique which has been used for the treatment of RVOs is the *peeling of the inner limiting membrane* off the macula to reduce macular edema (Saika et al., 2001; García-Arumí et al., 2004; Mandelcorn et al., 2004; Radetzky et al., 2004; Nkeme et al., 2006; Kumagai et al., 2007; Kumagai et al., 2007; Berker et al., 2008; Oh et al., 2008; Arai et al., 2009; DeCroos et al., 2009; Lu et al., 2009; Uemura et al., 2009)[116–128]. In view of the risk of surgical complications (such as the development of iatrogenic peripheral retinal defects with secondary retinal detachment or a iatrogenic damage to the paracentral retina by

the peeling of the inner limiting membrane), peeling of the inner limiting membrane may be reserved for clinical situations in which other modalities of treatment, namely the intravitreal injection of antiedematous (steroids) or anti-VEGF drugs, have failed in achieving a satisfactory improvement in vision, and in which the blood perfusion of the macula physiologically allows an increase in visual acuity.

The peeling of the inner limiting membrane of the retina is similar to the vitrectomy technique applied for diffuse diabetic macular edema associated with taut membranes (Lewis et al., 1992)[129]. The decrease in macular edema observed after vitrectomy could be the result of an increase in oxygen concentration in the macular area. Other hypotheses have been suggested to explain the positive effect of vitrectomy, such as a decompression from tangential tractions, removal of intravitreal proinflammatory and proangiogenic factors, collateral development stimulation, or specific Müller cell fibrosis (Mandelcorn et al., 2004;Stefánsson, 2009)[118, 130].

The positive action of vitrectomy seems durable, which differs from intravitreal injection. The combination of surgery and intravitreal injection of steroids could permit a more rapid and lasting action (Nkeme et al., 2006)[120]. Another surgical technique consists of vitrectomy combined with an injection of tissue plasminogen activator into the retinal vein (Weiss, 1998; Weiss et al., 2001)[131, 132]. This technique, however, has still not achieved wide distribution and application.

Ophthalmic: Intravitreal Drug
Intravitreal Steroids (Triamcinolone, Fluocinolone, Dexamethasone)

Intravitreal triamcinolone acetonide has been increasingly used in studies for treatment of various intraocular proliferative, edematous, and neovascular diseases, such as diffuse diabetic macular edema, proliferative diabetic retinopathy, neovascular glaucoma, persistent pseudophakic cystoid macular edema, CRVO (Greenberg et al., 2002; Jonas et al., 2002, 2005; Park et al., 2003)[133–136], and in other clinical situations. Systemic and local side effects reported include cataract, secondary ocular hypertension leading in some patients to secondary chronic open-angle glaucoma, and postinjection infectious endophthalmitis (Wingate et al., 1999; Bakri et al., 2003; Benz et al., 2003; Jonas et al., 2003; Jonas et al., 2003; Jonas et al., 2004)[137–142].

Due to its antiedematous and antiangiogenic effects, as shown in experimental investigations and clinical studies (Ishibashi et al., 1985; Wilson et al., 1992; Antoszyk et al., 1993; Penfold et al., 2001; Penfold et al., 2002)[143–147], *intravitreal triamcinolone acetonide* has additionally been used in studies on RVOs (Jonas et al., 2002; Bashshur et al., 2004; Ip et al., 2004; Jonas et al., 2004; Karacorlu et al., 2004; Karacorlu et al., 2005; Cekiç et al., 2005; Cekiç et al., 2005; Jonas et al., 2005; Jonas et al., 2005; Jonas et al., 2005; Lee et al., 2005; Chen et al., 2006; Goff et al., 2006; Gregori et al., 2006; Jonas, 2006; Ramezani et al., 2006; Bhavsar et al., 2007; Hirano et al., 2007; Jonas et al., 2007; Karacorlu et al., 2007; Pathai, 2007; Cakir et al., 2008; Chung et al., 2008; Park et al., 2008; Parodi et al., 2008; Patel et al., 2008; Riese et al., 2008; Roth et al., 2008; Cheng et al., 2009; Gewaily and Greenberg, 2009; McAllister et al., 2009; Scott et al., 2009; Wang et al., 2009; Wu et al., 2009)[148–182].

Although randomized trials on the intravitreal use of triamcinolone in particular and of steroids in general as treatment of RVO have been missing until recently, the available literature strongly suggests an antiedematous effect of intravitreal triamcinolone and an associated improvement in vision. Due to the limited duration of the intraocular availability of triamcinolone, the visual improvement is limited in its duration. It may depend on the dosage of triamcinolone used.

Prospective double-masked randomized trials have been published presenting leading knowledge on the intravitreal use of steroids for treatment of RVOs (Scott et al., 2009; Scott et al., 2009; Scott et al., 2009)[180, 183, 184]. The Standard Care versus Corticosteroid for Retinal Vein Occlusion (SCORE) study's multicenter clinical trial of 411 participants compared the efficacy and safety of 1-mg and 4-mg doses of preservative-free intravitreal triamcinolone with standard care (grid photocoagulation in eyes without dense macular hemorrhage and deferral of photocoagulation until hemorrhage clears in eyes with dense macular hemorrhage) for eyes with vision loss associated with macular edema secondary to BRVO. The drug used in this trial was prepared as a sterile, preservative-free, single-use, intravitreal injection (Trivaris®; Allergan Inc., Irvine, Calif., USA) in 1-mg and 4-mg doses, in a volume of 0.05 ml. The main outcome measure was the gain in visual acuity letter score of 15 or more from baseline to month 12. Twenty-nine, 26, and 27% of the participants achieved the primary outcome in the standard care, 1-mg, and 4-mg groups, respectively. None of the pairwise comparisons between the 3 groups was statistically significant at month 12. The rates of elevated intraocular pressure and cataract were similar for the standard care and 1-mg groups, but higher in the 4-mg group. The study group concluded that there was no difference identified in visual acuity at 12 months for the standard care group compared with the triamcinolone groups; however, rates of adverse events (particularly elevated intraocular pressure and cataract) were highest in the 4-mg group. The authors inferred that 'grid photocoagulation as applied in the SCORE study remained the standard care for patients with vision loss associated with macular edema secondary to BRVO who have characteristics similar to participants in the SCORE-BRVO trial. Grid photocoagulation should remain the benchmark against which other treatments are compared in clinical trials for eyes with vision loss associated with macular edema secondary to BRVO.' One may, however, also consider the limitation of the study. Central visual acuity and the paracentral visual field both contribute to the quality of vision. Paracentral laser coagulation in contrast to intravitreal triamcinolone leads to paracentral visual field defects. Since the paracentral visual field or reading ability was not examined, the conclusions of the SCORE-BRVO study may be valid for the outcome parameter of central visual acuity; however, it may remain questionable whether the results also refer to the quality of vision in general.

As mentioned in the natural course section, it is important to consider the *duration of the edema*. In the subgroup analysis in the SCORE-BRVO trial, patients with a duration of less than 3 months showed a trend to have more benefit with usual care. However, among those patients that had a macular edema of more than 3 months' duration, 34% in the 4-mg group showed a gain in visual acuity letter score of 15 or more, versus 15% in the photocoagulation group. According to the authors, these numbers were not significant but show the importance of the duration of the edema at the time of analyzing the results of the different trials, which may differ in the baseline characteristics. In the SCORE-BRVO trial, more than 50% of the patients had a macular edema with a duration of less than 3 months. If approximately 25% of patients with BRVO have a transient edema as a natural course (Gutman, 1977)[60], it is possible that in the SCORE-BRVO study approximately 12% of patients had transient macular edema with spontaneous resolution.

With respect to CRVO, the results of the SCORE-CRVO study differed from the findings in the SCORE-BRVO study. In the SCORE-CRVO study (Ip et al., 2009)[185], 271 participants with macular edema secondary to perfused CRVO were included. Seven, 27, and 26% of the participants achieved the primary outcome (i.e., gain in visual acuity letter score of 15 or more from baseline to month 12) in the observation, 1-mg, and 4-mg groups, respectively. The odds of achieving the primary outcome were 5.0 times greater in the 1-mg group than in the observation group (p = 0.001) and 5.0 times greater in the 4-mg group than in the observation group (p = 0.001). There was no difference identified between the 1-mg and 4-mg groups (p = 0.97). The rates of elevated intraocular pressure and cataract were similar for the observation and 1-mg groups, but higher in the 4-mg group.

The study group concluded that intravitreal triamcinolone was superior to observation for treating vision loss associated with macular edema secondary to CRVO in patients who had characteristics similar to those in the SCORE-CRVO trial. The 1-mg dose had a safety profile superior to that of the 4-mg dose. The authors suggested that intravitreal triamcinolone in a 1-mg dose, following the retreatment criteria applied in the SCORE study, should be considered for up to 1 year and possibly 2 years for patients with characteristics similar to those in the SCORE-CRVO trial. The formulation used in this study (Trivaris®) is not currently available.

Dexamethasone has been used for a long time as a potent corticosteroid that decreases inflammatory mediators implicated in macular edema. Due to its anti-edematous and antiangiogenic effects, intravitreal dexamethasone has been used in studies on RVOs. Previous data suggest fewer side effects than for other corticosteroids. Because of the short half-life of intravitreal injections of dexamethasone, an intravitreal dexamethasone implant (Ozurdex) was developed to deliver sustained levels of dexamethasone to the back of the eye in a 6-month randomized controlled clinical trial on macular edema associated with RVO, the GENEVA study. The objective of the GENEVA study was to evaluate an intravitreal dexamethasone drug delivery system (Ozurdex®) in patients with vision loss due to macular edema associated with RVO. The study design included two identical, randomized, prospective, multicenter, masked, sham-controlled, parallel groups. Phase III clinical trials were conducted in 2 periods of 6 months each. In the double-masked, initial treatment phase, patients were randomly assigned (1:1:1) to receive either a 350-μg or a 700-μg dexamethasone implant, or to receive sham treatment (needleless applicator). In the open-label phase (2nd injection), patients received a 700-µg dexamethasone implant. The primary endpoint was the time to achieve a ≥15-letter (3 Snellen lines) improvement in best-corrected visual acuity (BCVA), and key secondary endpoints included BCVA over the 6-month trial, central retinal thickness measured by OCT, and safety. To be eligible for the study, the patients had to be >18 years of age, have a >34- and <68-letter improvement in BCVA (20/200 to 20/50), and a macular edema with the following characteristics: (1) involvement of the fovea, (2) due to either BRVO or CRVO, (3) duration of macular edema of 6 weeks to 12 months for BRVO, (4) duration of macular edema of 6 weeks to 9 months for CRVO, (5) visual acuity decrease due to edema, and (6) retinal thickness of ≥300 µm in the central 1-mm macula subfield. The percentage of patients with BRVO or CRVO was similar in the 3 groups with about two thirds of BRVO patients (68.1% of BRVO patients for the dexamethasone 700-µg group) and one third of CRVO patients in each group (39.1% of CRVO patients for the dexamethasone 700-µg group). The duration of macular edema was similar in each group with about 15% of the patients having a macular edema of <3 months' duration, 50% with a macular edema duration between 3 and 6 months, and 30% with a macular edema duration >6 months (16.4% of the patients <3 months, 51.3% between 3 and 6 months, and 32.3% >6 months). Only 1.2% of patients in the dexamethasone 700-µg group and 1% of patient in the dexamethasone 350-µg group discontinued because of an ocular adverse event. It is noteworthy that only 15% of the patients had macular edema of less than 3 months' duration in comparison to more than 50% in the SCORE-BRVO trial, 51.5–53.8% in the BRAVO trial, and 51.5–61.5% in the CRUISE trial. This might affect the results and create difficulties when comparing trials, since spontaneous resolution is higher among those trials in which a large number of patients have a short duration of the macular edema. The proportion of patients

achieving at least a 15-letter or 10-letter improvement from baseline BCVA was significantly greater in the dexamethasone 700-µg group than in the sham group from day 30 through day 90. The greatest response was seen at day 60:

- 29% of patients in the dexamethasone 700-µg group achieved at least a 15-letter improvement from baseline as compared with 11% in the sham group
- 51% of patients in the dexamethasone 700-µg group achieved at least a 10-letter improvement from baseline as compared with 26% in the sham group
- Statistical differences between the dexamethasone groups and the sham group were no longer seen at day 180 in an analysis of all patients

The difference in mean change in BCVA from baseline between the dexamethasone 700-µg group and the sham group was statistically significant: (1) at all time points for all patients, (2) at all time points for BRVO patients, and (3) at days 30, 60, and 90 for CRVO patients. The main difference between the BRVO and CRVO subgroups was in the sham treatment group. Among patients with BRVO in the sham group, mean BCVA slowly improved over the course of the study. In contrast, mean BCVA slowly declined to below baseline levels among CRVO patients in the sham group.

Mean change from baseline in BCVA was similar following a second treatment with dexamethasone 700 or 350 µg. Patients who had received sham treatment in the initial treatment phase demonstrated a lower mean change from baseline in BCVA after receiving open-label treatment than patients who had received dexamethasone 700 or 350 µg during the initial treatment phase.

The percentage of patients in the dexamethasone groups reaching an intraocular pressure of ≥35 mm Hg (about 2–3% of the patients at day 60), ≥25 mm Hg (about 15% of the patients at day 60), and ≥10 mm Hg (about 15% of the patients at day 60) peaked at day 60 and returned to baseline by day 180. After 12 months (2 injections of dexamethasone), only 1.2% of the patients (n = 4) had an intraocular pressure procedure and 0.9% of patients (n = 3) a cataract surgery (for the 700-µg/700-µg group, patients injected twice). Adverse events in the initial treatment whose maximum severity increased during the open-label extension were reported for 2.6% of the patients (700-µg/700-µg group).

In summary, two identical, randomized, prospective, multicenter, masked, sham-controlled, parallel-group, phase III clinical trials showed a statistically significant effect and a rapid action, with a maximum effect at day 60 and a decrease of the effect beginning at day 90 but still persistent at day 180. The 2nd injection is effective, with an even slightly better effect than after the 1st injection. No adverse events were related to the injection, with a low cataract rate and low rates of persistent intraocular pressure increases. These results suggest that this slow-release device for the intraocular dexamethasone delivery could be considered as a first-choice therapy in both BRVO and CRVO retinal diseases.

Intravitreal Anti-VEGF Drugs

On the basis of the published results of prospective randomized controlled trials, intravitreal anti-VEGF drugs have been developed as front-line therapy for the treatment of ME associated with CRVOs42 and BRVOs (Campochiaro et al., 2010; Ho et al., 2016)[62, 186].

Bevacizumab. Since the landmark study on the intravitreal use of bevacizumab for treatment of exudative age-related macular degeneration (Rosenfeld et al., 2005)[187], bevacizumab has become a medication used worldwide for patients affected by various neovascular intraocular diseases including RVOs (Iturralde et al., 2006; Jaissle et al., 2006; Rosenfeld et al., 2006; Spandau et al., 2006; Costa et al., 2007; Matsumoto et al., 2007; Rabena et al., 2007)[188–194]. Most of the studies published so far agree that bevacizumab and ranibizumab appear to have improved vision in patients with RVOs.

Ranibizumab, Pegaptanib. Related to bevacizumab, the effect of *ranibizumab* and *pegaptanib* on macular edema in eyes with RVOs has been reported in several studies (Campochiaro et al., 2008; Pieramici et al., 2008; Spaide et al., 2009; Wroblewski et al., 2009)[195–198]. These studies all reported on a reduction in macular edema after the intravitreal injection of the anti-VEGF drugs. The first multicenter, randomized study on the effect of anti-VEGF therapy in the treatment of RVO was designed to evaluate the efficacy of pegaptanib sodium. The results have been reported at the Congress of the European Vitreo-Retinal Society in 2006. Patients with visual loss due to macular edema secondary to CRVO were randomly assigned to sham injection, 0.3, or 1 mg of pegaptanib sodium. The group treated with 1 mg of pegaptanib sodium showed a higher rate of visual gain superior to 5 letters and a lower rate of loss of 15 letters or more than the control group (p < 0.05 and p < 0.01, respectively). There was a difference of 13 letters in the change in visual acuity between the control group (sham injections) and the group treated with 1 mg of pegaptanib sodium.

Several retrospective and prospective case series illustrated that intravitreal bevacizumab resulted in improvement in visual acuity, concomitant with a reduction in central macular thickness (Epstein et al., 2012; Epstein et al., 2012; Zhang et al., 2011; Kriechbaum et al., 2008; Prager et al., 2009; Ding et al., 2011)[199–204]. Epstein and colleagues reported in a prospective controlled clinical trial the beneficial effect of intravitreal bevacizumab for the treatment of macular edema due to RVOs. These findings were confirmed by a recent relatively large series with a 2-year follow-up (Hikichi et al., 2014)[205]. Although bevacizumab has been reported to have a similar effect as ranibizumab in controlling macular edema of CRVO patients in various studies, its use in treating RVO-related macular edema is mainly off-label (Kriechbaum et al., 2008; Costa et al., 2007; Ferrara et al., 2007; Pai et al., 2007; Ehlers et al., 2011)[206–210].

Ranibizumab. The Ranibizumab for the Treatment of Macular Edema after Central Retinal Vein Occlusion (CRUISE) trials compared the effectiveness of ranibizumab 0.3 or 0.5 mg with sham in patients with macular edema secondary to CRVO. Both 6-month and 12-month results showed superiority of ranibizumab in terms of functional and anatomical improvement (Brown et al., 2010; Campochiaro et al., 2011)[211, 212]. After the CRUISE trial, the 0.5-mg ranibizumab dose was marketed for treatment of ME resulting from CRVO. Long-term treatment outcomes were provided in the HORIZON cohort and the RETAIN study, confirming the results with respect to functional and anatomical improvement in the ranibizumab study group (Campochiaro et al., 2014)[213]. The effects of ranibizumab on CRVO and BRVO patients were further ascertained by a post hoc analysis study regarding the data obtained by CRUISE and BRAVO (Thach et al., 2014)[61]. The improvement in visual acuity could be observed as early as 7 days after the injection and were maintained up to 12 months by the as-needed doses.

Aflibercept. GALILEO and COPERNICUS were two sister, phase III randomized double-masked multicenter clinical studies, which aimed to evaluate the intravitreal VEGF aflibercept in patients with CRVO-related macular edema (Boyer et al., 2012; Brown et al., 2013)[214, 215]. It revealed that the study group with aflibercept showed a significantly better functional and morphological outcome as compared to the control group. It was also concluded that visual acuity gain achieved by intravitreally applied aflibercept could be maintained with less frequent doses of aflibercept after a loading period. In the GALILEO study, significantly more aflibercept-treated patients gained >15 letters by week 24 than those receiving sham injections (Holz et al., 2013)[216].

Systemic Therapy

Several studies have suggested a beneficial effect of hemodilution as a therapy of the early phase of RVOs. Hemodilution is expected to prevent the slowdown of blood circulation and its complications by dramatically lowering blood viscosity. Some randomized studies have been published on the topic showing a statistically significant difference between treated and nontreated patients (Hansen et al., 1989; Hansen et al., 1989; Wolf et al., 1994; Hattenbach et al., 1999; Glacet-Bernard et al., 2001)[217–221]. These monocenter studies were conducted in the 1980s and 1990s, and used different treatment protocols. A more recent multicenter controlled randomized study using erythrocyte-apheresis, an automated method of hemodilution, confirmed the beneficial effect of isovolumic hemodilution administered early in the course of the CRVO (Glacet-Bernard et al., 2011)[222]. For economic and pharmaceutical reasons, however, this treatment becomes less readily available.

Prevention

Only a few studies have addressed the prevention of a recurrence of an RVO in the same eye or the development of an RVO in the contralateral eye. So far, none of these studies have shown a release device, and intravitreal anti-VEGF drugs (bevacizumab, ranibizumab, aflibercept, pegaptanib) may at least temporarily reduce any benefit. In particular, thrombocyte aggregation inhibitors and anticoagulant drugs were not shown to be of benefit (Koizumi et al., 2007; McIntosh et al., 2007)[56, 223].

Potential Future Developments

Future developments may include new intraocular drug delivery systems (comparable to the dexamethasone posterior segment drug delivery system (Ozurdex®) for intraocular delivery of steroids (Kuppermann et al., 2007; Williams et al., 2009)[224, 225]. Other future developments are combination treatments of steroids with anti-VEGF drugs, other slow-release devices for the intraocular steroid delivery (Ramchandran et al., 2008)[226], and addressing aspects of retinal protection and reopening of occluded retinal capillaries (Otani et al., 2004; Harris et al., 2006; Smith, 2006; Jonas et al., 2008; Jonas et al., 2009; Ma et al., 2009)[227–232].

Conclusion

RVOs belong to the most frequently encountered retinal vascular diseases in all ethnic groups. If the macula is involved, central visual acuity drops, depending on the amount of foveal edema and macular ischemia. It is essential to differentiate between the nonischemic type, which has a relatively good prognosis without treatment, and the ischemic type, which has a relatively poor prognosis. Known risk factors for RVOs include systemic arterial hypertension and glaucomatous optic neuropathy.

Generally vision can be improved as much as it was decreased by macular edema. The amount of vision loss due to capillary nonperfusion cannot currently be markedly increased. Recent case series studies and prospective randomized trials have suggested that intravitreal steroids (triamcinolone, fluocinolone, dexamethasone in a slow-release device) and intravitreal anti-VEGF drugs (bevacizumab, ranibizumab, aflibercept, pegaptanib) may at least temporarily reduce foveal edema and correspondingly improve visual function. The duration of edema is also crucial. Some patients may have transient macular edema with spontaneous visual acuity recovery. Alternatively, when macular edema is persistent, the earlier the treatment the better the chances of visual response.

Since most studies, particularly those on the use of retinal laser coagulation, performed so far have addressed mainly central visual acuity and have not taken into account the pericentral visual field, and since pericentral laser coagulation in contrast to an intravitreal drug therapy deteriorates the pericentral visual field, the clinical value of a pericentral laser treatment in comparison with intravitreal drug therapy has remained unclear.

A preventive therapy to avoid a recurrence of RVOs or the development of an RVO in the contralateral eye has not yet been shown.

Key Messages

- The diagnosis of macular edema from RVO is facilitated by OCT, which allows retinal thickness to be quantified, and is a useful tool to evaluate the treatment.
- FA or OCT-based angiography remains essential to differentiate perfused macular edema from ischemic macular edema.
- In CRVO, intravitreal injections of steroids or antiangiogenic drugs seem to demonstrate a benefit compared to the natural course. Ongoing studies are expected to confirm these preliminary results.
- Some patients may have transient macular edema with spontaneous visual acuity recovery, but when macular edema is persistent, the earlier the treatment the better the chances of visual response.

References

1 Hayreh SS: Occlusion of the central retinal vessels. Br J Ophthalmol 1965;49: 626–645.
2 Hayreh SS: An experimental study of the central retinal vein occlusion. Trans Ophthalmol Soc UK 1964;84:586–595.
3 Coscas G, Dhermy P: Occlusions veineuses rétiniennes. Paris, Masson, 1978, pp 283–346.
4 Hayreh SS: Classification of central retinal vein occlusion. Ophthalmology 1983;90:458–474.
5 The Central Vein Occlusion Study. Baseline and early natural history report. Arch Ophthalmol 1993;111:1087–1095.
6 The Central Vein Occlusion Study Group M report. Evaluation of grid pattern photocoagulation for macular edema in central vein occlusion. Ophthalmology 1995;102:1425–1433.

7 The Central Vein Occlusion Study Group N report. A randomized clinical trial of early panretinal photocoagulation for ischemic central vein occlusion. Ophthalmology 1995;102:1434–1444.

8 Hayreh SS, Klugman MR, Beri M, Kimura AE, Podhajsky P: Differentiation of ischemic from non-ischemic central retinal vein occlusion during the early acute phase. Graefes Arch Clin Exp Ophthalmol 1990;228:201–217.

9 Coscas G, Gaudric A: Natural course of nonaphakic cystoid macular edema. Surv Ophthalmol 1984;28(suppl):471–484.

10 Liebreich R: Ueber die Farbe des Augenhintergrundes. Albrecht Von Graefes Arch Ophthalmol 1855;1:333–358.

11 Klein R, Klein BE, Moss SE, Meuer SM: The epidemiology of retinal vein occlusion: the Beaver Dam Eye Study. Trans Am Ophthalmol Soc 2000;98:133–141.

12 Mitchell P, Smith W, Chang A: Prevalence and associations of retinal vein occlusion in Australia. The Blue Mountains Eye Study. Arch Ophthalmol 1996; 114:1243–1247.

13 Wong TY, Larsen EK, Klein R, Mitchell P, Couper DJ, Klein BE, Hubbard LD, Siscovick DS, Sharrett AR: Cardiovascular risk factors for retinal vein occlusion and arteriolar emboli: the Atherosclerosis Risk in Communities & Cardiovascular Health studies. Ophthalmology 2005; 112:540–547.

14 Liu W, Xu L, Jonas JB: Vein occlusion in Chinese subjects. Ophthalmology 2007; 114:1795–1796.

15 Zhou JQ, Xu L, Wang S, Wang YX, You QS, Tu Y, Yang H, Jonas JB: The 10-year incidence and risk factors of retinal vein occlusion: the Beijing Eye Study. Ophthalmology 2013;120:803–808.

16 Cheung N, Klein R, Wang JJ, Cotch MF, Islam AF, Klein BE, Cushman M, Wong TY: Traditional and novel cardiovascular risk factors for retinal vein occlusion: the multiethnic study of atherosclerosis. Invest Ophthalmol Vis Sci 2008;49: 4297–4302.

17 Lim LL, Cheung N, Wang JJ, Islam FM, Mitchell P, Saw SM, Aung T, Wong TY: Prevalence and risk factors of retinal vein occlusion in an Asian population. Br J Ophthalmol 2008;92:1316–1319.

18 Jonas JB, Nangia V, Khare A, Sinha A, Lambat S: Prevalence of retinal vein occlusion. The Central India Eye and Medical Study. Retina 2013;33:152–159.

19 Hayreh SS, Zimmerman B, McCarthy MJ, Podhajsky P: Systemic diseases associated with various types of retinal vein occlusion. Am J Ophthalmol 2001; 131:61–77.

20 O'Mahoney PR, Wong DT, Ray JG: Retinal vein occlusion and traditional risk factors for atherosclerosis. Arch Ophthalmol 2008;126:692–699.

21 Hayreh S: Prevalent misconceptions about acute retinal vascular occlusive disorders. Prog Retin Eye Res 2005;24: 493–519.

22 McIntosh R, Mohamed Q, Saw S, Wong T: Interventions for branch retinal vein occlusion. Ophthalmology 2006;114: 835–854.

23 Mohamed Q, McIntosh R, Saw S, Wong T: Interventions for central retinal vein occlusion: an evidence-based systematic review. Ophthalmology 2006;114:507–519.

24 Rogers S, McIntosh RL, Cheung N, Lim L, Wang JJ, Mitchell P, Kowalski JW, Nguyen H, Wong TY; International Eye Disease Consortium: The prevalence and number of people with retinal vein occlusion: pooled data from population-based studies from the US, Europe, Australia and Asia. Ophthalmology 2010; 117:313–319.e1.

25 Leenen FH, Dumais J, McInnis NH, Turton P, Stratychuk L, Nemeth K, Moy Lum-Kwong M, Fodor G: Results of the Ontario survey on the prevalence and control of hypertension. CMAJ 2008; 178:1441–1449.

26 Read JG, Gorman BK: Racial/ethnic differences in hypertension and depression among US adult women. Ethn Dis 2007; 17:389–396.

27 Giles T, Aranda JMJ, Suh DC, Choi IS, Preblick R, Rocha R, Frech-Tamas F: Ethnic/racial variations in blood pressure awareness, treatment, and control. J Clin Hypertens 2007;9:345–354.

28 Ostchega Y, Hughes JP, Wright JD, McDowell MA, Louis T: Are demographic characteristics, health care access and utilization, and comorbid conditions associated with hypertension among US adults? Am J Hypertens 2008;21:159–165.

29 Hayreh SS, Zimmerman MB, Podhajsky P: Hematological abnormalities associated with various types of retinal vein occlusion. Graefes Arch Clin Exp Ophthalmol 2002;240:180–196.

30 Risk factors for branch retinal vein occlusion. The Eye Disease Case-Control Study Group. Am J Ophthalmol 1993; 116:286–296.

31 Cugati S, Wang JJ, Knudtson MD, Rochtchina E, Klein R, Klein BE, Wong TY, Mitchell P: Retinal vein occlusion and vascular mortality: pooled data analysis of 2 population-based cohorts. Ophthalmology 2007;114:520–524.

32 Xu L, Liu W, Wang Y, Yang H, Jonas JB: Retinal vein occlusions and mortality. The Beijing Eye Study. Am J Ophthalmol 2007;144:972–973.

33 Girmens JF, Scheer S, Heron E, Sahel JA, Tournier-Lasserve E, Paques M: Familial central retinal vein occlusion. Eye 2008;22:308–310.

34 Natural history and clinical management of central retinal vein occlusion. The Central Vein Occlusion Study Group. Arch Ophthalmol 1997;115:486–491.

35 Glacet-Bernard A, Bayani N, Chretien P, Cochard C, Lelong F, Coscas G: Antiphospholipid antibodies in retinal vascular occlusions. A prospective study of 75 patients. Arch Ophthalmol 1994;112: 790–795.

36 Arsène S, Delahousse B, Regina S, Le Lez ML, Pisella PJ, Gruel Y: Increased prevalence of factor V Leiden in patients with retinal vein occlusion and under 60 years of age. Thromb Haemost 2005;94: 101–106.

37 Kuhli C, Scharrer I, Koch F, Ohrloff C, Hattenbach LO: Factor XII deficiency: a thrombophilic risk factor for retinal vein occlusion. Am J Ophthalmol 2004;137: 459–464.

38 Kuhli C, Hattenbach LO, Scharrer I, Koch F, Ohrloff C: High prevalence of resistance to APC in young patients with retinal vein occlusion. Graefes Arch Clin Exp Ophthalmol 2002;240:163–168.

39 Pinna A, Carru C, Solinas G, Zinellu A, Carta F: Glucose-6-phosphate dehydrogenase deficiency in retinal vein occlusion. Invest Ophthalmol Vis Sci 2007;48: 2747–2752.

40 Jonas JB, Wang N, Wang YX, You QS, Yang D, Xie X, Xu L: Incident retinal vein occlusions and estimated cerebrospinal fluid pressure. The Beijing Eye Study. Acta Ophthalmol 2015;93:e522–e526.

41 Berdahl JP, Fleischman D, Zaydlarova J, Stinnett S, Allingham RR, Fautsch MP: Body mass index has a linear relationship with cerebrospinal fluid pressure. Invest Ophthalmol Vis Sci 2012;53: 1422–1427.

42 Ren R, Wang N, Zhang X, Tian G, Jonas JB: Cerebrospinal fluid pressure correlated with body mass index. Graefes Arch Clin Exp Ophthalmol 2013;250: 445–446.

43 Jonas JB, Wang N, Wang S, Wang YX, You QS, Yang D, Wei WB, Xu L: Retinal vessel diameter and estimated cerebrospinal fluid pressure in arterial hypertension. The Beijing Eye Study. Am J Hypertens 2014;27:1170–1178.

44 Glacet-Bernard A, les Jardins GL, Lasry S, Coscas G, Soubrane G, Souied E, Housset B: Obstructive sleep apnea among patients with retinal vein occlusion. Arch Ophthalmol 2010;128:1533–1538.

45 Chou K-T, Huang C-C, Tsai DC, Chen YM, Perng DW, Shiao GM, Lee YC, Leu HB: Sleep apnea and risk of retinal vein occlusion: a nationwide population-based study of Taiwanese. Am J Ophthalmol 2012;154:200–205.

46 Paques M, Massin P, Sahel JA, Gaudric A, Bergmann JF, Azancot S, Lévy BI, Vicaut E: Circadian fluctuations of macular edema in patients with morning vision blurring: correlation with arterial pressure and effect of light deprivation. Invest Ophthalmol Vis Sci 2005;46: 4707–4711.

47 Gupta B, Grewal J, Adewoyin T, Pelosini L, Williamson TH: Diurnal variation of macular oedema in CRVO: prospective study. Graefes Arch Clin Exp Ophthalmol 2009;247:593–596.

48 Usui S, Ikuno Y, Akiba M, Maruko I, Sekiryu T, Nishida K, Iida T: Circadian changes in subfoveal choroidal thickness and the relationship with circulatory factors in healthy subjects. Invest Ophthalmol Vis Sci 2012;53:2300–2307.

49 Tan CS, Ouyang Y, Ruiz H, Sadda SR: Diurnal variation of choroidal thickness in normal, healthy subjects measured by spectral domain optical coherence tomography. Invest Ophthalmol Vis Sci 2012;53:261–266.

50 Jonas JB, Wang N, Yang D, Ritch R, Panda-Jonas S: Facts and myths of cerebrospinal fluid pressure for the physiology of the eye. Prog Retin Eye Res 2015; 46:67–83.

51 Jonas JB, Wang N, Wang YX, You QS, Yang D, Xie X, Wei WB, Xu L: Subfoveal choroidal thickness and cerebrospinal fluid pressure. The Beijing Eye Study 2011. Invest Ophthalmol Vis Sci 2014; 55:1292–1928.

52 Du KF, Xu L, Shao L, Chen CX, Zhou JQ, Wang YX, You QS, Jonas JB, Wei WB: Subfoveal choroidal thickness in retinal vein occlusion. The Beijing Eye Study 2011. Ophthalmology 2013;120:2749–2750.

53 Tsuiki E, Suzuma K, Ueki R, Maekawa Y, Kitaoka T: Enhanced depth imaging optical coherence tomography of the choroid in central retinal vein occlusion. Am J Ophthalmol 2013;156:543–547.

54 Xu L, You QS, Jonas JB: Central corneal thickness and retinal vein occlusions: the Beijing Eye Study. Graefes Arch Clin Exp Ophthalmol 2010;248:759–760.

55 Xu L, You QS, Liu W, Jonas JB: Smoking and retinal vein occlusions. The Beijing Eye Study. Graefes Arch Clin Ophthalmol 2010;248:1046–1046.

56 Koizumi H, Ferrara DC, Bruè C, Spaide RF: Central retinal vein occlusion case-control study. Am J Ophthalmol 2007; 144:858–863.

57 Glacet-Bernard A, Coscas G, Chabanel A, Zourdani A, Lelong F, Samama MM: Prognostic factors for retinal vein occlusion: prospective study of 175 cases. Ophthalmology 1996;103:551–560.

58 Browning DJ: Patchy ischemic retinal whitening in acute central retinal vein occlusion. Ophthalmology 2002;109: 2154–2159.

59 Paques M, Gaudric A: Perivenous macular whitening during central retinal vein occlusion. Arch Ophthalmol 2003;121: 1488–1491.

60 Gutman FA: Macular edema in branch retinal vein occlusion: prognosis and management. Trans Am Acad Ophthalmol Otolaryngol 1977;83:488–495.

61 Thach AB, Yau L, Hoang C, Tuomi L: Time to clinically significant visual acuity gains after ranibizumab treatment for retinal vein occlusion: BRAVO and CRUISE trials. Ophthalmology 2014; 121:1059–1066.

62 Campochiaro PA, Heier JS, Feiner L, Gray S, Saroj N, Rundle AC, Murahashi WY, Rubio RG; BRAVO Investigators: Ranibizumab for macular edema following branch retinal vein occlusion: six month primary end point results of a phase III study. Ophthalmology 2010; 117:1102–1112.

63 Haller JA, Bandello F, Belfort R Jr, Blumenkranz MS, Gillies M, Heier J, Loewenstein A, Yoon YH, Jacques ML, Jiao J, Li XY, Whitcup SM; OZURDEX GENEVA Study Group: Randomized, sham-controlled trial of dexamethasone intravitreal implant in patients with macular edema due to retinal vein occlusion. Ophthalmology 2010;117:1134–1146.

64 Haller JA, Bandello F, Belfort R Jr, Blumenkranz MS, Gillies M, Heier J, Loewenstein A, Yoon YH, Jiao J, Li XY, Whitcup SM; Ozurdex GENEVA Study Group, Li J: Dexamethasone intravitreal implant in patients with macular edema related to branch or central retinal vein occlusion twelve-month study results. Ophthalmology 2011;118:2453–2460.

65 Hayreh SS, Hayreh MS: Hemi-central retinal vein occlusion. Pathogenesis, clinical features, and natural history. Arch Ophthalmol 1980;98:1600–1609.

66 Paques M, Girmens JF, Riviere E, Sahel J: Dilation of the minor arterial circle of the iris preceding rubeosis iridis during retinal vein occlusion. Am J Ophthalmol 2004;138:1083–1086.

67 Casselholmde Salles M, Kvanta A, Amrén U, Epstein D: Optical coherence tomography angiography in central retinal vein occlusion: correlation between the foveal avascular zone and visual acuity. Invest Ophthalmol Vis Sci 2016; 57:OCT242–OCT246.

68 Coscas F, Glacet-Bernard A, Miere A, Caillaux V, Uzzan J, Lupidi M, Coscas G, Souied EH: Optical coherence tomography angiography in retinal vein occlusion: evaluation of superficial and deep capillary plexa. Am J Ophthalmol 2016; 161:160–171.

69 Abri Aghdam K, Reznicek L, Soltan Sanjari M, Framme C, Bajor A, Klingenstein A, Kernt M, Seidensticker F: Peripheral retinal non-perfusion and treatment response in branch retinal vein occlusion. Int J Ophthalmol 2016;9:858–862.

70 Kashani AH, Lee SY, Moshfeghi A, Durbin MK, Puliafito CA: Optical coherence tomography angiography of retinal venous occlusion. Retina 2015;35:2323–2331.

71 Suzuki N, Hirano Y, Yoshida M, Tomiyasu T, Uemura A, Yasukawa T, Ogura Y: Microvascular abnormalities on optical coherence tomography angiography in macular edema associated with branch retinal vein occlusion. Am J Ophthalmol 2016;161:126–132.

72 Laatikainen L, Kohner EM: Fluorescein angiography and its prognostic significance in central retinal vein occlusion. Br J Ophthalmol 1976;60:411–418.

73 Catier A, Tadayoni R, Paques M, Erginay A, Haouchine B, Gaudric A, Massin P: Characterization of macular edema from various etiologies by optical coherence tomography. Am J Ophthalmol 2005;140:200–206.

74 Ota M, Tsujikawa A, Kita M, Miyamoto K, Sakamoto A, Yamaike N, Kotera Y, Yoshimura N: Integrity of foveal photoreceptor layer in central retinal vein occlusion. Retina 2008;28:1502–1508.

75 Shroff D, Mehta DK, Arora R, Narula R, Chauhan D: Natural history of macular status in recent-onset branch retinal vein occlusion: an optical coherence tomography study. Int Ophthalmol 2008;28:261–268.

76 Wei E, Jia Y, Tan O, Potsaid B, Liu JJ, Choi W, Fujimoto JG, Huang D: Parafoveal retinal vascular response to pattern visual stimulation assessed with OCT angiography. PLoS One 2013;8:e81343.

77 Wang X, Jia Y, Spain R, Potsaid B, Liu JJ, Baumann B, Hornegger J, Fujimoto JG, Wu Q, Huang D: Optical coherence tomography angiography of optic nerve head and parafovea in multiple sclerosis. Br J Ophthalmol 2014;98:1368–1373.

78 Jia Y, Wei E, Wang X, Zhang X, Morrison JC, Parikh M, Lombardi LH, Gattey DM, Armour RL, Edmunds B, Kraus MF, Fujimoto JG, Huang D: Optical coherence tomography angiography of optic disc perfusion in glaucoma. Ophthalmology 2014;121:1322–1332.

79 Jia Y, Bailey ST, Hwang TS, McClintic SM, Gao SS, Pennesi ME, Flaxel CJ, Lauer AK, Wilson DJ, Hornegger J, Fujimoto JG, Huang D: Quantitative optical coherence tomography angiography of vascular abnormalities in the living human eye. Proc Natl Acad Sci USA 2015; 112:E2395–E2402.

80 Yu J, Jiang C, Wang X, Zhu L, Gu R, Xu H, Jia Y, Huang D, Sun X: Macular perfusion in healthy Chinese: an optical coherence tomography angiogram study. Invest Ophthalmol Vis Sci 2015; 56:3212–3217.

81 Pechauer AD, Jia Y, Liu L, Gao SS, Jiang C, Huang D: Optical coherence tomography angiography of peripapillary retinal blood flow response to hyperoxia. Invest Ophthalmol Vis Sci 2015;56: 3287–3291.

82 Glacet-Bernard A, Sellam A, Coscas F, Coscas G, Souied EH: Optical coherence tomography angiography in retinal vein occlusion treated with dexamethasone Implant: a new test for follow-up evaluation. Eur J Ophthalmol 2016;26:460–468.

83 Sellam A, Glacet-Bernard A, Coscas F, Miere A, Coscas G, Souied E: Qualitative and quantitative follow-up using optical coherence tomography angiography of retinal vein occlusion treated with anti-VEGF: optical coherence tomography angiography follow-up of retinal vein occlusion. Retina 2016, Epub ahead of print.

84 Hitchings RA, Spaeth GL: Chronic retinal vein occlusion in glaucoma. Br J Ophthalmol 1976;60:694–699.

85 Jonas JB: Reproducibility of ophthalmodynamometric measurements of the central retinal artery and vein collapse pressure. Br J Ophthalmol 2003;87:577–579.

86 Jonas JB: Ophthalmodynamometric assessment of the central retinal vein collapse pressure in eyes with retinal vein stasis or occlusion. Graefes Arch Clin Exp Ophthalmol 2003;241:367–370.

87 Jonas JB: Central retinal artery and vein pressure in patients with chronic open-angle glaucoma. Br J Ophthalmol 2003; 87:949–951.

88 Jonas JB: Ophthalmodynamometric determination of the central retinal vessel collapse pressure correlated with systemic blood pressure. Br J Ophthalmol 2004;88:501–504.

89 Harder B, Jonas JB: Frequency of spontaneous pulsations of the central retinal vein in normal eyes. Br J Ophthalmol 2007;91:401–402.

90 Jonas JB, Harder B: Ophthalmodynamometric differences between ischemic versus non-ischemic retinal vein occlusion. Am J Ophthalmol 2007;143:112–116.

91 Hayreh SS, Klugman MR, Podhajsky P, Servais GE, Perkins ES: Argon laser panretinal photocoagulation in ischemic central retinal vein occlusion. A 10-year prospective study. Graefes Arch Clin Exp Ophthalmol 1990;228:281–296.

92 Argon laser photocoagulation for macular edema in branch vein occlusion. The Branch Vein Occlusion Study Group. Am J Ophthalmol 1984;98:271–282.

93 Argon laser scatter photocoagulation for prevention of neovascularization and vitreous hemorrhage in branch vein occlusion. A randomized clinical trial. Branch Vein Occlusion Study Group. Arch Ophthalmol 1986;104:34–41.

94 Hayreh SS, Rubenstein L, Podhajsky P: Argon laser scatter photocoagulation in treatment of branch retinal vein occlusion. A prospective clinical trial. Ophthalmologica 1993;206:1–14.

95 Arnarsson A, Stefánsson E: Laser treatment and the mechanism of edema reduction in branch retinal vein occlusion. Invest Ophthalmol Vis Sci 2000; 41:877–879.

96 Maár N, Luksch A, Graebe A, Ergun E, Wimpissinger B, Tittl M, Vécsei P, Stur M, Schmetterer L: Effect of laser photocoagulation on the retinal vessel diameter in branch and macular vein occlusion. Arch Ophthalmol 2004;122: 987–991.

97 Ohashi H, Oh H, Nishiwaki H, Nonaka A, Takagi H: Delayed absorption of macular edema accompanying serous retinal detachment after grid laser treatment in patients with branch retinal vein occlusion. Ophthalmology 2004;111:2050–2056.

98 Esrick E, Subramanian ML, Heier JS, Devaiah AK, Topping TM, Frederick AR, Morley MG: Multiple laser treatments for macular edema attributable to branch retinal vein occlusion. Am J Ophthalmol 2005;139:653–657.

99 Parodi MB, Spasse S, Iacono P, Di Stefano G, Canziani T, Ravalico G: Subthreshold grid laser treatment of macular edema secondary to branch retinal vein occlusion with micropulse infrared (810 nanometer) diode laser. Ophthalmology 2006;113:2237–2242.

100 Hayreh SS: Management of central retinal vein occlusion. Ophthalmologica 2003;217:167–188.

101 Opremcak EM, Bruce RA: Surgical decompression of branch retinal vein occlusion via arteriovenous crossing sheathotomy: a prospective review of 15 cases. Retina 1999;19:1–5.

102 Shah GK, Sharma S, Fineman MS, Federman J, Brown MM, Brown GC: Arteriovenous adventitial sheathotomy for the treatment of macular edema associated with branch retinal vein occlusion. Am J Ophthalmol 2000;129: 104–106.

103 Le Rouic JF, Bejjani RA, Rumen F, Caudron C, Bettembourg O, Renard G, Chauvaud D: Adventitial sheathotomy for decompression of recent onset branch retinal vein occlusion. Graefes Arch Clin Exp Ophthalmol 2001;239: 747–751.

104 Cahill MT, Kaiser PK, Sears JE, Fekrat S: The effect of arteriovenous sheathotomy on cystoid macular oedema secondary to branch retinal vein occlusion. Br J Ophthalmol 2003;87: 1329–1332.

105 Fujii GY, de Juan E Jr, Humayun MS: Improvements after sheathotomy for branch retinal vein occlusion documented by optical coherence tomography and scanning laser ophthalmoscope. Ophthalmic Surg Lasers Imaging 2003;34:49–52.

106 Mason J 3rd, Feist R, White M Jr, Swanner J, McGwin G Jr, Emond T: Sheathotomy to decompress branch retinal vein occlusion: a matched control study. Ophthalmology 2004;111: 540–545.

107 Charbonnel J, Glacet-Bernard A, Korobelnik JF, Nyouma-Moune E, Pournaras CJ, Colin J, Coscas G, Soubrane G: Management of branch retinal vein occlusion with vitrectomy and arteriovenous adventitial sheathotomy, the possible role of surgical posterior vitreous detachment. Graefes Arch Clin Exp Ophthalmol 2004;242:223–228.

108 Yamaji H, Shiraga F, Tsuchida Y, Yamamoto Y, Ohtsuki H: Evaluation of arteriovenous crossing sheathotomy for branch retinal vein occlusion by fluorescein videoangiography and image analysis. Am J Ophthalmol 2004; 137:834–841.

109 Yamamoto S, Saito W, Yagi F, Takeuchi S, Sato E, Mizunoya S: Vitrectomy with or without arteriovenous adventitial sheathotomy for macular edema associated with branch retinal vein occlusion. Am J Ophthalmol 2004;138: 907–914.

110 Opremcak EM, Bruce RA, Lomeo MD, Ridenour CD, Letson AD, Rehmar AJ: Radial optic neurotomy for central retinal vein occlusion: a retrospective pilot study of 11 consecutive cases. Retina 2001;215:408–415.

111 García-Arumí J, Boixadera A, Martinez-Castillo V, Castillo R, Dou A, Corcostegui B: Chorioretinal anastomosis after radial optic neurotomy for central retinal vein occlusion. Arch Ophthalmol 2003;121:1385–1391.

112 Weizer JS, Stinnett SS, Fekrat S: Radial optic neurotomy as treatment for central retinal vein occlusion. Am J Ophthalmol 2003;136:814–819.

113 Spaide RF, Klancnik JM Jr, Gross NE: Retinal choroidal collateral circulation after radial optic neurotomy correlated with the lessening of macular edema. Retina 2004;243:356–359.

114 Arevalo JF, Garcia RA, Wu L, Rodriguez FJ, Dalma-Weiszhausz J, Quiroz-Mercado H, Morales-Canton V, Roca JA, Berrocal MH, Graue-Wiechers F, Robledo V; Pan-American Collaborative Retina Study Group: Radial optic neurotomy for central retinal vein occlusion: results of the Pan-American Collaborative Retina Study Group (PA-CORES). Retina 2008;288:1044–1052.

115 Hayreh SS: Radial optic neurotomy for central retinal vein occlusion. Retina 2002;226:827.

116 Saika S, Tanaka T, Miyamoto T, Ohnishi Y: Surgical posterior vitreous detachment combined with gas/air tamponade for treating macular edema associated with branch retinal vein occlusion: retinal tomography and visual outcome. Graefes Arch Clin Exp Ophthalmol 2001;239:729–732.

117 García-Arumí J, Martinez-Castillo V, Boixadera A, Blasco H, Corcostegui B: Management of macular edema in branch retinal vein occlusion with sheathotomy and recombinant tissue plasminogen activator. Retina 2004;24:530–540.

118 Mandelcorn MS, Nrusimhadevara RK: Internal limiting membrane peeling for decompression of macular edema in retinal vein occlusion: a report of 14 cases. Retina 2004;24:348–355.

119 Radetzky S, Walter P, Fauser S, Koizumi K, Kirchhof B, Joussen AM: Visual outcome of patients with macular edema after pars plana vitrectomy and indocyanine green-assisted peeling of the internal limiting membrane. Graefes Arch Clin Exp Ophthalmol 2004; 242:273–278.

120 Nkeme J, Glacet-Bernard A, Gnikpingo K, Zourdani A, Mimoun G, Mahiddine H, Gkoritsa A, Tchamo A, Coscas G, Soubrane G: Surgical treatment of persistent macular edema in retinal vein occlusion (in French). J Fr Ophthalmol 2006;29:808–814.

121 Kumagai K, Furukawa M, Ogino N, Uemura A, Larson E: Long-term outcomes of vitrectomy with or without arteriovenous sheathotomy in branch retinal vein occlusion. Retina 2007;27: 49–54.

122 Kumagai K, Furukawa M, Ogino N, Larson E, Uemura A: Long-term visual outcomes after vitrectomy for macular edema with foveal hemorrhage in branch retinal vein occlusion. Retina 2007;27:584–588.

123 Berker N, Batman C: Surgical treatment of central retinal vein occlusion. Acta Ophthalmol 2008;86:245–252.

124 Oh IK, Kim S, Oh J, Huh K: Long-term visual outcome of arteriovenous adventitial sheathotomy on branch retinal vein occlusion induced macular edema. Korean J Ophthalmol 2008;22: 1–5.

125 Arai M, Yamamoto S, Mitamura Y, Sato E, Sugawara T, Mizunoya S: Efficacy of vitrectomy and internal limiting membrane removal for macular edema associated with branch retinal vein occlusion. Ophthalmologica 2009; 223:172–176.

126 DeCroos FC, Shuler RK Jr, Stinnett S, Fekrat S: Pars plana vitrectomy, internal limiting membrane peeling, and panretinal endophotocoagulation for macular edema secondary to central retinal vein occlusion. Am J Ophthalmol 2009;147:627–633.e1.

127 Lu N, Wang NL, Wang GL, Li XW, Wang Y: Vitreous surgery with direct central retinal artery massage for central retinal artery occlusion. Eye 2009; 23:867–872.

128 Uemura A, Yamamoto S, Sato E, Sugawara T, Mitamura Y, Mizunoya S: Vitrectomy alone versus vitrectomy with simultaneous intravitreal injection of triamcinolone for macular edema associated with branch retinal vein occlusion. Ophthalmic Surg Lasers Imaging 2009;40:6–12.

129 Lewis H, Abrams GW, Blumenkranz MS, Campo RV: Vitrectomy for diabetic macular traction and edema associated with posterior hyaloidal traction. Ophthalmology 1992;99:753–759.

130 Stefánsson E: Physiology of vitreous surgery. Graefes Arch Clin Exp Ophthalmol 2009;247:147–163.

131 Weiss JN: Treatment of central retinal vein occlusion by injection of tissue plasminogen activator into a retinal vein. Am J Ophthalmol 1998;126:142–144.

132 Weiss JN, Bynoe LA: Injection of tissue plasminogen activator into a branch retinal vein in eyes with central retinal vein occlusion. Ophthalmology 2001; 108:2249–2257.

133 Greenberg PB, Martidis A, Rogers AH, Duker JS, Reichel E: Intravitreal triamcinolone acetonide for macular oedema due to central retinal vein occlusion. Br J Ophthalmol 2002;86: 247–248.

134 Jonas JB, Kreissig I, Degenring RF: Intravitreal triamcinolone acetonide as treatment of macular oedema in central retinal vein occlusion. Graefes Arch Clin Exp Ophthalmol 2002;240: 782–783.

135 Park CH, Jaffe GJ, Fekrat S: Intravitreal triamcinolone acetonide in eyes with cystoid macular edema associated with central retinal vein occlusion. Am J Ophthalmol 2003;136:419–425.

136 Jonas JB: Intravitreal triamcinolone acetonide for treatment of intraocular oedematous and neovascular diseases. Acta Ophthalmol 2005;83:645–663.

137 Wingate RJ, Beaumont PE: Intravitreal triamcinolone and elevated intraocular pressure. Aust NZ J Ophthalmol 1999; 27:431–432.

138 Bakri SJ, Beer PM: The effect of intravitreal triamcinolone acetonide on intraocular pressure. Ophthalmic Surg Lasers Imaging 2003;34:386–390.

139 Benz MS, Murray TG, Dubovy SR, Katz RS, Eifrig CW: Endophthalmitis caused by *Mycobacterium chelonae* abscessus after intravitreal injection of triamcinolone. Arch Ophthalmol 2003;121: 271–273.

140 Jonas JB, Kreissig I, Degenring RF: Endophthalmitis after intravitreal injection of triamcinolone acetonide. Arch Ophthalmol 2003;121:1663–1664.

141 Jonas JB, Kreissig I, Degenring R: Intraocular pressure after intravitreal injection of triamcinolone acetonide. Br J Ophthalmol 2003;87:24–27.

142 Jonas JB, Bleyl U: Morphallaxia-like ocular histology after intravitreal triamcinolone acetonide. Br J Ophthalmol 2004;88:839–840.

143 Ishibashi T, Miki K, Sorgente N, Patterson R, Ryan SJ: Effects of intravitreal administration of steroids on experimental subretinal neovascularization in the subhuman primate. Arch Ophthalmol 1985;103: 708–711.

144 Wilson CA, Berkowitz BA, Sato Y, Ando N, Handa JT, de Juan E Jr: Treatment with intravitreal steroid reduces blood-retinal barrier breakdown due to retinal photocoagulation. Arch Ophthalmol 1992;110:1155–1159.

145 Antoszyk AN, Gottlieb JL, Machemer R, Hatchell DL: The effects of intravitreal triamcinolone acetonide on experimental pre-retinal neovascularization. Graefes Arch Clin Exp Ophthalmol 1993;231:34–40.

146 Penfold PL, Wong JG, Gyory J, Billson FA: Effects of triamcinolone acetonide on microglial morphology and quantitative expression of MHC-II in exudative age-related macular degeneration. Clin Exp Ophthalmol 2001;29:188–192.

147 Penfold PL, Wen L, Madigan MC, King NJ, Provis JM: Modulation of permeability and adhesion molecule expression by human choroidal endothelial cells. Invest Ophthalmol Vis Sci 2002; 43:3125–3130.

148 Jonas JB, Kreissig I, Degenring RF: Intravitreal triamcinolone acetonide as treatment of macular edema in central retinal vein occlusion. Graefes Arch Clin Exp Ophthalmol 2002;240:782–783.

149 Bashshur ZF, Ma'luf RN, Allam S, Jurdi FA, Haddad RS, Noureddin BN: Intravitreal triamcinolone for the management of macular edema due to nonischemic central retinal vein occlusion. Arch Ophthalmol 2004;122: 1137–1140.

150 Ip MS, Gottlieb JL, Kahana A, Scott IU, Altaweel MM, Blodi BA, Gangnon RE, Puliafito CA: Intravitreal triamcinolone for the treatment of macular edema associated with central retinal vein occlusion. Arch Ophthalmol 2004;122: 1131–1136.

151 Jonas JB, Degenring R, Kamppeter B, Kreissig I, Akkoyun I: Duration of the effect of intravitreal triamcinolone acetonide as treatment of diffuse diabetic macular edema. Am J Ophthalmol 2004;138:158–160.

152 Karacorlu M, Ozdemir H, Karacorlu S: Intravitreal triamcinolone acetonide for the treatment of central retinal vein occlusion in young patients. Retina 2004;24:324–327.

153 Karacorlu M, Ozdemir H, Karacorlu SA: Resolution of serous macular detachment after intravitreal triamcinolone acetonide treatment of patients with branch retinal vein occlusion. Retina 2005;25:856–860.

154 Cekiç O, Chang S, Tseng JJ, Barile GR, Weissman H, Del Priore LV, Schiff WM, Weiss M, Klancnik JM Jr: Intravitreal triamcinolone treatment for macular edema associated with central retinal vein occlusion and hemiretinal vein occlusion. Retina 2005;25:846–850.

155 Cekiç O, Chang S, Tseng JJ, Barile GR, Del Priore LV, Weissman H, Schiff WM, Ober MD: Intravitreal triamcinolone injection for treatment of macular edema secondary to branch retinal vein occlusion. Retina 2005;25:851–855.

156 Jonas JB, Akkoyun I, Kamppeter B, Kreissig I, Degenring RF: Branch retinal vein occlusion treated by intravitreal triamcinolone acetonide. Eye 2005;19: 65–71.

157 Jonas JB, Akkoyun I, Kamppeter B, Kreissig I, Degenring RF: Intravitreal triamcinolone acetonide for treatment of central retinal vein occlusion. Eur J Ophthalmol 2005;15:751–758.

158 Jonas JB, Kreissig I, Degenring R: Intravitreal triamcinolone acetonide for treatment of intraocular proliferative, exudative, and neovascular diseases. Prog Retin Eye Res 2005;24:587–611.

159 Lee H, Shah GK: Intravitreal triamcinolone as primary treatment of cystoid macular edema secondary to branch retinal vein occlusion. Retina 2005;25: 551–555.

160 Chen SD, Sundaram V, Lochhead J, Patel CK: Intravitreal triamcinolone for the treatment of ischemic macular edema associated with branch retinal vein occlusion. Am J Ophthalmol 2006; 141:876–883.

161 Goff MJ, Jumper JM, Yang SS, Fu AD, Johnson RN, McDonald HR, Ai E: Intravitreal triamcinolone acetonide treatment of macular edema associated with central retinal vein occlusion. Retina 2006;26:896–901.

162 Gregori NZ, Rosenfeld PJ, Puliafito CA, Flynn HW Jr, Lee JE, Mavrofrides EC, Smiddy WE, Murray TG, Berrocal AM, Scott IU, Gregori G: One-year safety and efficacy of intravitreal triamcinolone acetonide for the management of macular edema secondary to central retinal vein occlusion. Retina 2006;26: 889–895.

163 Jonas JB: Intravitreal triamcinolone acetonide: a change in a paradigm. Ophthalmic Res 2006;38:218–245.

164 Ramezani A, Entezari M, Moradian S, Tabatabaei H, Kadkhodaei S: Intravitreal triamcinolone for acute central retinal vein occlusion; a randomized clinical trial. Graefes Arch Clin Exp Ophthalmol 2006;244:1601–1606.

165 Bhavsar AR, Ip MS, Glassman AR; DR-CRnet and the SCORE Study Groups: The risk of endophthalmitis following intravitreal triamcinolone injection in the DRCRnet and SCORE clinical trials. Am J Ophthalmol 2007;144:454–456.

166 Hirano Y, Sakurai E, Yoshida M, Ogura Y: Comparative study on efficacy of a combination therapy of triamcinolone acetonide administration with and without vitrectomy for macular edema associated with branch retinal vein occlusion. Ophthalmic Res 2007;39:207–212.

167 Jonas JB, Rensch F: Decreased retinal vein diameter after intravitreal triamcinolone for retinal vein occlusions. Br J Ophthalmol 2007;91:1711–1712.

168 Karacorlu M, Karacorlu SA, Ozdemir H, Senturk F: Intravitreal triamcinolone acetonide for treatment of serous macular detachment in central retinal vein occlusion. Retina 2007;27:1026–1030.

169 Pathai S: Intravitreal triamcinolone acetonide for treatment of persistent macular oedema in branch retinal vein occlusion. Eye 2007;21:255–256.

170 Cakir M, Dogan M, Bayraktar Z, Bayraktar S, Acar N, Altan T, Kapran Z, Yilmaz OF: Efficacy of intravitreal triamcinolone for the treatment of macular edema secondary to branch retinal vein occlusion in eyes with or without grid laser photocoagulation. Retina 2008;28:465–472.

171 Chung EJ, Lee H, Koh HJ: Arteriovenous crossing sheathotomy versus intravitreal triamcinolone acetonide injection for treatment of macular edema associated with branch retinal vein occlusion. Graefes Arch Clin Exp Ophthalmol 2008;246:967–974.

172 Park SP, Ahn JK: Changes of aqueous vascular endothelial growth factor and interleukin-6 after intravitreal triamcinolone for branch retinal vein occlusion. Clin Exp Ophthalmol 2008;36:831–835.

173 Parodi MB, Iacono P, Ravalico G: Intravitreal triamcinolone acetonide combined with subthreshold grid laser treatment for macular oedema in branch retinal vein occlusion: a pilot study. Br J Ophthalmol 2008;92:1046–1050.

174 Patel PJ, Zaheer I, Karia N: Intravitreal triamcinolone acetonide for macular oedema owing to retinal vein occlusion. Eye 2008;22:60–64.

175 Riese J, Loukopoulos V, Meier C, Timmermann M, Gerding H: Combined intravitreal triamcinolone injection and laser photocoagulation in eyes with persistent macular edema after branch retinal vein occlusion. Graefes Arch Clin Exp Ophthalmol 2008;246:1671–1676.

176 Roth DB, Cukras C, Radhakrishnan R, Feuer WJ, Yarian DL, Green SN, Wheatley HM, Prenner J: Intravitreal triamcinolone acetonide injections in the treatment of retinal vein occlusions. Ophthalmic Surg Lasers Imaging 2008;39:446–454.

177 Cheng KC, Wu WC, Lin CJ: Intravitreal triamcinolone acetonide for patients with macular oedema due to central retinal vein occlusion in Taiwan. Eye 2009;23:849–857.

178 Gewaily D, Greenberg PB: Intravitreal steroids versus observation for macular edema secondary to central retinal vein occlusion. Cochrane Database Syst Rev 2009;1:CD007324.

179 McAllister IL, Vijayasekaran S, Chen SD, Yu DY: Effect of triamcinolone acetonide on vascular endothelial growth factor and occludin levels in branch retinal vein occlusion. Am J Ophthalmol 2009;147:838–846.

180 Scott IU, Ip MS, VanVeldhuisen PC, Oden NL, Blodi BA, Fisher M, Chan CK, Gonzalez VH, Singerman LJ, Tolentino M; SCORE Study Research Group: A randomized trial comparing the efficacy and safety of intravitreal triamcinolone with standard care to treat vision loss associated with macular edema secondary to branch retinal vein occlusion: the Standard Care vs Corticosteroid for Retinal Vein Occlusion (SCORE) study report 6. Arch Ophthalmol 2009;127:1115–1128.

181 Wang L, Song H: Effects of repeated injection of intravitreal triamcinolone on macular oedema in central retinal vein occlusion. Acta Ophthalmol 2009;87:285–289.

182 Wu WC, Cheng KC, Wu HJ: Intravitreal triamcinolone acetonide vs bevacizumab for treatment of macular oedema due to central retinal vein occlusion. Eye (Lond) 2009;23:2215–2222.

183 Scott IU, VanVeldhuisen PC, Oden NL, Ip MS, Blodi BA, Jumper JM, Figueroa M, SCORE Study Investigator Group: SCORE Study report 1: baseline associations between central retinal thickness and visual acuity in patients with retinal vein occlusion. Ophthalmology 2009;116:504–512.

184 Scott IU, Blodi BA, Ip MS, Vanveldhuisen PC, Oden NL, Chan CK, Gonzalez V; SCORE Study Investigator Group: SCORE Study Report 2: interobserver agreement between investigator and reading center classification of retinal vein occlusion type. Ophthalmology 2009;116:756–761.

185 Ip MS, Scott IU, VanVeldhuisen PC, Oden NL, Blodi BA, Fisher M, Singerman LJ, Tolentino M, Chan CK, Gonzalez VH; SCORE Study Research Group: A randomized trial comparing the efficacy and safety of intravitreal triamcinolone with observation to treat vision loss associated with macular edema secondary to central retinal vein occlusion: the Standard Care vs Corticosteroid for Retinal Vein Occlusion (SCORE) study report 5. Arch Ophthalmol 2009;127:1101–1114.

186 Ho M, Liu DT, Lam DS, Jonas JB: Retinal vein occlusions, from basics to the latest treatment. Retina 2016;36:432–448.

187 Rosenfeld PJ, Moshfeghi AA, Puliafito CA: Optical coherence tomography findings after an intravitreal injection of bevacizumab (Avastin) for neovascular age-related macular degeneration. Ophthalmic Surg Lasers Imaging 2005;36:331–335.

188 Iturralde D, Spaide RF, Meyrele CB, Klancnik JM, Yannuzzi LA, Fisher YL, Sorenson J, Slakter JS, Freund KB, Cooney M, Fine HF: Intravitreal bevacizumab (Avastin) treatment of macular edema in central retinal vein occlusion: a short-term study. Retina 2006;26:279–284.

189 Jaissle GB, Ziemssen F, Petermeier K, Szurman P, Ladewig M, Gelisken F, Völker M, Holz FG, Bartz-Schmidt KU: Bevacizumab zur Therapie des sekundären Makulaödems nach venösen Gefässverschlüssen. Ophthalmologe 2006;103:471–475.

190 Rosenfeld PJ, Fung AE, Pulifito CA: Optical coherence tomography findings after an intravitreal injection of bevacizumab (Avastin) for macular edema from central retinal vein occlusion. Ophthalmic Surg Lasers Imaging 2006;36:336–339.

191 Spandau UH, Ihloff AK, Jonas JB: Intravitreal bevacizumab treatment of macular oedema due to central retinal vein occlusion. Acta Ophthalmol 2006; 84:555–556.

192 Costa RA, Jorge R, Calucci D, Melo LA Jr, Cardillo JA, Scott IU: Intravitreal bevacizumab (Avastin) for central and hemicentral retinal vein occlusions: IBeVO study. Retina 2007;27:141–149.

193 Matsumoto Y, Freund KB, Peiretti E, Cooney MJ, Ferrara DC, Yannuzzi LA: Rebound macular edema following bevacizumab (Avastin) therapy for retinal venous occlusive disease. Retina 2007;27:426–431.

194 Rabena MD, Pieramici DJ, Castellarin AA, Nasir MA, Avery RL: Intravitreal bevacizumab (Avastin) in the treatment of macular edema secondary to branch retinal vein occlusion. Retina 2007;27:419–425.

195 Campochiaro PA, Hafiz G, Shah SM, Nguyen QD, Ying H, Do DV, Quinlan E, Zimmer-Galler I, Haller JA, Solomon SD, Sung JU, Hadi Y, Janjua KA, Jawed N, Choy DF, Arron JR: Ranibizumab for macular edema due to retinal vein occlusions: implication of VEGF as a critical stimulator. Mol Ther 2008;16:791–799.

196 Pieramici DJ, Rabena M, Castellarin AA, Nasir M, See R, Norton T, Sanchez A, Risard S, Avery RL: Ranibizumab for the treatment of macular edema associated with perfused central retinal vein occlusions. Ophthalmology 2008; 115:e47–e54.

197 Spaide RF, Chang LK, Klancnik JM, Yannuzzi LA, Sorenson J, Slakter JS, Freund KB, Klein R: Prospective study of intravitreal ranibizumab as a treatment for decreased visual acuity secondary to central retinal vein occlusion. Am J Ophthalmol 2009;147: 298–306.

198 Wroblewski JJ, Wells JA 3rd, Adamis AP, Buggage RR, Cunningham ET Jr, Goldbaum M, Guyer DR, Katz B, Altaweel MM; Pegaptanib in Central Retinal Vein Occlusion Study Group: Pegaptanib sodium for macular edema secondary to central retinal vein occlusion. Arch Ophthalmol 2009;127:374–380.

199 Epstein DL, Algvere PV, von Wendt G, Seregard S, Kvanta A: Bevacizumab for macular edema in central retinal vein occlusion: a prospective, randomized, double-masked clinical study. Ophthalmology 2012;119:1184–1189.

200 Epstein DL, Algvere PV, von Wendt G, Seregard S, Kvanta A: Benefit from bevacizumab for macular edema in central retinal vein occlusion: twelve-month results of a prospective, randomized study. Ophthalmology 2012; 119:2587–2591.

201 Zhang H, Liu ZL, Sun P, Gu F: Intravitreal bevacizumab for treatment of macular edema secondary to central retinal vein occlusion: eighteen-month results of a prospective trial. J Ocul Pharmacol Ther 2011;27:615–621.

202 Kriechbaum K, Michels S, Prager F, Georgopoulos M, Funk M, Geitzenauer W, Schmidt-Erfurth U: Intravitreal Avastin for macular oedema secondary to retinal vein occlusion: a prospective study. Br J Ophthalmol 2008;92:518–522.

203 Prager F, Michels S, Kriechbaum K, Georgopoulos M, Funk M, Geitzenauer W, Polak K, Schmidt-Erfurth U: Intravitreal bevacizumab (Avastin) for macular oedema secondary to retinal vein occlusion: 12-month results of a prospective clinical trial. Br J Ophthalmol 2009;93:452–456.

204 Ding X, Li J, Hu X, Yu S, Pan J, Tang S: Prospective study of intravitreal triamcinolone acetonide versus bevacizumab for macular edema secondary to central retinal vein occlusion. Retina 2011;31:838–845.

205 Hikichi T, Higuchi M, Matsushita T, Kosaka S, Matsushita R, Takami K, Ohtsuka H, Kitamei H, Shioya S: Two-year outcomes of intravitreal bevacizumab therapy for macular oedema secondary to branch retinal vein occlusion. Br J Ophthalmol 2014;98:195–199.

206 Kriechbaum K, Michels S, Prager F, et al: Intravitreal avastin for macular oedema secondary to retinal vein occlusion: a prospective study. Br J Ophthalmol 2008;92:518–522.

207 Costa RA, Jorge R, Calucci D, et al: Intravitreal bevacizumab (avastin) for central and hemicentral retinal vein occlusions: IBeVO study. Retina 2007; 27:141–149.

208 Ferrara DC, Koizumi H, Spaide RF: Early bevacizumab treatment of central retinal vein occlusion. Am J Ophthalmol 2007;144:864–871.

209 Pai SA, Shetty R, Vijayan PB, et al: Clinical, anatomic, and electrophysiologic evaluation following intravitreal bevacizumab for macular edema in retinal vein occlusion. Am J Ophthalmol 2007;143:601–606.

210 Ehlers JP, Decroos FC, Fekrat S: Intravitreal bevacizumab for macular edema secondary to branch retinal vein occlusion. Retina 2011;31:1856–1862.

211 Brown DM, Campochiaro PA, Singh RP, Li Z, Gray S, Saroj N, Rundle AC, Rubio RG, Murahashi WY; CRUISE Investigators: Ranibizumab for macular edema following central retinal vein occlusion: six-month primary end point results of a phase III study. Ophthalmology 2010;117:1124–1133.

212 Campochiaro PA, Brown DM, Awh CC, Lee SY, Gray S, Saroj N, Murahashi WY, Rubio RG: Sustained benefits from ranibizumab for macular edema following central retinal vein occlusion: twelve-month outcomes of a phase III study. Ophthalmology 2011; 118:2041–2049.

213 Campochiaro PA, Sophie R, Pearlman J, Brown DM, Boyer DS, Heier JS, Marcus DM, Feiner L, Patel A; RETAIN Study Group: Long-term outcomes in patients with retinal vein occlusion treated with ranibizumab: the RETAIN study. Ophthalmology 2014;121:209–219.

214 Boyer D, Heier J, Brown DM, Clark WL, Vitti R, Berliner AJ, Groetzbach G, Zeitz O, Sandbrink R, Zhu X, Beckmann K, Haller JA: Vascular endothelial growth factor Trap-Eye for macular edema secondary to central retinal vein occlusion: six-month results of the phase 3 COPERNICUS study. Ophthalmology 2012;119:1024–1032.

215 Brown DM, Heier JS, Clark WL, Boyer DS, Vitti R, Berliner AJ, Zeitz O, Sandbrink R, Zhu X, Haller JA: Intravitreal aflibercept injection for macular edema secondary to central retinal vein occlusion: 1-year results from the phase 3 COPERNICUS study. Am J Ophthalmol 2013;155:429–437.

216 Holz FG, Roider J, Ogura Y, Korobelnik JF, Simader C, Groetzbach G, Vitti R, Berliner AJ, Hiemeyer F, Beckmann K, Zeitz O, Sandbrink R: VEGF Trap-Eye for macular oedema secondary to central retinal vein occlusion: 6-month results of the phase III GALILEO study. Br J Ophthalmol 2013;97:278–284.

217 Hansen LL, Wiek J, Schade M, Müller-Stolzenburg N, Wiederholt M: Effect and compatibility of isovolaemic haemodilution in the treatment of ischaemic and non-ischaemic central retinal vein occlusion. Ophthalmologica 1989;199:90–99.

218 Hansen LL, Wiek J, Wiederholt M: A randomised prospective study of treatment of non-ischaemic central retinal vein occlusion by isovolaemic haemodilution. Br J Ophthalmol 1989;73:895–899.

219 Wolf S, Arend O, Bertram B, Remky A, Schulte K, Wald KJ, Reim M: Hemodilution therapy in central retinal vein occlusion. One-year results of a prospective randomized study. Graefes Arch Clin Exp Ophthalmol 1994;232:33–39.

220 Hattenbach LO, Wellermann G, Steinkamp GW, Scharrer I, Koch FH, Ohrloff C: Visual outcome after treatment with low-dose recombinant tissue plasminogen activator or hemodilution in ischemic central retinal vein occlusion. Ophthalmologica 1999;2136:360–366.

221 Glacet-Bernard A, Zourdani A, Milhoub M, Maraqua N, Coscas G, Soubrane G: Effect of isovolemic hemodilution in central retinal vein occlusion. Graefes Arch Clin Exp Ophthalmol 2001;239:909–914.

222 Glacet-Bernard A, Atassi M, Fardeau C, Romanet JP, Tonini M, Conrath J, Denis P, Mauget-Faÿsse M, Coscas G, Soubrane G, Souied E: Hemodilution therapy using automated erythrocytapheresis in central retinal vein occlusion: results of a multicenter randomized controlled study. Graefes Arch Clin Exp Ophthalmol 2011;249:505–512.

223 McIntosh RL, Mohamed Q, Saw SM, Wong TY: Interventions for branch retinal vein occlusion: an evidence-based systematic review. Ophthalmology 2007;114:835–854.

224 Kuppermann BD, Blumenkranz MS, Haller JA, Williams GA, Weinberg DV, Chou C, Whitcup SM; Dexamethasone DDS Phase II Study Group: Randomized controlled study of an intravitreous dexamethasone drug delivery system in patients with persistent macular edema. Arch Ophthalmol 2007;125:309–317.

225 Williams GA, Haller JA, Kuppermann BD, Blumenkranz MS, Weinberg DV, Chou C, Whitcup SM; Dexamethasone DDS Phase II Study Group: Dexamethasone posterior-segment drug delivery system in the treatment of macular edema resulting from uveitis or Irvine-Gass syndrome. Am J Ophthalmol 2009;1476:1048–1054.

226 Ramchandran RS, Fekrat S, Stinnett SS, Jaffe GJ: Fluocinolone acetonide sustained drug delivery device for chronic central retinal vein occlusion: 12-month results. Am J Ophthalmol 2008;146:285–291.

227 Otani A, Dorrell MI, Kinder K, Otero FJ, Schimmel P, Friedlander M: Rescue of retinal degeneration by intravitreally injected adult bone marrow-derived lineage-negative hematopoietic stem cells. J Clin Invest 2004;114:765–774.

228 Harris JR, Brown GA, Jorgensen M, Kaushal S, Ellis EA, Grant MB, Scott EW: Bone marrow-derived cells home to and regenerate retinal pigment epithelium after injury. Invest Ophthalmol Vis Sci 2006;47:2108–2113.

229 Smith LE: Bone marrow-derived stem cells preserve cone vision in retinitis pigmentosa. J Clin Invest 2006;114:755–757.

230 Jonas JB, Witzens-Harig M, Arseniev L, Ho AD: Intravitreal autologous bone marrow derived mononuclear cell transplantation: a feasibility report. Acta Ophthalmol 2008;86:225–226.

231 Jonas JB, Witzens-Harig M, Arseniev L, Ho AD: Intravitreal autologous bonemarrow-derived mononuclear cell transplantation. Acta Ophthalmol 2010;88:e131–e132.

232 Ma K, Xu L, Zhang H, Zhang S, Pu M, Jonas JB: Effect of brimonidine on retinal ganglion cell survival in an optic nerve crush model. Am J Ophthalmol 2009;147:326–331.

Prof. Jost B. Jonas
Universitäts-Augenklinik
Theodor-Kutzer-Ufer 1–3
DE–68167 Mannheim (Germany)
E-Mail jost.jonas@medma.uni-heidelberg.de

Coscas G (ed): Macular Edema. 2nd, revised and extended edition.
Dev Ophthalmol. Basel, Karger, 2017, vol 58, pp 168–177 (DOI: 10.1159/000455279)

Insights into the Physiopathology of Inflammatory Macular Edema

Marc D. de Smet[a, b]

[a] MicroInvasive Ocular Surgery Center, Lausanne, Switzerland; [b] Department of Ophthalmology, Leiden University, Leiden, The Netherlands

Abstract

Macular edema is one of the most common causes of permanent vision loss in patients with uveitis. The current understanding of water balance and metabolism within the retina has given us better insight into the mechanisms underlying macular edema arising from both acute and chronic inflammation. Uveitic macular edema (UME) occurs when the equilibrium between water influx and efflux is lost, and more importantly when compensatory mechanisms are overwhelmed. While in the acute setting, control of inflammation can reestablish homeostasis, chronic inflammation can lead to alternate pathways to establish a water balance. To understand UME, one must understand the regulation and consequences of inflammation at the tissular level. A fine interplay exists between inflammation and the retina replete with compensatory mechanisms, bystander effects, and structural sequelae once inflammation subsides. This understanding may allow us to develop new therapeutic strategies for the treatment of inflammatory macular edema.

Macular edema is one of the most common causes of permanent loss of vision in patients with uveitis. It may be present in up to 60% of patients with birdshot retinochoroiditis, sarcoidosis, or intermediate uveitis with a duration of more than 1 year (Lardenoye et al., 2006; Monnet et al., 2007; Johnson, 2009; de Smet and Okada, 2010)[1–4]. Even in children, its prevalence increases as a function of duration. It is present in 17% of cases at 1 year and in 35% of cases at 5 years (Smith et al., 2009)[5]. Uveitic macular edema (UME) is a consequence of chronic inflammation. The recent understanding on the mechanisms of water balance and metabolism within the retina has given insights into the mechanisms underlying macular edema arising from chronic inflammation. UME occurs when the equilibrium between water influx and efflux is lost, or more importantly when compensatory mechanisms are overwhelmed, which in chronic inflammation may be irremediably damaged. Hence, control of inflammation, which is paramount in the acute phase of the disease, is not necessarily as critical in chronic stages when atrophy and fibrosis may be more important contributors to UME, at which point a different therapeutic strategy must be adopted.

To understand UME, one must understand the regulation and consequences of inflammation at a tissular level. A fine interplay exists between inflammation and the retina replete with compensatory mechanisms, activation processes, bystander effects and sequelae once inflammation subsides. This understanding may allow us to develop new therapeutic strategies for the treatment of macular edema arising from ocular inflammation.

The Role of Inflammation

The immune response is characterized by two complementary mechanisms. The innate response is a primary, rapid, and programmed response, but it lacks memory. The adaptive response is slower but directed at specific local targets. It is capable of eliminating a pathogen in a precise and effective manner, and it can mount a rapid and specific immune response if faced with the same situation a second time. The innate immune system is primarily responsible for homeostasis and functions through three primary receptors: (1) lectins and C-reactive proteins which activate complement, (2) endocytic receptors such as Toll-like receptors which initiate a rapid immune response when activated, and (3) by recognizing alarmins, endogenous molecular proteins generated by damaged or necrotic cells (Oppenheim et al., 2005; Medzhitov and Janeway, 2002; Chovatiya and Medzhitov, 2014; Dumitriu et al., 2005)[6–9]. This latter mechanism allows the immune system to intervene in the absence of an infection and on stressed or damaged tissues, as well as favor healing or at least a return to homeostasis. Alarmins are secreted in higher amounts in the presence of free radicals, nitrous oxides and hyperglycemia. They bind to TLF and IL-1r, and induce the activation of NF-κB.

Infection and trauma are two extreme conditions that are capable of activating the innate immune pathways, but to a variable level depending on the severity of the aggression. Hence, exogenous and endogenous stressors initiate a common immune response. The level and duration of

this response will result in a reparative process (parainflammatory process) or permanent damage: The higher the oxidative stress level, the more intense the immune response. In both the brain and the retina, this response leads to an alteration in the fine homeostatic environment needed for its function. From a clinical standpoint, the observed phenotype, for example on optical coherence tomography (OCT), will depend on the degree and nature of the insult. Macular edema can be limited to the outer nuclear layer (around the Müller cell body) or extend either more superficially or into the deeper retina before it affects all retinal layers (Munk, 2014)[10]. It could lead to retinal pigment epithelium (RPE) dysfunction causing a serous retinal detachment (Ouyang et al., 2014; Tran et al., 2008)[11, 12]. It can also take more specific forms such as in the case of multiple sclerosis where a diffuse microcystic edema is observed in the inner plexiform layer (Gelfand et al., 2012)[13]. In all cases, the phenotype results from a summation of cytotoxic and vasogenic effects resulting from the immune aggression.

Cellular Components of the Retinal Immune Response and Their Regulation

Neurons, glial cells, microglia, and blood vessels are organized across the nervous system (including the retina) in neurovascular units. These are characterized by intimate physical contact and functional integration which allows a rapid, adapted physiologic response to a rapidly evolving environment. The neurovascular unit modulates and responds to the metabolic requirements and synaptic activity by adapting the influx of blood and nutrients and the evacuation of byproducts, and by responding to tissue levels of glutamate, nitrous oxide, and metabolites such as arachidonic acid (Stem and Gardner, 2013; Kur et al. 2012)[14, 15].

Immunity is mainly directed towards immunosuppression. Müller cells (the retina's glial cells) are responsible for maintaining the extracellular homeostasis in balance. Direct synaptic connections with blood vessels facilitate vascular autoregulation (Petzold and Murthy, 2011)[16], while membrane-bound aquaporin 4 (AQP4) and the potassium-rectifying channel (KIR4.1) allow a direct regulation of the electrolyte levels within the extracellular space and hence the transmembrane potentials required for nerve transmission (Koferl et al., 2014)[17]. Microglial cells monitor the cellular integrity of the retina and its synaptic activity (Schafer et al., 2012)[18]. It prunes the synaptic terminals of neuronal cells and disposes of any senescent cells. There are multiple effects of having inflammatory mediators in this fine equilibrium.

Macular edema arises when there is either an overwhelming influx of fluid inside the retina, or when the drainage mechanisms for water and electrolytes are inadequate. Both components are subject to the influences of inflammation. A breach in the blood-retinal barrier will increase oncotic pressure leading to vasogenic edema; however, in the absence of a visible leak on angiography or in the presence of a serous retinal detachment, we are witness to a disequilibrium in the drainage mechanisms, in particular to a dysfunction in the pump function of the RPE and more specifically to transmembrane ionic channels (Na^+, K^+, Cl^-, HCO_3^-) and AQP1 (Koferl et al., 2014; Stamer et al., 2003; Wimmers et al., 2007)[17, 19, 20].

Microglial and Dendritic Cells
Microglial cells as well as retinal dendritic cells are responsible for immune surveillance within the retina. In their resting state, their immunologic profile is directed towards tolerance and immunosuppression, but they can be converted to a proinflammatory response (Forrester et al., 2010)[21]. Microglial cells originate during fetal development, as their brain homologues, from the allantoic sac, and once located in the retina replicate locally for the remainder of a person's life

(Brendecke and Prinz, 2015; Prinz et al., 2014)[22, 23]. Tissue macrophages derived from bone marrow are found adjacent to blood vessels. However, these may also repopulate the retina as shown experimentally when microglial cells are depleted, or possibly following a major breech of the immune system (Xu et al., 2007)[24].

In a resting state, microglial cells are dendritic in shape. They modify their shape as a function of their degree of immunologic activation (Xu et al., 2009)[25]. In an activated state, they take on an amoeboid form and migrate to the subretinal space as observed in diabetes, retinal detachments, and inflammatory states (Xu et al., 2009; Omri et al., 2011; Hollborn et al., 2008)[25–27]. Their presence in the subretinal space is not necessarily deleterious to retinal function. Indeed, in the elderly, they are observed without causing a change in the morphology of the retina. However, in diabetes, their accumulation above the RPE is linked to cellular dysfunction (Omri et al., 2011)[26]. Under normal circumstances, microglial cells are evacuated through the RPE to the choroid through a mechanism of transcellular migration, similar to that observed in vascular endothelium elsewhere in the body (Dejana, 2006)[28]. In diabetes, this mechanism becomes progressively dysfunctional, leading to an accumulation of activated cells in the subretinal space. A similar mechanism has not yet been identified for other ocular inflammatory states, but is likely present. Once beyond the blood-retinal barrier, the course of microglial cells has not been clearly established. However, within the choroid, an extensive plexus of regulatory cells can be found adjacent to the RPE.

Whether the antigenic stimulus is exogenous or of local origin, microglial cells, once activated, will multiply and express surface markers typical of proinflammatory-presenting cells. Their numbers will increase throughout the retina, in particular adjacent to blood vessels. Expressed markers will vary from species to species, according to age, health, and prior immune status (Kettenmann et al., 2011; Meeuwsen et al., 2004)[29, 30]. At a minimum, one can expect an increase in the expression of HLA-DR, CD45, and CD68 (Zeng et al., 2008; Rungger-Brändle et al., 2000)[31, 32], chemokines CCL2 (MCP-1), CX3CR1 (Rangasamy et al., 2014; Zhang et al., 2009; Zhang et al., 2012)[33–35]. The secretion of cytokines such as IL-8 and IL-1 also increases, but the degree and nature of the secreted cytokines remains to be defined and varies depending on the specifics of the immune stressors (Meeuwsen et al., 2004)[30]. Once inflammation is present, these various soluble factors will profoundly influence Müller cells and their ability to regulate the extracellular space (Kettenmann et al., 2011; Abcouwer, 2013; Saijo and Glass, 2011)[29, 36, 37].

Müller Cells
Müller cells are the most important retinal macroglial cells insuring important physiologic functions. They ensure structural integrity and provide a functional link between neural elements and the vascular network. They form a metabolic symbiosis with neural elements and participate in the processing (transmission) of visual information. They facilitate the transfer of nutrients from the blood to the neural circuity as well as evacuate metabolic by-products. Homeostasis within the retinal extracellular space is ensured by active transport mechanisms located within their cell membranes (Bringmann et al., 2006)[38]. In a resting state, Müller cells are an important source of pigment epithelium-derived factor (PEDF), thereby playing a role in the regulation of retinal angiogenesis. This situation changes under conditions of stress, at which point they can secrete important amounts of vascular endothelial growth factor (VEGF), leading to an increase in vascular permeability and possibly neovascularization (Bringmann et al., 2006; Bai et al., 2009)[38, 39]. Müller cells swell in the presence of inflammatory stimuli, contributing to the formation of edema. In endotoxin-induced uveitis, this swelling can persist for several days following the removal of the inciting antigen (Pannicke et al., 2005)[40]. Swelling has also been observed in the presence of arachidonic acid and prostaglandin E_2, both of which are known as causes of inflammatory macular edema, particularly following surgery (Pannicke et al., 2005; Miyake and Ibaraki, 2002)[40, 41].

Under normal circumstances, Müller cells do not express HLA class II antigens and do not participate in immunosurveillance. In a nonactivated state, they are immunosuppressive (Caspi and Roberge, 1989)[42]. However, in the presence of activated T-helper cells, INFγ, or major oxidative stresses, they transform themselves into efficient presenting cells, thus promoting inflammation. In the presence of certain viruses, they synthesize a number of inflammatory cytokines including IL-6, TNFα, INFα, INFβ, INFγ, and IL-8 (Reichenbach and Bringmann, 2010; Roberge et al., 1988; Bringmann and Wiedemann, 2012)[43–45], as well as chemokines such as CCL2 (Zhang et al., 2009; Rutar et al., 2015)[34, 46]. This proinflammatory state only persists under conditions of continued stimulation. Once the inflammatory stimulus is gone, the Müller cells return to their immunosuppressive state.

Retinal Pigment Epithelial Cells
Given its position at the interface between the retina and choroid, the RPE has an important adjunctive regulatory role, though it is not strictly speaking part of the immune system. Its physiologic role in the egress of microglial cells out of the retina and into the choroid has already been mentioned earlier. Ingress of inflammatory cells from the choriocapillaris to the retina is prevented by the tight junctions present between RPE cells, and the absence of a transcellular pathway in this direction. The RPE normally secretes a number of suppressive soluble factors such as TGFβ, somatostatin, and thrombospondin (Zamiri et al., 2007)[47]. It helps modulate T-regulatory cells toward an immunosuppressive profile (Zamiri et al., 2007; Sugita et al., 2008)[47, 48].

In the presence of inflammation, however, RPE participates in the amplification of the response through the expression of Toll-like receptors, in particular 3 and 9. These are particularly important in innate immunity directed to viruses, as well as the secretion of IFNβ, IL-1, IL-6, IL-8, and MCP-1 (Kumar et al., 2004; Ebihara et al., 2007)[49, 50]. Oxidative stress, lipopolysaccharide, and age can lead to the secretion of inflammatory factors such as IL-8 (Xu et al., 2009)[25]. Once activated, the RPE favors the maturation of monocytes and macrophages, and gains the ability to present antigens to the immune system (Percopo et al., 1990)[51]. With increased levels of IL-1, IL-2, and TNFα in its vicinity, synthesis of cyclooxygenases, in particular COX-2, is initiated. The latter is responsible for the synthesis of prostaglandin E_2 and prostaglandin $F_{2\alpha}$, which are well known for their role in inflammatory macular edema (Chin et al., 2001)[52].

Tight junctions between RPE cells maintain the outer blood retinal barrier and slow the transepithelial diffusion of proteins and water. Increases in TNFα levels on the apical side of the barrier will lead to an increase in permeability (Peng et al., 2012)[53]. Much less response is observed to other modulators such as IL-1β and INFγ, which are usually active at the level of endothelial tight junctions, indicative of the specificity of the RPE tissue (Peng et al., 2012; Abe et al., 2003)[53, 54].

Mechanistic Pathways of Inflammatory Macular Edema

Cytotoxic Macular Edema
Optimal function of the retinal neurovascular unit requires a rapid adaptation to a highly variable neural activity, which necessitates a rapid flux of H_2O and ions. Neural depolarization leads to a rapid inward migration of sodium and calcium into nerve cells, while potassium is excreted. A buffer for excess extracellular potassium is provided by Müller cells. Potassium-rectifying channels Kir4.1 and Kir2.1 ensure a rapid transfer of K^+ into the intracellular space of Müller. In a noninflamed state, Kir2.1 is expressed in proximity to cells involved in the neural signal transmission (these are bidirectional K^+ channels), while Kir4.1 is found close to retinal capillaries where it promotes in conjunction with AQP4 the extrusion of water and K^+ ions to the blood circulation (Kofuji et al., 2002)[55]. Under normal conditions, water and ionic flow are in the direction of retinal capillaries through ATP-dependent active transport mechanisms (Kusaka and Puro, 1997)[56].

A very different picture is found in the presence of inflammation. The distribution of Kir4.1 receptors is more diffuse along the surface of cells with a certain preponderance for the apical surface of the Müller cell close to the external limiting membrane. However, the overall synthesis of Kir channels is decreased (Pannicke et al., 2005; Liu et al., 2007)[40, 57]. These alterations favor the formation of intracellular edema and the accumulation of subretinal fluid, both of which are characteristic of UME (Tran et al., 2008)[12]. These functional alterations in Müller cells are seen as fundamental mechanisms leading to the formation of cytotoxic macular edema. In its pure form, this edema is characterized by the absence of leakage on fluorescein angiography despite manifest edema on the OCT. It is more commonly observed in older individuals, possibly because Müller cells are less able to excrete water and potassium ions as a result of a progressive loss of Kir proteins with age (Bringmann et al., 2003)[58].

Earlier we mentioned the role of microglial cells in immune surveillance and cellular homeostasis. As mentioned, when they express class II antigens, they become antigen-presenting cells. They also secrete multiple cytokines such as IL-1, IL-8, CCL2, and CX3CR1, which lead to activation of Müller cells, escalating the development of edema (Zeng et al., 2008; Rungger-Brändle et al., 2000; Rangasamy et al., 2014; Zhang et al., 2009; Zhang et al., 2012)[31–35].

Vasogenic Macular Edema
In most cases of inflammatory macular edema, there is an important vasogenic component. Activated Müller and microglial cells secrete VEGF, TNFα, IL-1β, and prostaglandins, which leads to a loss of integrity of the blood-retinal barrier as desmosomes present between capillary endothelial cells and between cells of the RPE are lost (Wang et al., 2015; Wang et al., 2010; Claudio et al., 1994; Luna et al., 1997; Derevjanik et al., 2002)[59–63]. Other proteins present in the complement or coagulation cascades also have an effect on edema, in particular thrombin and fibrinogen (Pollreisz et al., 2013; Joshi et al., 2013)[64, 65]. In response to tissue injury caused for example by vitreoretinal traction, these appear in the extracellular space where they favor the appearance of breaks in the blood-retinal barrier as well as favor the secretion of VEGF (Bian, 2007)[66].

Retinal capillaries are surrounded by Müller cells. A breach in the blood-retinal barrier leads to a rapid activation of Müller cells during an ischemic or inflammatory insult (Rungger-Brändle et al., 2000)[32]. The maintenance of an intact blood-retinal barrier is favored by the secretion of soluble factors such as GDNF, thrombospondin-1, TGFβ, and PEDF by retinal tissue macrophages and microglial and Müller cells (Igarashi et al., 2000; Yafai et al., 2013)[67, 68]. PEDF regulates the secretion of VEGF (Aymerich et al., 2001)[69]. PEDF is itself regulated by retinoic acid levels and 17β-estradiol produced by endothelial cells (Yafai et al., 2007)[70]. A drop in the secretion of PEDF in the presence of inflammation leads to an increase in the secretion of VEGF with an associated increase in capillary permeability (Yafai et al., 2007; Zhang et al., 2006)[70, 71]. Parallel to its VEGF secretion, inflamed Müller cells produce matrix metalloproteases such as MMP-9, leading to the proteolysis of occludin and the loss of blood-retinal barrier integrity (Behzadian et al., 2001; Giebel et al., 2005; De Groef et al., 2015)[72–74]. Modulation of the MMP secretion is mediated by levels of TNFα and basic fibroblast factor.

Other Contributing Factors
When actively involved in retinal traction, epiretinal membranes can contribute to macular edema. Mechanical stress concentrated onto a limited number of Müller cells can induce the secretion of inflammatory and vasogenic factors (Schubert, 1989)[75]. Few studies have analyzed the interplay between inflammation and membrane formation. We know that inflammation contributes to the formation of membranes (Joshi et al., 2013)[65], but these do not progress in the absence of inflammatory factors (Nazari and Rao, 2013)[76]. A distinctive finding in inflammatory membranes is the presence of a significant number of microglial cells, macrophages, and Müller cell extensions (Snead et al., 2008; Sheybani et al., 2012)[77, 78]. Soluble inflammatory factors often found in association with such membranes are TNFα, activated complement (both classic and alternative pathways), fibrinogen, and constitutive elements of the innate immune response (Pollreisz et al., 2013; Harada et al., 2006)[64, 79]. Hence, inflammation can lead to the appearance or the exacerbation of tractional epiretinal membranes (Harada et al., 2006; Theocharis, 2010; Wynn and Ramalingam, 2012)[79–81]. The growth of preexisting membranes can be interpreted as a sign of active inflammation, indicating the possible need for a therapeutic intervention – either medical or surgical.

Macular ischemia is often present in inflammatory macular edema (de Smet and Okada, 2010; Forooghian et al., 2009)[4, 82]. It is more often present in Behçet's disease, collagenopathies, granulomatous uveitis, and ocular sacoïdosis (de Smet and Okada, 2010; Forooghian et al., 2009; Bentley et al., 1993)[4, 82, 83]. Retinal ischemia leads to an increase in the levels of extracellular glutamate which initially leads to swelling of ganglion cells, which may on occasion been seen on OCT as small lacunae within the ganglion cell layer (Burggraaff et al., 2014)[84]. In a more advanced stage, Müller cells swell, leading to the swelling of the internal nuclear layer and the appearance of lacunae on OCT within this layer (Burggraaff et al., 2014; Saidha et al., 2012; Kaur et al., 2007; Da and Verkman, 2004)[84–87]. An alteration in the transport mechanisms for water and ions is at the source of these manifestations, and these can be blocked by normalizing the expression of AQP4 and Kir4.1 (Da and Verkman, 2004; Rehak et al., 2009)[87, 88]. By adding corticosteroids, Müller cell swelling is reduced, though different steroids will have diverging effects on the cell surface expression of these channels (Zhao et al., 2011; Pannicke et al., 2006; Uckermann et al., 2005)[89–91]. A therapeutic effect in this context is not necessarily linked to an anti-inflammatory effect, but to a better regulation of water balance, often required in the presence of chronic macular edema both experimentally and clinically. Better water regulation is not limited to Müller cells, but also extends to the efficacy of the pump present in the RPE (Reichenbach and Bringmann, 2010)[92].

Late Consequences of Macular Edema
Chronic edema leads to significant structural changes in the retina. Yanoff observed that some cases of chronic macular edema was associated with the presence of large cysts, and the swelling of endothelial cells leading to a near complete obstruction of the vascular lumen (Yanoff et al., 1984)[93]. Leakage from the perifoveal capillary network in the absence of retinal inflammation has been observed on fluorescein angiography in several cases, sometimes accompanied by late staining of the optic nerve (de Smet and Okada, 2010; Pelitli Gürlü et al., 2007)[4, 94]. Loss of Müller cells by apoptosis in more chronic states leads to the formation of large cysts, often in association with swelling of neighboring surviving Müller cells (Wolter, 1981)[95]. It is possible to predict residual acuity by the density of residual Müller cells on transverse OCT (Pelosini et al., 2011)[96]. Even at this late stage, it is possible to recover some visual function by eliminating residual edema and increasing the pump function of Müller cells and the RPE pump (de Smet and Okada, 2010)[4].

References

1 Lardenoye CW, van Kooij B, Rothova A: Impact of macular edema on visual acuity in uveitis. Ophthalmology 2006;113: 1446–1449.

2 Monnet D, et al: Longitudinal cohort study of patients with birdshot chorioretinopathy. III. Macular imaging at baseline. Am J Ophthalmol 2007;144: 818–828.

3 Johnson MW: Etiology and treatment of macular edema. Am J Ophthalmol 2009; 147:11–21.e1.

4 de Smet MD, Okada AA: Cystoid macular edema in uveitis. Dev Ophthalmol 2010;47:136–147.

5 Smith JA, et al: Epidemiology and course of disease in childhood uveitis. Ophthalmology 2009;116:1544–1551.

6 Oppenheim JJ, et al: Autoantigens act as tissue-specific chemoattractants. J Leukoc Biol 2005;77:854–861.

7 Medzhitov R, Janeway CA Jr: Decoding the patterns of self and nonself by the innate immune system. Science 2002; 296:298–300.

8 Chovatiya R, Medzhitov R: Stress, inflammation, and defense of homeostasis. Mol Cell 2014;54:281–288.

9 Dumitriu IE, Baruah P, Manfredi AA, Bianchi ME, Rovere-Quierini P: HMGB1: guiding immunity from within. Trends Immunol 2005;26:381–387.

10 Munk MR, et al: Influence of the vitreomacular interface on the efficacy of intravitreal therapy for uveitis-associated cystoid macular oedema. Acta Ophthalmol 2015;93:e561–e567.

11 Ouyang Y, et al: Evaluation of cystoid change phenotypes in ocular toxoplasmosis using optical coherence tomography. PLoS One 2014;9:e86626.

12 Tran TH, et al: Uveitic macular oedema: correlation between optical coherence tomography patterns with visual acuity and fluorescein angiography. Br J Ophthalmol 2008;92:922–927.

13 Gelfand JM, Nolan R, Schwartz DM, Graves J, Green AJ: Microcystic macular oedema in multiple sclerosis is associated with disease severity. Brain 2012; 135:1786–1793.

14 Stem MS, Gardner TW: Neurodegeneration in the pathogenesis of diabetic retinopathy: molecular mechanisms and therapeutic implications. Curr Med Chem 2013;20:3241–3250.

15 Kur J, Newman EA, Chan-Ling T: Cellular and physiological mechanisms underlying blood flow regulation in the retina and choroid in health and disease. Prog Retin Eye Res 2012;31:377–406.

16 Petzold GC, Murthy VN: Role of astrocytes in neurovascular coupling. Neuron 2011;71:782–797.

17 Koferl P, et al: Effects of arteriolar constriction on retinal gene expression and Müller cell responses in a rat model of branch retinal vein occlusion. Graefes Arch Clin Exp Ophthalmol 2014;252:257–265.

18 Schafer DP, et al: Microglia sculpt postnatal neural circuits in an activity and complement-dependent manner. Neuron 2012;74:691–705.

19 Stamer WD, Bok D, Hu J, Jaffe GJ, McKay BS: Aquaporin-1 channels in human retinal pigment epithelium: role in transepithelial water movement. Invest Ophthalmol Vis Sci 2003;44:2803.

20 Wimmers S, Karl MO, Strauss O: Ion channels in the RPE. Prog Retin Eye Res 2007;26:263–301.

21 Forrester JV, Xu H, Kuffová L, Dick AD, McMenamin PG: Dendritic cell physiology and function in the eye. Immunol Rev 2010;234:282–304.

22 Brendecke SM, Prinz M: Do not judge a cell by its cover – diversity of CNS resident, adjoining and infiltrating myeloid cells in inflammation. Semin Immunopathol 2015;37:591–605.

23 Prinz M, Tay TL, Wolf Y, Jung S: Microglia: unique and common features with other tissue macrophages. Acta Neuropathol 2014;128:319–331.

24 Xu H, Chen M, Mayer EJ, Forrester JV, Dick AD: Turnover of resident retinal microglia in the normal adult mouse. Glia 2007;55:1189–1198.

25 Xu H, Chen M, Forrester JV: Para-inflammation in the aging retina. Prog Retin Eye Res 2009;28:348–368.

26 Omri S, et al: Microglia/macrophages migrate through retinal epithelium barrier by a transcellular route in diabetic retinopathy: role of PKCζ in the Goto Kakizaki rat model. Am J Pathol 2011;179:942–953.

27 Hollborn M, et al: Early activation of inflammation- and immune response-related genes after experimental detachment of the porcine retina. Invest Ophthalmol Vis Sci 2008;49:1262–1273.

28 Dejana E: The transcellular railway: insights into leukocyte diapedesis. Nat Cell Biol 2006;8:105–107.

29 Kettenmann H, Hanisch UK, Noda M, Verkhratsky A: Physiology of microglia. Physiol Rev 2011;91:461–553.

30 Meeuwsen S, Bsibsi M, Persoon-Deen C, Ravid R, van Noort JM: Cultured human adult microglia from different donors display stable cytokine, chemokine and growth factor gene profiles but respond differently to a pro-inflammatory stimulus. Neuroimmunomodulation 2004;12:235–245.

31 Zeng HY, Green WR, Tso MO: Microglial activation in human diabetic retinopathy. Arch Ophthalmol 2008;126:227–232.

32 Rungger-Brändle E, Dosso AA, Leuenberger PM: Glial reactivity, an early feature of diabetic retinopathy. Invest Ophthalmol Vis Sci 2000;41:1971–1980.

33 Rangasamy S, et al: Chemokine mediated monocyte trafficking into the retina: role of inflammation in alteration of the blood-retinal barrier in diabetic retinopathy. PLoS One 2014;9:e108508.

34 Zhang W, et al: NAD(P)H oxidase-dependent regulation of CCL2 production during retinal inflammation. Invest Ophthalmol Vis Sci 2009;50:3033–3040.

35 Zhang M, Xu G-T, Liu W, Ni Y, Zhou W: Role of fractalkine/CX3CR1 interaction in light-induced photoreceptor degeneration through regulating retinal microglial activation and migration. PLoS One 2012;7:e35446.

36 Abcouwer SF: Angiogenic factors and cytokines in diabetic retinopathy. J Clin Cell Immunol 2013; Suppl 1: DOI: 10.4172/2155-9899.

37 Saijo K, Glass CK: Microglial cell origin and phenotypes in health and disease. Nat Rev Immunol 2011;11:775–787.

38 Bringmann A, et al: Müller cells in the healthy and diseased retina. Prog Retin Eye Res 2006;25:397–424.

39 Bai Y, et al: Müller cell-derived VEGF is a significant contributor to retinal neovascularization. J Pathol 2009;219:446–454.

40 Pannicke T, et al: Ocular inflammation alters swelling and membrane characteristics of rat Müller glial cells. J Neuroimmunol 2005;161:145–154.

41 Miyake K, Ibaraki N: Prostaglandins and cystoid macular edema. Surv Ophthalmol 2002;47:S203–S218.

42 Caspi RR, Roberge FG: Glial cells as suppressor cells: characterization of the inhibitory function. J Autoimmunity 1989;2:709–722.

43 Reichenbach A, Bringmann A: Immunomodulatory role of Müller cells; in: Müller Cells in the Healthy and Diseased Retina. Heidelberg, Springer, 2010, pp 249–251.

44 Roberge FG, Caspi RR, Nussenblatt RB: Glial retinal Müller cells produce IL-1 activity and have a dual effect on autoimmune T helper lymphocytes. Antigen presentation manifested after removal of suppressive activity. J Immunol 1988;140:2193–2196.

45 Bringmann A, Wiedemann P: Müller glial cells in retinal disease. Ophthalmologica 2012;227:1–19.

46 Rutar M, Natoli R, Chia R, Valter K, Provis JM: Chemokine-mediated inflammation in the degenerating retina is coordinated by Müller cells, activated microglia, and retinal pigment epithelium. J Neuroinflammation 2015;12:8.

47 Zamiri P, Sugita S, Streilein JW: Immunosuppressive properties of the pigmented epithelial cells and the subretinal space. Chem Immunol Allergy 2007;92:86–93.

48 Sugita S, et al: Retinal pigment epithelium-derived CTLA-2 alpha induced TGFbeta-producing T regulatory cells. J Immunol 2008;181:7525–7536.

49 Kumar MV, Nagineni CN, Chin MS, Hooks JJ, Detrick B: Innate immunity in the retina: Toll-like receptor (TLR) signaling in human retinal pigment epithelial cells. J Neuroimmunol 2004;153:7–15.

50 Ebihara N, et al: Distinct functions between toll-like receptors 3 and 9 in retinal pigment epithelial cells. Ophthalmic Res 2007;39:155–163.

51 Percopo CM, Hooks JJ, Shinohara T, Caspi RR, Detrick B: Cytokine-mediated activation of a neuronal retinal resident cell provokes antigen presentation. J Immunol 1990;145:4101–4107.

52 Chin MS, Nagineni CN, Hooper LC, Detrick B, Hooks JJ: Cyclooxygenase-2 gene expression and regulation in human retinal pigment epithelial cells. Invest Ophthalmol Vis Sci 2001;42:2338–2346.

53 Peng S, Gan G, Rao VS, Adelman RA, Rizzolo LJ: Effects of proinflammatory cytokines on the claudin-19 rich tight junctions of human retinal pigment epithelium. Invest Ophthalmol Vis Sci 2012;53:5016–5028.

54 Abe T, Sugano E, Saigo Y, Tamai M: Interleukin-1 beta and barrier function of retinal pigment epithelial cells (ARPE-19): aberrant expression of junctional complex molecules. Invest Ophthalmol Vis Sci 2003;44:4097–4104.

55 Kofuji P, et al: Kir potassium channel subunit expression in retinal glial cells: implications for spatial potassium buffering. Glia 2002;39:292–303.

56 Kusaka S, Puro DG: Intracellular ATP activates inwardly rectifying K$^+$ channels in human and monkey retinal Müller (glial) cells. J Physiol 1997;500:593–604.

57 Liu XQ, Kobayashi H, Jin ZB, Wada A, Nao-I N: Differential expression of Kir4.1 and aquaporin 4 in the retina from endotoxin-induced uveitis rat. Mol Vis 2007;13:309–317.

58 Bringmann A, Kohen L, Wolf S, Wiedemann P, Reichenbach A: Age-related decrease in potassium currents in human retinal glial (Müller) cells. Can J Ophthalmol 2003;38:464–468.

59 Wang JJ, Zhu M, Le YZ: Functions of Müller cell-derived vascular endothelial growth factor in diabetic retinopathy. World J Diabetes 2015;6:726–733.

60 Wang J, Xu X, Elliott MH, Zhu M, Le YZ: Müller cell-derived VEGF is essential for diabetes-induced retinal inflammation and vascular leakage. Diabetes 2010;59:2297–2305.

61 Claudio L, Martiney LA, Brosnan CF: Ultrastructural studies of the blood-retina barrier after exposure to interleukin-1 beta or tumor necrosis factor-alpha. Lab Invest 1994;70:850–861.

62 Luna JD, et al: Blood-retinal barrier (BRB) breakdown in experimental autoimmune uveoretinitis: comparison with vascular endothelial growth factor, tumor necrosis factor α, and interleukin-1β-mediated breakdown. J Neurosci Res 1997;49:268–280.

63 Derevjanik NL, et al: Quantitative assessment of the integrity of the blood-retinal barrier in mice. Invest Ophthalmol Vis Sci 2002;43:2462–2467.

64 Pollreisz A, et al: Quantitative proteomics of aqueous and vitreous fluid from patients with idiopathic epiretinal membranes. Exp Eye Res 2013;108:48–58.

65 Joshi M, Agrawal S, Christoforidis JB: Inflammatory mechanisms of idiopathic epiretinal membrane formation. Mediators Inflamm 2013;2013:192582.

66 Bian ZM, Elner SG, Elner VM: Thrombin-induced VEGF expression in human retinal pigment epithelial cells. Invest Ophthalmol Vis Sci 2007;48:2738–2746.

67 Igarashi Y, et al: Expression of receptors for glial cell line-derived nerotrophic factor (GNDF) and neurturin in the inner blood-retinal barrier of rats. Cell Struct Funct 2000;25:237–241.

68 Yafai Y, et al: Basic fibroblast growth factor contributes to a shift in the angioregulatory activity of retinal glial (Müller) cells. PLoS One 2013;8:e68773.

69 Aymerich MS, Alberdi EM, Martinez A, Becerra SP: Evidence for pigment epithelium-derived factor receptors in the neural retina. Invest Ophthalmol Vis Sci 2001;42:3287–3293.

70 Yafai Y, Lange J, Wiedemann P, Reichenbach A, Eichler W: Pigment epithelium-derived factor acts as an opponent of growth-stimulatory factors in retinal glial-endothelial cell interactions. Glia 2007;55:642–651.

71 Zhang SX, et al: Pigment epithelium-derived factor (PEDF) is an endogenous antiinflammatory factor. FASEB J 2006;20:323–325.

72 Behzadian MA, Wang XL, Windsor LJ, Ghaly N, Caldwell RB: TGF-beta increases retinal endothelial cell permeability by increasing MMP-9: possible role of glial cells in endothelial barrier function. Invest Ophthalmol Vis Sci 2001;42:853–859.

73 Giebel SJ, Menicucci G, McGuire PG, Das A: Matrix metalloproteinases in early diabetic retinopathy and their role in the alteration of the blood-retinal barrier. Lab Invest 2005;85:597–607.

74 De Groef L, et al: Decreased TNF levels and improved retinal ganglion cell survival in MMP-2 null mice suggest a role for MMP-2 as TNF Sheddase. Mediators Inflamm 2015;2015:108617.

75 Schubert HD: Cystoid macular edema: the apparent role of mechanical factors. Prog Clin Biol Res 1989;312:277–291.

76 Nazari H, Rao N: Longitudinal morphometric analysis of epiretinal membrane in patients with uveitis. Ocul Immunol Inflamm 2013;21:2–7.

77 Snead DR, James S, Snead MP: Pathological changes in the vitreoretinal junction 1: epiretinal membrane formation. Eye (Lond) 2008;22:1310–1317.

78 Sheybani A, Harocopos GJ, Rao PK: Immunohistochemical study of epiretinal membranes in patients with uveitis. J Ophthalmic Inflamm Infect 2012;2:243–248.

79 Harada C, Mitamura Y, Harada T: The role of cytokines and trophic factors in epiretinal membranes: involvement of signal transduction in glial cells. Prog Retin Eye Res 2006;25:149–164.

80 Theocharis IP: Fibrinogen and rhegmatogenous retinal detachment: a pilot prospective study. Clin Ophthalmol 2010;4:73–76.

81 Wynn TA, Ramalingam TR: Mechanisms of fibrosis: therapeutic translation for fibrotic disease. Nat Med 2012;18:1028–1040.

82 Forooghian F, Yeh S, Faia LJ, Nussenblatt RB: Uveitis foveal atrophy. Arch Ophthalmol 2009;127:179–186.

83 Bentley CR, Stanford MR, Shilling JS, Sanders MD, Graham EM: Macular ischemia in posterior uveitis. Eye 1993;7:411–414.

84 Burggraaff MC, Trieu J, de Vries-Knoppert WA, Balk L, Petzold A: The clinical spectrum of microcystic macular edema. Invest Ophthalmol Vis Sci 2014;55:952–961.

85 Saidha S, et al: Microcystic macular oedema, thickness of the inner nuclear layer of the retina, and disease characteristics in multiple sclerosis: a retrospective study. Lancet Neurol 2012;11:963–972.

86 Kaur C, et al: Blood-retinal barrier disruption and ultrastructural changes in the hypoxic retina in adult rats: the beneficial effect of melatonin administration. J Pathol 2007;212:429–439.

87 Da T, Verkman AS: Aquaporin-4 gene disruption in mice protects against impaired retinal function and cell death after ischemia. Invest Ophthalmol Vis Sci 2004;45:4477–4483.

88 Rehak M, et al: Retinal gene expression and Muller cell responses after branch retinal vein occlusion in the rat. Invest Ophthalmol Vis Sci 2009;50:2359–2367.

89 Zhao M, et al: Differential regulations of AQP4 and Kir4.1 by triamcinolone acetonide and dexamethasone in the healthy and inflamed retina. Invest Ophthalmol Vis Sci 2011;52:6340–6347.

90 Pannicke T, et al: Diabetes alters osmotic swelling characteristics and membrane conductance of glial cells in rat retina. Diabetes 2006;55:633–639.

91 Uckermann O, et al: The glucocorticoid triamcinolone acetonide inhibits osmotic swelling of retinal glial cells via stimulation of endogenous adenosine signaling. J Pharmacol Exp Ther 2005;315:1036–1045.

92 Reichenbach A, Bringmann A: Müller cells in the diseased retina; in: Müller Cells in the Healthy and Diseased Retina. Heidelberg, Springer, 2010. pp 215–301.

93 Yanoff M, Fine BS, Brucker AJ, Eagle RC Jr: Pathology of human cystoid macular edema. Surv Ophthalmol 1984;28:505–511.

94 Pelitli Gürlü V, Alimgil ML, Esgin H: Fluorescein angiographic findings in cases with intermediate uveitis in the inactive phase. Can J Ophthalmol 2007;42:107–109.

95 Wolter JR: The histopathology of cystoid macular edema. Albrecht Von Graefes Arch Clin Exp Ophthalmol 1981;216:85–101.

96 Pelosini L, et al: Optical coherence tomography may be used to predict visual acuity in patients with macular edema. Invest Ophthalmol Vis Sci 2011;52:2741–2748.

Marc D. de Smet, MD, CM, PhD, FRCSC, FMH, FEBO
MicroInvasive Ocular Surgery Center
Avenue du Léman 32
CH–1003 Lausanne (Switzerland)
E-Mail mddesmet1@mac.com

Coscas G (ed): Macular Edema. 2nd, revised and extended edition.
Dev Ophthalmol. Basel, Karger, 2017, vol 58, pp 178–190 (DOI: 10.1159/000455280)

Postsurgical Cystoid Macular Edema

Dinah Zur · Anat Loewenstein

Division of Ophthalmology, Tel Aviv Sourasky Medical Center, Sackler Faculty of Medicine, Tel Aviv University, Tel Aviv, Israel

Abstract

Cystoid macular edema (CME) is a primary cause of reduced vision following both cataract and successful vitreoretinal surgery. The incidence of clinical CME following
modern cataract surgery is 0.1–2.35%. Preexisting conditions such as diabetes mellitus and uveitis as well as intraoperative complications can raise the risk of postsurgical
CME. The etiology of CME is not completely understood.
Prolapsed or incarcerated vitreous and postoperative inflammatory processes have been proposed as causative
agents. Pseudophakic CME is characterized by poor postoperative visual acuity. Fluorescein angiography shows
the classical perifoveal petaloid staining pattern and late
leakage of the optic disk. Optical coherence tomography
is a useful diagnostic tool, which displays cystic spaces in
the outer nuclear layer. The most important differential
diagnoses include age-related macular degeneration and
other causes of CME such as diabetic macular edema.
Most cases of pseudophakic CME resolve spontaneously.
The value of prophylactic treatment is doubtful. First-line
treatment of postsurgical CME should include topical
nonsteroidal anti-inflammatory drugs and corticosteroids. Oral carbonic anhydrase inhibitors can be considered complementary. In cases of resistant CME, periocular
or intraocular corticosteroids present an option. Antiangiogenic agents, though experimental, should be considered for nonresponsive persistent CME. Surgical options
should be reserved for special indications.

© 2017 S. Karger AG, Basel

Definition and Epidemiology

Cystoid macular edema (CME) is a primary cause of
reduced vision following both successful cataract
(Gass and Norton, 1966; Irvine, 1976)[1, 2] and vitreoretinal surgeries (Gass and Norton, 1966)[1].[a] Postsurgical CME (PCME) appears as a distressing problem
also following neodymium:yttrium-aluminum-gar-
net (Nd:YAG) capsulotomy, penetrating kerato-
plasty, scleral buckling, filtering procedures, and
panretinal photocoagulation (Shimura et al., 2009)[3].

The introduction of phacoemulsification has
led to a significant decrease of pseudophakic
CME. Still, it remains the most frequent postoperative complication resulting in impaired vision.
Although mostly self-limited, persisting cases
present a therapeutic challenge to ophthalmologists and are associated with substantial costs for
the health care system (Schmier et al., 2007)[4].

[a] Usually named Irvine-Gass syndrome, CME could more appropriately be named Hruby-Irvine-Gass Syndrome since Irvine did
not notice the foregoing biomicroscopic observations of K. Hruby.

The incidence of clinical CME following modern cataract surgery is reported as 0.1–2.35% (Henderson et al., 2007)[5]. A recent database study on 81,984 eyes found an incidence of 1.17–4.04% (Chu et al., 2015)[6]. The great variance of incidence can be explained by presence of diabetes, copathologic features, and intraoperative complications (see Risk Factors).

The appearance of angiographic CME (see below) is much more frequent, with varying incidence up to 70% in some studies (Flach, 1998)[7]. The incidence of subclinical pseudophakic CME diagnosed by optical coherence tomography (OCT) varies between 4 and 10.9% (Perente et al., 2007; Bélair et al., 2009; Vukicevic et al., 2012)[8–10].

Pathology and Pathophysiology

Histopathological Features

Histopathological specimens of CME following cataract surgery display retinal capillary dilation, serous fluid in the outer plexiform and inner nuclear layer, and inflammatory cells in the iris-ciliary perivascular complex (Neal et al., 2005)[11]. Intraretinal accumulation of fluid causes formation of perifoveal cysts, which may combine to form larger cysts and give rise to lamellar holes. In severe cases, the edema involves most of the retinal layers.

Pathophysiology

The pathogenesis of PCME is multifactorial, but remains unclear. Alterations of the retinal microenvironment contribute to the development of PCME (Hruby, 1985)[12].

Vitreous Traction

Direct macular traction from prolapsed vitreous or incarcerated iris or vitreous has been proposed as being responsible for the development of CME. The presence of fine strands of vitreous connecting the posterior vitreous face and the macular area support this theory (Tolentino and Schepens, 1965)[13].

Inflammation

The current main theory suggests a major role for inflammatory processes and increased levels of intraocular prostaglandins and other inflammatory mediators released during surgical trauma. The association of severe anterior ocular inflammation and PCME accords with this thesis (Rossetti and Autelitano, 2000)[14]. There is considerable alteration in the protein composition of the vitreous fluid after cataract extraction as compared to phakic eyes. Patients with clinical pseudophakic CME have significantly more aqueous flare than pseudophakic and phakic eyes without CME (Ersoy et al., 2013)[15]. Flare values were reported to be high in the postoperative period and decline thereafter. Following cataract surgery, inflammatory mediators like prostaglandins, cytokines, and other vasopermeability factors disrupt the blood-retinal barrier, increasing permeability of the perifoveal capillaries, resulting in perifoveal intraretinal fluid accumulation (Miyake and Ibaraki, 2002)[16].

The occasional accumulation of subretinal fluid indicates a disruption of normal apposition between the retinal pigment epithelium and photoreceptors, in contrast to the usual disruption of cell-cell contacts within the retina.

Light Damage

Phototoxicity has been suggested as another cause of CME. Light from the operating microscope was thought to increase the proportion of relatively short wavelength light entering the eye and subsequently releasing prostaglandin and advancing CME. However, this theory has been disproved (Iliff, 1985)[17].

Risk Factors

Identifying risk factors for PCME is crucial for prevention and adequate treatment. Systemic diseases, intraoperative complications, and preexisting ocular conditions influence the development of CME.

Systemic Factors
Diabetes mellitus promotes the development of CME even in the absence of diabetic retinopathy (Pollack et al., 1992)[18]. Two large database studies reported an increased rate for CME incidence after cataract extraction between 1.73 and 3.05% (RR 1.80) (Schmier et al., 2007; Chu et al., 2015)[4, 6].

Systemic hypertension apparently increases the incidence of PCME (Flach, 1998)[7]. Furthermore, it is a risk factor for retinal vein occlusion, which itself promotes development of PCME.

Complicated Surgery
Advancements in surgical techniques have significantly reduced the rate of PCME over the last decades. Intracapsular cataract extraction was much more frequently associated with PCME than extracapsular cataract extraction. Nowadays, pseudophakic CME occurs primarily in patients following uncomplicated surgery. Still, surgical complications raise the risk for PCME. Rupture of the posterior capsule (risk ratio 2.61) (Chu et al., 2015)[6] as well as secondary capsulotomy, including YAG capsulotomy, are associated with a higher rate of PCME. Remarkably, a well-designed study showed an increase in angiographic CME but no significant difference in vision following capsulotomy (Kraff et al., 1984)[19]. Vitreous loss increases the prevalence of CME by 10–20%. Vitreous prolapse to the wound prolongs CME and can be associated with a poorer prognosis (Flach, 1998)[7]. Iris incarceration, an additional risk factor for CME, may have a more important association with poor vision in patients with chronic PCME than with other intraoperative complications. Specific intraocular lenses (IOLs) are associated with increased occurrence of CME. A meta-analysis showed that the prevalence of CME is highest with implantation of an iris-fixated IOL. Anterior chamber IOLs raise the risk more than posterior chamber IOLs.

Review of patients with CME following pars plana vitrectomy for retained lens fragments revealed that 8% of eyes with a sulcus-fixated posterior chamber IOL and 46% of eyes left aphakic or with an anterior chamber IOL developed CME (Cohen et al., 2006)[20].

Preexisting Conditions
Several preexisting ocular conditions may compromise the integrity of the blood-retinal barrier and boost inflammatory activity.

In patients with uveitis, CME is the most important cause for poor visual outcome following cataract surgery, especially in the long term (Bélair et al., 2009)[9]. Uveitic eyes have an increased relative risk for the development of pseudophakic CME (RR 2.88) (Chu et al., 2015)[6]. Implantation of an IOL in cases of anterior and intermediate uveitis is controversial. As stated before, diabetes mellitus even in the absence of diabetic retinopathy increases the risk of onset for PCME. The presence of any grade of diabetic retinopathy increases the relative risk for PCME (Henderson et al., 2007; Iliff, 1985)[5, 17] up to 6.23, with a linear trend proportional to the severity of the retinopathy (Chu et al., 2015)[6].

A history of retinal vein occlusion and epiretinal membrane (ERM) also increase the risk for development of CME (Henderson et al., 2007)[5] (RR 4.47 and 5.60, respectively) (Chu et al., 2015)[6]. Caution is advised since ERM can induce macular edema without cataract surgery, and CME itself is associated with generation of ERM. Previous retinal detachment repair is another risk factor for the development of pseudophakic CME (RR 2.61) (Chu et al., 2015)[6].

The topical use of prostaglandin analogues in glaucoma patients has been reported in association with pseudophakic CME (Warwar et al., 1998)[21]. In a randomized controlled study latanoprost was shown to enhance disruption of the blood-aqueous barrier in early postoperative pseudophakia (Miyake et al., 1999)[22]. Remarkably, a retrospective database study of almost 82,000 eyes undergoing cataract surgery did not identify preoperative prostaglandin use as a risk

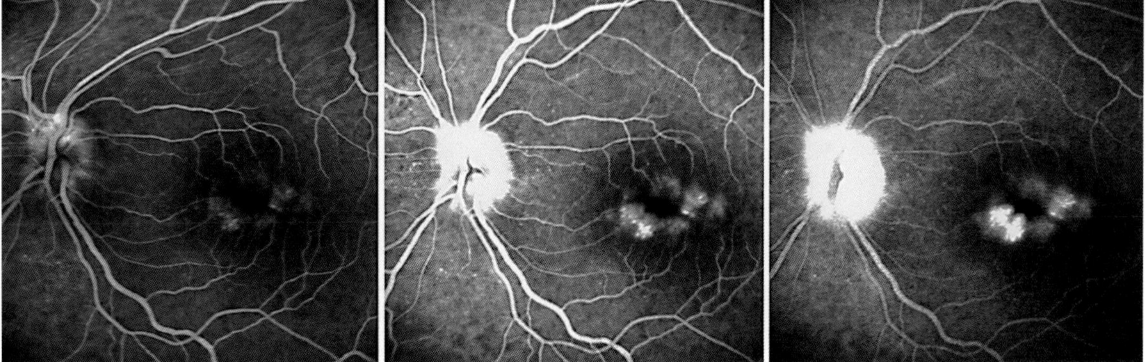

Fig. 1. FA of a patient with PCME. Note macular hyperfluorescence, which increases in size and intensity and accumulates in a petaloid shape and late staining of the optical nerve.

factor (Chu et al., 2015)[6]. However, PCME appearing under prostaglandin analogue treatment usually resolves after discontinuation of treatment and therapy with nonsteroidal anti-inflammatory drugs (NSAIDs).

Diagnosis

Clinical Findings

The most frequent sign of CME is poor postoperative visual acuity. Onset of clinically significant CME is generally 4–12 weeks after surgery and reaches its peak at 4–6 weeks postoperatively. Patients typically complain of impaired vision after an initial postoperative period of improvement. Less common complaints are positive central scotoma, metamorphopsia, low-grade eye redness, photophobia, and ocular irritation. Reduced contrast sensitivity is an early sign of diabetic macular edema that may present similarly in PCME.

In biomicroscopy, the loss of foveal depression is the most common sign of CME. The perifoveal area appears yellow xanthophyllic colored. Intraretinal cystoid spaces can be detected. Small splinter retinal hemorrhages may appear as well. In about 10% of the cases, ERMs are present. Optic nerve head swelling is frequently seen. In cases of chronic CME, small cystoid spaces fuse to foveal cysts. These patients have worse visual acuity and a worse prognosis.

Imaging
Fluorescein Angiography
Clinical examination was shown to miss the diagnosis of clinical significant CME in 5–10% of cases (Tolentino and Schepens, 1965)[13]. Fluorescein angiography (FA) is highly valuable for diagnosing CME, especially in uncertain cases. In the early phase of FA, capillary dilation and leakage from small perifoveal capillaries are visible. In later phases, pooling in the outer plexiform layer results in the classic perifoveal 'petaloid' staining pattern. In addition, late leakage and staining of the optic nerve due to capillary leakage can be seen. Improvement in CME correlates with decreased optic nerve staining. In severe CME, cystoid spaces may have a honeycomb appearance in FA, which correlates with large cystoid spaces, extending outside the immediate perifoveal region (fig. 1, 2).

Optical Coherence Tomography
OCT is an accurate and useful tool for detecting PCME. Central foveal thickness and thickness in all other macular quadrants was shown to be increased after cataract surgery and returns to pre-

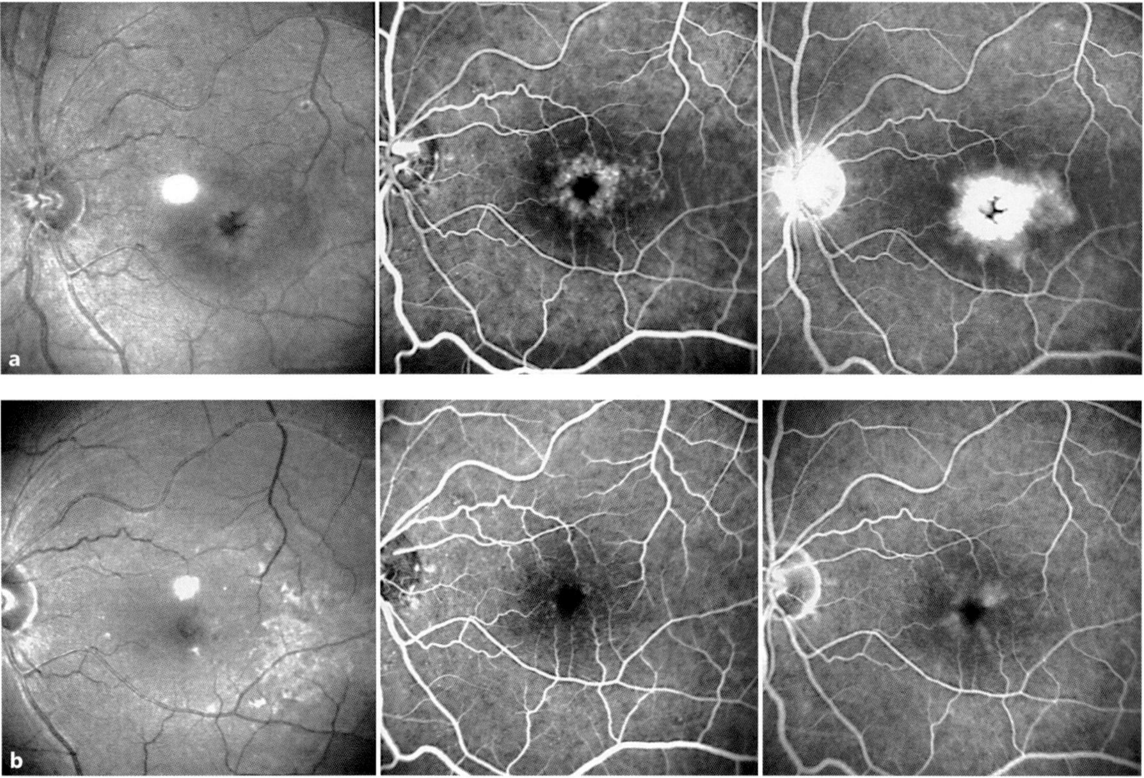

Fig. 2. Fluorescein angiogram showing the classical petaloid appearance of CME (visual acuity 20/80) (top line). The same patient after treatment with topical corticosteroids and NASIDs (visual acuity 20/25) (bottom line). Note almost complete resolution of macular hyperfluorescence and no staining of the optical nerve.

operative values 6 months postoperatively (Vukicevic et al., 2012)[10]. The peak incidence of CME, when detected by OCT, is 4 weeks after cataract surgery. Foveal thickness was found to increase significantly and correlate with decreased visual acuity, whereas control groups of pseudophakic eyes without CME showed only a minimal increase in foveal thickness and improvement in visual acuity.

Intraretinal cystoid hydration appears initially in the inner nuclear layer and proceeds to involve the outer plexiform layer; finally, accumulation of fluid in the subretinal space can be found (fig. 3) (Sigler et al., 2015)[23].

OCT provides several advantages over FA in the diagnosis of PCME: it is a noninvasive tool, avoiding injection of fluorescein and potential complications. OCT allows quantitative evaluation of structural retinal changes and is of prognostic value (fig. 4). Intactness of the photoreceptor layer and external limiting membrane is a prognostic factor for good visual outcome. Recently, Munk et al. (2015)[24] used OCT successfully in order to differentiate between diabetic and pseudophakic CME.

Functional Testing (Electrophysiology)
In electrophysiological studies – for scientific rather than for clinical use – aphakic CME is characterized by reduced amplitudes of oscillatory potentials with normal a-wave and b-wave responses.

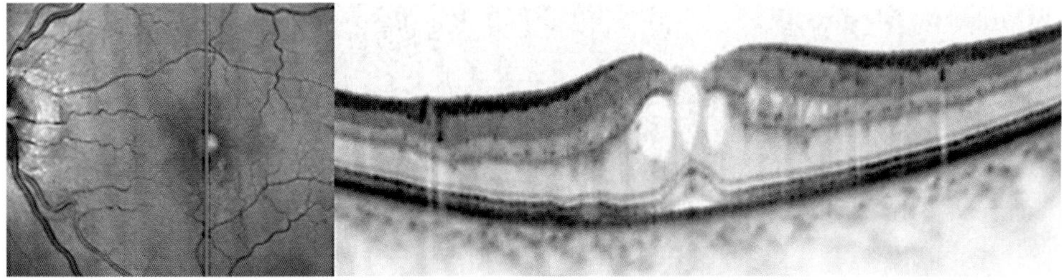

Fig. 3. OCT of a patient with CME following cataract surgery shows intraretinal fluid accumulation in cystoid spaces in the outer nuclear and inner plexiform layers and subretinal fluid.

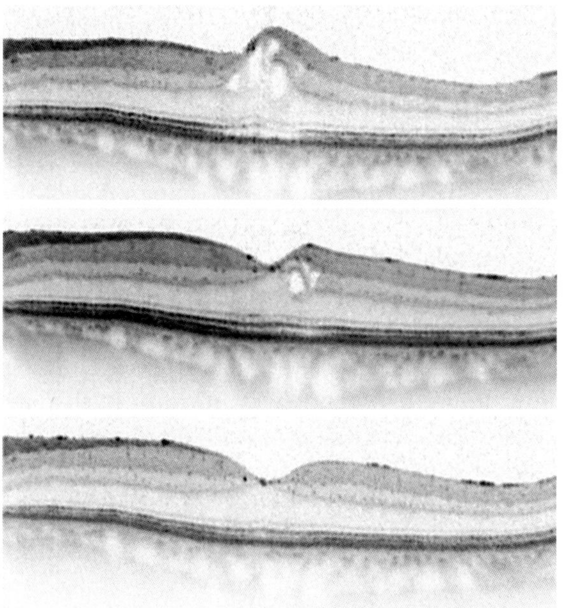

Fig. 4. Left eye OCT in a patient with pseudophakic CME shows intraretinal fluid accumulation in the outer nuclear and inner plexiform layer (top). The patient was treated with topical prednisolone and nepafenac. After 4 weeks there is reduction in retinal thickness and partial resorption of intraretinal fluid (middle), and after an additional 4 weeks all fluid is resolved (bottom). Note development of a mild ERM.

Staging and Classification

Angiographic CME
Angiographic CME is defined as the presence of fluorescein leakage in FA. It is classified by four levels: in level 1, the edema is less than 360° perifoveal; in level 2, minimal but 360° perifoveal edema is seen; level 3 is associated with moderate perifoveal edema; and level 4 is characterized by severe perifoveal edema.

Angiographic CME is mostly asymptomatic. Decreased visual acuity does not correlate with the extension of leakage. Therefore, the grading system has little clinical importance (Tolentino and Schepens, 1965)[13].

Clinical CME
Clinically significant macular edema presents with decreased vision and is diagnosed by biomicroscopy. The exact relationship between angiographic CME and clinically significant CME is uncertain. Patients with clinically significant CME may have a chronic form of angiographic CME. Otherwise, both may be separate conditions on a histologic or pathophysiologic level – not differentiable using conventional FA.

Classification
The following classifications are used:
1 Acute: acute CME appears within 4 months of surgery
2 Late onset: late onset occurs after more than 4 months postoperatively
3 Chronic: chronic CME lasts more than 6 months
4 Recurrent.

Differential Diagnosis

Differentiation between PCME and other ocular pathologies has important implications for treatment. Conversely, several ocular and systemic diseases themselves are associated with CME.

It is important to distinguish postsurgical macular edema in diabetic patients from diabetic macular edema. Frequently, preexisting diabetic macular edema worsens considerably after surgery. On the other hand, the prevalence of PCME in diabetic patients is increased (Henderson et al., 2007; Chu et al., 2015)[5, 6]. The clinical presentation of diabetic macular edema is accompanied by microaneurysms, intraretinal hemorrhages, and lipid deposits. FA is helpful for differential diagnosis. Diabetic macular edema presents with diffuse leakage that may not be localized only at the foveal area. Since disk leakage is absent in diabetic macular edema, its presence should raise suspicion for PCME (Arcieri et al., 2005)[25].

In acute retinal vein occlusion, biomicroscopy shows intraretinal hemorrhages and edema according to the distribution of the affected vein. CME can accompany these findings. FA shows delayed venous filling and increasing leakage of dye. In some cases, hypofluorescent areas of retinal ischemia may be present at the periphery. Again, history of retinal vein occlusion itself is predictive for the development of PCME.

CME also occurs as a component of hypertensive retinopathy. A history of chronic systemic hypertension and additional signs such as cotton wool spots, retinal hemorrhages, hyperemic optic disk, and exudates will also be present.

Preexisting ERM is a risk factor for developing PCME. Secondary ERM, which can occur after every vitreoretinal procedure, may be confused with CME. Both conditions present with decreased vision and metamorphopsia. In ERM, biomicroscopy reveals an irregular light reflex or thickening of the macula, distortion of blood vessels, and retinal wrinkling, which is best seen in red-free light. FA may be an auxiliary tool in detecting the extent of vessel distortion and the associated leakage of dye.

Retinitis pigmentosa presenting with nyctalopia is also associated with CME. Onset is generally during the third decade, an untypical age for cataract surgery. CME occurs relatively late in the course of this disease and is usually accompanied by the typical signs in fundus examination.

Age-related macular degeneration is the most common cause of choroidal neovascularization and mostly affects the same age group as cataracts. Choroidal neovascularization can be mistaken for PCME. Exudative maculopathy caused by choroidal neovascularization presents with intraretinal and subretinal hemorrhages, retinal pigment epithelium detachments, and hard exudates, which are not found in postoperative CME. Furthermore, it is important to distinguish PCME from CME caused by occult choroidal neovascularization. In FA, occult choroidal neovascularization is seen with gradually increasing irregular hyperfluorescence and leakage of dye from the retinal pigment epithelium in the late phase. An elevated area of hyperfluorescence marks the region of the fibrovascular retinal pigment epithelium detachment. Disk leakage does not appear in occult choroidal neovascularization.

Macular edema is sometimes a component of radiation retinopathy. A history of ocular or facial radiotherapy should prompt this differential diagnosis when diagnosing PCME.

Management

Angiographic CME does not necessarily portend a poor visual outcome. Most cases of PCME resolve spontaneously, with only a small portion reaching clinical relevance. Available therapeutic interventions, both for prophylaxis and for treatment of CME, are based on theories regarding the pathogenesis of the condition. Studies testing the efficacy of these interventions have generally not been well designed or conducted, and results have been inconsistent. Thus, there is no widely accepted treatment algorithm. However, all treatment strategies aim to decrease macular edema and thereby improve visual acuity.

Medical Treatment

NSAIDs

Topical administration of NSAIDs shows better ocular penetration than systemic administration and achieves higher aqueous levels. Furthermore, there are fewer adverse effects. Systemic indomethacin is ineffective in the treatment of PCME.

A lot of information is available on topical 0.5% ketorolac tromethamine. Its application decreases the breakdown of the blood-aqueous barrier (Flach et al., 1988)[26]. Topical ketorolac (Heier et al., 2000; Flach et al., 1987; Flach et al., 1991)[27–29] and indomethacin (Peterson et al., 1992)[30] cause significant improvement of visual acuity in acute and chronic PCME. Diclofenac sodium 0.1% is as effective as ketorolac in reducing the severity and duration of acute PCME (Rho, 2003)[31]. The newer NSAID nepafenac 0.1% is highly effective (Warren and Fox, 2007)[32], better tolerated than indomethacin, and requires only 3 instead of 4 times instillation daily. The addition of topical nepafenac or bromfenac caused an additional benefit to intravitreal and steroid treatment in cases of chronic PCME (Warren et al., 2010)[33].

When prescribing NSAIDs for CME, one should be aware of the 'on-off' phenomena, occurring with cessation and resumption of treatment (Rossetti et al., 1998)[34].

Steroids

Well-controlled trials comparing topical steroid treatment to placebo are lacking. Topical prednisolone has been studied in comparison to or in combination with topical NSAIDS. For acute CME, therapy combining topical ketorolac and prednisolone is superior to either treatment alone

(Heier et al., 2000; Singal and Hopkins, 2004)[27, 35]. Combination treatment caused improvement of 3.8 Snellen lines and a quicker response, compared to 1.6 Snellen lines with ketorolac and 1.1 lines with prednisolone.

Intravitreal triamcinolone acetonide (IVTA) has been used successfully to treat macular edema associated with retinal vein occlusion, uveitis, and diabetic maculopathy (Ip et al., 2009; Diabetic Retinopathy Clinical Research Network, 2009; Shin and Yu, 2015)[36–38]. Small case series have shown high efficacy of IVTA for refractory PCME with significant improvement in visual acuity and retinal thickness (Conway et al., 2003; Benhamou et al., 2003; Boscia et al., 2005; Koutsandrea et al., 2007)[39–42]. However, IVTA caused intraocular pressure rise in a third of cases; still, most can be well controlled with topical IOP lowering therapy (Conway et al., 2003; Koutsandrea et al., 2007)[39, 42].

Dexamethasone is a more potent corticosteroid, available as a biocompatible intravitreal implant (Ozurdex©), slowly releasing 0.7 mg over up to 6 months. Intraocular pressure rise is less frequent and more moderate than after triamcinolone injection. Small case series and case reports showed good efficacy in the treatment of PCME (Khurana et al., 2015; Brynskov et al., 2013; Meyer and Schonfeld, 2011)[43–45]. A comparison between IVTA and Ozurdex in diabetic patients with PCME showed equal efficacy regarding visual acuity and retinal thickness (Dang et al., 2014)[46]. However, 40% needed a repeated ITVA injection within 6 months. Intraocular hypertension was more frequent and more prolonged after IVTA injection.

Injection of periocular corticosteroids is a viable option for CME resistant to topical medication. Both retrobulblar and subtenon injections are efficient to treat refractory PCME and improve visual acuity with a similar small rate of intraocular tension rise (Thach et al., 1997)[47].

Systemic steroid treatment was shown to be effective for PCME refractory to topical treatment with a quick response and resolution of edema (Abe et al., 1999; Stern et al., 1981)[48, 49]. Due to a high rate of systemic side effects, this is not considered an accepted treatment option.

Carbonic Anhydrase Inhibitors

The rationale for treatment of macular edema with systemic carbonic anhydrase inhibitors (CAIs) is improvement of the pumping function of the retinal pigment epithelium in order to reduce intra- and subretinal fluid. Furthermore, CAIs induce acidification of the subretinal space and thereby increase fluid resorption from the retina through the retinal pigment epithelium into the choroid. CAIs demonstrated effectiveness in the treatment of macular edema secondary to uveitis or inherited outer retinal diseases such as retinitis pigmentosa (Farber et al., 1994; Liew et al., 2015)[50, 51]. Although case reports have shown the effectiveness of acetazolamide for PCME (Ismail et al., 2008; Tripathi et al., 1991; Weene, 1992)[52–54], randomized controlled clinical trials demonstrating a sustained positive effect on PCME do not exist. If choosing CAI, the treating physician should be aware of potential adverse effects such as metabolic acidosis and hypokalemia. Close follow-up with electrolyte studies is important.

Antiangiogenic Agents

Vascular endothelial growth factor (VEGF) is a mediator in inflammatory macular edema. Bevacizumab, a monoclonal antibody against all isoforms of VEGF, has been used off-label to treat various neovascular eye diseases. Retrospective studies have shown safety and efficacy for intravitreal bevacizumab injections in refractory PCME (Barone et al., 2009; Arevalo et al., 2009)[55, 56]. However, there were various durations and intensities of prior treatments and were not reported in detail. In some of the cases, improvement after the bevacizumab injection may have been the expression of the natural course of the disease with self-limited course. Others did not find a beneficial effect of bevacizumab injections (Spitzer et al., 2008)[57].

Laser Treatment

Vitreous incarceration in the cataract incision wound complicates CME and prolongs its healing. The Nd:YAG laser has shown promising results for such cases (Steinert and Wasson, 1989)[58]. Interpretation of these results, however, is difficult for several reasons: since anti-inflammatory drops were often prescribed after laser treatment, the therapeutic effect could have been a combination of both Nd:YAG laser and anti-inflammatory drops. The study had no control groups. Moreover, treatment was started early and spontaneous resolution may have interfered.

Though an advantage of YAG laser vitreolysis is avoidance of invasive surgery, rare but severe complications, such as elevation of intraocular pressure and retinal detachment, may occur (Aslam et al., 2003)[59].

Grid laser photocoagulation was described as a therapeutic option in a few patients with mixed results (Lardenoye et al., 1998)[60]. Controlled clinical trials investigating its efficacy and safety have not been conducted.

Surgical Treatments

There are several rationales for performing vitrectomy in PCME: removal of vitreous adhesions, reduction of inflammatory mediators in the vitreous, and greater access of topical steroids to the posterior pole.

A large multicenter prospective, randomized, controlled study investigated the efficacy of vitrectomy in patients with chronic aphakic CME and vitreous incarceration to a corneoscleral wound (Fung, 1985)[61]. Since spontaneous resolution of CME in patients with a visual acuity of 20/80 or better is almost 30%, surgery was performed only in cases with lower and long-standing decreased vision. The group that underwent vitrectomy demonstrated visual improvement.

However, treatment of this group and not the control group with corticosteroids may have influenced the results. The pars plana approach seemed superior to the limbal approach. Nowadays, aphakia is rare and aphakic CME has become less important.

A retrospective study of 24 patients with chronic pseudophakic CME and vitreous adhesions or iris capture of the IOL unresponsive to medical treatment investigated the effect of pars plana vitrectomy (Harbour et al., 1995)[62]. Patients gained 4.7 Snellen lines postoperatively, unrelated to the time interval between cataract surgery and secondary vitrectomy. The presence of an anterior or posterior chamber IOL was irrelevant. It is noteworthy that patients received topical corticosteroids after vitrectomy.

Using modern cataract surgery, vitreous incarceration is a relatively uncommon complication. Well-designed studies of visual improvement following vitrectomy are lacking. In any case, current opinion does not consider surgery as a first-line treatment for postoperative CME. Still, in cases unresponsive to medical treatment for more than 1 year, vitrectomy may present an alternative.

Former types of IOLs were more frequently associated with CME due to particular technical and anatomical properties. Small-scale studies have shown a slight visual benefit after removal or replacement of the lens (Shepard, 1979)[63]. Improved quality of modern IOLs has considerably diminished their impact on CME development over recent decades. In cases of PCME and coexisting problems that can be attributed to the presence of the IOL (i.e., pseudobullous keratopathy, chronic inflammation), removal or exchange of the IOL still presents a therapeutic option (Price and Whitson, 1990)[64].

Prevention
Surgical Technique in Primary Surgery
Atraumatic surgery is a primary means of preventing CME. Some operative factors significantly influence the development of CME. Extracapsular cataract extraction reduces the risk compared to intracapsular cataract extraction. Posterior chamber IOLs should be preferred to anterior chamber IOL. Iris clip lenses are associated with the highest risk of all IOLs. Special care should be taken to keep the posterior capsule intact.

Medical Prophylaxis
Topical steroids and NSAIDs are the two drug groups currently available to prevent postoperative inflammation and PCME.

A meta-analysis by Rossetti et al. (1998)[34] included randomized controlled trials that compared prophylactic treatment with steroids or NSAIDs and placebo. The authors concluded that prophylactic intervention with steroids and NSAIDS was beneficial for preventing angiographic CME (Demco et al., 1997; el-Harazi et al., 1998)[65, 66]. Combined data of the relevant studies showed a statistically significant benefit in terms of achieving a final visual acuity of 20/40 or better (Rossetti et al., 1998)[34]. This meta-analysis was published in 1998. The vast majority of cited studies reported ICCE operations and in 37% of the studies, eyes were left aphakic. Hence, this data does not reflect common clinical practice nowadays. A recent systematic review compared the preventive efficacy of topical steroids with that of topical NSAIDs (Kessel et al., 2014)[67]. The authors report high-quality evidence that with use of topical steroids, pseudophakic CME was 6–7 times more prevalent than in patients using topical NSAIDs (Kessel et al., 2014; Asano et al., 2008)[67, 68]. Two prospective randomized trials compared the use of the newer NSAID nepafenac ophthalmic suspension 0.1% to placebo (Singh et al., 2012; Tzelikis et al., 2015)[69, 70]. In patients with diabetic retinopathy, there was a significantly lower rate of PCME and a lower percentage of patients with vision loss >5 letters in the treatment group (Singh et al., 2012)[69]. In contrast, in nondiabetic eyes there was no benefit with treatment

(Tzelikis et al., 2015)[70]. In conclusion, long-term visual advantage from prophylactic treatment remains doubtful.

Key Messages

Ways to Prevent PCME
Prevention of PCME starts with a thorough preoperative evaluation of the patient to identify treatable risk factors and preexisting anatomic conditions that can complicate cataract surgery. Patients with known preexisting conditions or complicated surgery should be followed up closely postoperatively for early detection of CME.

Explicit recommendations for prophylactic treatment are not relevant due to a lack of well-founded information. Currently, medical prophylaxis is not approved for normal eyes without previous problems. In diabetic patients, cases of postoperative CME in the fellow eye, or complicated operations, prophylactic treatment should be considered and offered for a period of 1 month after surgery.

Main Treatment Modalities of CME
First-line treatment of PCME should include topical NSAIDs and corticosteroids. In cases of resistant CME, periocular or intraocular corticosteroids present an option. Antiangiogenic agents, though experimental, may be considered for nonresponsive persistent CME. Surgical options should be reserved for special indications.

Best Sequential Management

We propose the following flow chart for best sequential management:
1 Topical NSAIDs × 3–4/day + topical corticosteroids × 4/day
2 Sub-Tenon triamcinolone
3 Intravitreal corticosteroids (possibly intravitreal anti-VEGF agents)
4 Vitreous incarceration → consider surgery
5 Persistent inflammatory reaction → consider IOL removal or vitrectomy

References

1 Gass JD, Norton EW: Fluorescein studies of patients with macular edema and papilledema following cataract extraction. Trans Am Ophthalmol Soc 1966; 64:232–249.
2 Irvine AR: Cystoid maculopathy. Surv Ophthalmol 1976;21:1–17.
3 Shimura M, Yasuda K, Nakazawa T, et al: Panretinal photocoagulation induces pro-inflammatory cytokines and macular thickening in high-risk proliferative diabetic retinopathy. Graefes Arch Clin Exp Ophthalmol 2009;247:1617–1624.
4 Schmier JK, Halpern MT, Covert DW, Matthews GP: Evaluation of costs for cystoid macular edema among patients after cataract surgery. Retina 2007;27: 621–628.
5 Henderson BA, Kim JY, Ament CS, Ferrufino-Ponce ZK, Grabowska A, Cremers SL: Clinical pseudophakic cystoid macular edema. Risk factors for development and duration after treatment. J Cataract Refract Surg 2007;33:1550–1558.
6 Chu CJ, Johnston RL, Buscombe C, Sallam AB, Mohamed Q, Yang YC: Risk Factors and incidence of macular edema after cataract surgery. Ophthalmology 2015;123:1–8.
7 Flach AJ: The incidence, pathogenesis and treatment of cystoid macular edema following cataract surgery. Trans Am Ophthalmol Soc 1998;96:557–634.
8 Perente I, Utine CA, Ozturker C, et al: Evaluation of macular changes after uncomplicated phacoemulsification surgery by optical coherence tomography. Curr Eye Res 2007;32:241–247.
9 Bélair M, Kim SJ, Thorne JE, et al: Incidence of cystoid macular edema after cataract surgery in patients with and without uveitis using optical coherence tomography. Am J Ophthalmol 2009; 148:128–135.e2.
10 Vukicevic M, Gin T, Al-Qureshi S: Prevalence of optical coherence tomography-diagnosed postoperative cystoid macular oedema in patients following uncomplicated phaco-emulsification cataract surgery. Clin Exp Ophthalmol 2012;40:282–287.
11 Neal RE, Bettelheim FA, Lin C, Winn KC, Garland DL, Zigler JS Jr: Alterations in human vitreous humour following cataract extraction. Exp Eye Res 2005; 80:337–347.
12 Hruby K: The first description of the Irvine syndrome (in German). Klin Monbl Augenheilkd 1985;187:549–550.

13 Tolentino FI, Schepens CL: Edema of posterior pole after cataract extraction. A biomicroscopic study. Arch Ophthalmol 1965;74:781–786.

14 Rossetti L, Autelitano A: Cystoid macular edema following cataract surgery. Curr Opin Ophthalmol 2000;11:65–72.

15 Ersoy L, Caramoy A, Ristau T, Kirchhof B, Fauser S: Aqueous flare is increased in patients with clinically significant cystoid macular oedema after cataract surgery. Br J Ophthalmol 2013;97:862–865.

16 Miyake K, Ibaraki N: Prostaglandins and CYSTOID MACULAR EDEMA. 2002; 47(suppl 1):S203–S218.

17 Iliff WJ: Aphakic cystoid macular edema and the operating microscope: is there a connection? Trans Am Ophthalmol Soc 1985;83:476–500.

18 Pollack A, Leiba H, Bukelman A, Oliver M: Cystoid macular oedema following cataract extraction in patients with diabetes. Br J Ophthalmol 1992;76:221–224.

19 Kraff MC, Sanders DR, Jampol LM, Lieberman HL: Effect of primary capsulotomy with extracapsular surgery on the incidence of pseudophakic cystoid macular edema. Am J Ophthalmol 1984; 98:166–170.

20 Cohen SM, Davis A, Cukrowski C: Cystoid macular edema after pars plana vitrectomy for retained lens fragments. J Cataract Refract Surg 2006;32:1521–1526.

21 Warwar RE, Bullock JD, Ballal D: Cystoid macular edema and anterior uveitis associated with latanoprost use. Experience and incidence in a retrospective review of 94 patients. Ophthalmology 1998;105:263–268.

22 Miyake K, Ota I, Maekubo K, Ichihashi S, Miyake S: Latanoprost accelerates disruption of the blood-aqueous barrier and the incidence of angiographic cystoid macular edema in early postoperative pseudophakias. Arch Ophthalmol 1999;117:34–40.

23 Sigler EJ, Randolph JC, Kiernan DF: Longitudinal analysis of the structural pattern of pseudophakic cystoid macular edema using multimodal imaging. Graefes Arch Clin Exp Ophthalmol 2015;43–51.

24 Munk MR, Jampol LM, Simader C, et al: Differentiation of diabetic macular edema from pseudophakic cystoid macular edema by spectral-domain optical coherence tomography. Invest Ophthalmol Vis Sci 2015;56:6724–6733.

25 Arcieri ES, Santana A, Rocha FN, et al: Blood-aqueous barrier changes after the use of prostaglandin analogues in patients with pseudophakia and aphakia. Arch Ophthalmol 2005;123:186–192.

26 Flach AJ, Graham J, Kruger LP, Stegman RC, Tanenbaum L: Quantitative assessment of postsurgical breakdown of the blood-aqueous barrier following administration of 0.5% ketorolac tromethamine solution. A double-masked, paired comparison with vehicle-placebo solution study. Arch Ophthalmol 1988; 106:344–347.

27 Heier JS, Topping TM, Baumann W, Dirks MS, Chern S: Ketorolac versus prednisolone versus combination therapy in the treatment of acute pseudophakic cystoid macular edema. Ophthalmology 2000;107:2034–2038.

28 Flach AJ, Dolan BJ, Irvine AR: Effectiveness of ketorolac tromethamine 0.5% ophthalmic solution for chronic aphakic and pseudophakic cystoid macular edema. Am J Ophthalmol 1987;103:479–486.

29 Flach AJ, Jampol LM, Weinberg D, et al: Improvement in visual acuity in chronic aphakic and pseudophakic cystoid macular edema after treatment with topical 0.5% ketorolac tromethamine. Am J Ophthalmol 1991;112:514–519.

30 Peterson M, Yoshizumi MO, Hepler R, Mondino B, Kreiger A: Topical indomethacin in the treatment of chronic cystoid macular edema. Graefes Arch Clin Exp Ophthalmol 1992;230:401–405.

31 Rho DS: Treatment of acute pseudophakic cystoid macular edema: diclofenac versus ketorolac. J Cataract Refract Surg 2003;29:2378–2384.

32 Warren KA, Fox JE: Topical nepafenac as an alternative for cystoid macular edema in steroid responsive patients. Retina 2007;28:1427–1434.

33 Warren KA, Bahrani H, Fox JE: NSAIDS in combination therapy for the treatment of chronic edema. Retina 2010;30: 260–266.

34 Rossetti L, Chaudhwi J, Dickersin K: Medical prophylaxis and treatment of cystoid macular edema after cataract surgery. The results of a meta-analysis. Ophthalmology 1998;105:397–405.

35 Singal N, Hopkins J: Pseudophakic cystoid macular edema: ketorolac alone vs. ketorolac plus prednisolone. Can J Ophthalmol 2004;39:245–250.

36 Ip MS, Scott IU, VanVeldhuisen PC, et al: A randomized trial comparing the efficacy and safety of intravitreal triamcinolone with observation to treat vision loss associated with macular edema secondary to central retinal vein occlusion: the Standard Care vs Corticosteroid for Retinal Vein Occlusion (SCORE) study report 5. Arch Ophthalmol 2009;127:1101–1114.

37 Diabetic Retinopathy Clinical Research Network (DRCR.net), Beck RW, Edwards AR, et al: Three-year follow-up of a randomized trial comparing focal/grid photocoagulation and intravitreal triamcinolone for diabetic macular edema. Arch Ophthalmol 2009;127:245–251.

38 Shin JY, Yu HG: Intravitreal triamcinolone injection for uveitic macular edema: a randomized clinical study. Ocul Immunol Inflamm 2015;23:430–436.

39 Conway MD, Canakis C, Livir-Rallatos C, Peyman GA: Intravitreal triamcinolone acetonide for refractory chronic pseudophakic cystoid macular edema. J Cataract Refract Surg 2003;29:27–33.

40 Benhamou N, Massin P, Haouchine B, Audren F, Tadayoni R, Gaudric A: Intravitreal triamcinolone for refractory pseudophakic macular edema. Am J Ophthalmol 2003;135:246–249.

41 Boscia F, Furino C, Dammacco R, Ferreri P, Sborgia L, Sborgia C: Intravitreal triamcinolone acetonide in refractory pseudophakic cystoid macular edema: functional and anatomic results. Eur J Ophthalmol 2005;15:89–95.

42 Koutsandrea C, Moschos MM, Brouzas D, Loukianou E, Apostolopoulos M, Moschos M: Intraocular triamcinolone acetonide for pseudophakic cystoid macular edema: optical coherence tomography and multifocal electroretinography study. Retina 2007;27:159–164.

43 Khurana RN, Palmer JD, Porco TC, Wieland MR: Dexamethasone intravitreal implant for pseudophakic cystoid macular edema in patients with diabetes. Ophthalmic Surg Lasers Imaging Retina 2015;46:56–61.

44 Brynskov T, Laugesen CS, Halborg J, Kemp H, Sorensen TL: Longstanding refractory pseudophakic cystoid macular edema resolved using intravitreal 0.7 mg dexamethasone implants. Clin Ophthalmol 2013;7:1171–1174.

45 Meyer LM, Schonfeld C-L: Cystoid macular edema after complicated cataract surgery resolved by an intravitreal dexamethasone 0.7-mg Implant. Case Rep Ophthalmol 2011;2:319–322.

46 Dang Y, Mu Y, Li L, et al: Comparison of dexamethasone intravitreal implant and intravitreal triamcinolone acetonide for the treatment of pseudophakic cystoid macular edema in diabetic patients. Drug Des Devel Ther 2014;8:1441–1449.

47 Thach AB, Dugel PU, Flindall RJ, Sipperley JO, Sneed SR: A comparison of retrobulbar versus sub-Tenon's corticosteroid therapy for cystoid macular edema refractory to topical medications. Ophthalmology 1997;104:2003–2008.

48 Abe T, Hayasaka S, Nagaki Y, Kadoi C, Matsumoto M, Hayasaka Y: Pseudophakic cystoid macular edema treated with high-dose intravenous methylprednisolone. J Cataract Refract Surg 1999;25:1286–1288.

49 Stern AL, Taylor DM, Dalburg LA, Cosentino RT: Pseudophakic cystoid maculopathy: a study of 50 cases. Ophthalmology 1981;88:942–946.

50 Farber MD, Lam S, Tessler HH, Jennings TJ, Cross A, Rusin MM: Reduction of macular oedema by acetazolamide in patients with chronic iridocyclitis: a randomised prospective crossover study. Br J Ophthalmol 1994;78:4–7.

51 Liew G, Moore AT, Webster AR, Michaelides M: Efficacy and prognostic factors of response to carbonic anhydrase inhibitors in management of cystoid macular edema in retinitis pigmentosa. Invest Ophthalmol Vis Sci 2015;56:1531–1536.

52 Ismail RA, Sallam A, Zambarakji HJ: Pseudophakic macular edema and oral acetazolamide: an optical coherence tomography measurable, dose-related response. Eur J Ophthalmol 2008;18:1011–1013.

53 Tripathi RC, Fekrat S, Tripathi BJ, Ernest JT: A direct correlation of the resolution of pseudophakic cystoid macular edema with acetazolamide therapy. Ann Ophthalmol 1991;23:127–129.

54 Weene LE: Cystoid macular edema after scleral buckling responsive to acetazolamide. Ann Ophthalmol 1992;24:423–424.

55 Barone A, Russo V, Prascina F, Noci ND: Short-term safety and efficacy of intravitreal bevacizumab for edema. Retina 2009;29:33–37.

56 Arevalo JF, Maia M, Garcia-Amaris RA, et al: Intravitreal bevacizumab for refractory pseudophakic cystoid macular edema: the Pan-American Collaborative Retina Study Group results. Ophthalmology 2009;116:1481–1487.

57 Spitzer MS, Ziemssen F, Yoeruek E, Petermeier K, Aisenbrey S, Szurman P: Efficacy of intravitreal bevacizumab in treating postoperative pseudophakic cystoid macular edema. J Cataract Refract Surg 2008;34:70–75.

58 Steinert RF, Wasson PJ: Neodymium:YAG laser anterior vitreolysis for Irvine-Gass cystoid macular edema. J Cataract Refract Surg 1989;15:304–307.

59 Aslam TM, Devlin H, Dhillon B: Use of Nd:YAG laser capsulotomy. Surv Ophthalmol 2003;48:594–612.

60 Lardenoye CW, van Schooneveld MJ, Frits Treffers W, Rothova A: Grid laser photocoagulation for macular oedema in uveitis or the Irvine-Gass syndrome. Br J Ophthalmol 1998;82:1013–1016.

61 Fung WE: Vitrectomy for chronic aphakic cystoid macular edema. Results of a national, collaborative, prospective, randomized investigation. Ophthalmology 1985;92:1102–1111.

62 Harbour JW, Smiddy WE, Rubsamen PE, Murray TG, Davis JL, Flynn HW Jr: Pars plana vitrectomy for chronic pseudophakic cystoid macular edema. Am J Ophthalmol 1995;120:302–307.

63 Shepard DD: The fate of eyes from which intraocular lenses have been removed. Ophthalmic Surg 1979;10:58–60.

64 Price FW Jr, Whitson WE: Natural history of cystoid macular edema in pseudophakic bullous keratopathy. J Cataract Refract Surg 1990;16:163–169.

65 Demco TA, Sutton H, Demco CJ, Raj PS: Topical diclofenac sodium compared with prednisolone acetate after phacoemulsification-lens implant surgery. Eur J Ophthalmol 1997;7:236–240.

66 el-Harazi SM, Ruiz RS, Feldman RM, Villanueva G, Chuang AZ: A randomized double-masked trial comparing ketorolac tromethamine 0.5%, diclofenac sodium 0.1%, and prednisolone acetate 1% in reducing post-phacoemulsification flare and cells. Ophthalmic Surg Lasers 1998;29:539–544.

67 Kessel L, Tendal B, Jørgensen KJ, et al: Post-cataract prevention of inflammation and macular edema by steroid and nonsteroidal anti-inflammatory eye drops: a systematic review. Ophthalmology 2014;121:1915–1924.

68 Asano S, Miyake K, Ota I, et al: Reducing angiographic cystoid macular edema and blood-aqueous barrier disruption after small-incision phacoemulsification and foldable intraocular lens implantation. Multicenter prospective randomized comparison of topical diclofenac 0.1% and betamethason. J Cataract Refract Surg 2008;34:57–63.

69 Singh R, Alpern L, Jaffe GJ, et al: Evaluation of nepafenac in prevention of macular edema following cataract surgery in patients with diabetic retinopathy. Clin Ophthalmol 2012;6:1259–1269.

70 Tzelikis PF, Vieira M, Hida WT, et al: Comparison of ketorolac 0.4% and nepafenac 0.1% for the prevention of cystoid macular oedema after phacoemulsification: prospective placebo-controlled randomised study. 2015;99:654–658.

Prof. Anat Loewenstein
Division of Ophthalmology, Tel Aviv Sourasky Medical Center
Sackler Faculty of Medicine, Tel Aviv University
6, Weizman St.
Tel Aviv 64239 (Israel)
E-Mail anatl@tlvmc.gov.il

Coscas G (ed): Macular Edema. 2nd, revised and extended edition.
Dev Ophthalmol. Basel, Karger, 2017, vol 58, pp 191–201 (DOI: 10.1159/000455281)

Retinitis Pigmentosa and Other Dystrophies

Sarah Mrejen[b] · Isabelle Audo[a, b] · Sébastien Bonnel[b] · José-Alain Sahel[a–d]

[a] Sorbonne Universités, UPMC Univ Paris 06, INSERM, CNRS, Institut de la Vision, [b] CHNO des Quinze-Vingts, DHU Sight Restore, INSERM-DGOS CIC 1423, and [c] Fondation Ophtalmologique Rothschild, Paris, France; [d] Department of Ophthalmology, The University of Pittsburgh School of Medicine, Pittsburgh, PA, USA

Abstract

Retinitis pigmentosa (RP) is a heterogeneous group of inherited retinal degenerations characterized by progressive degeneration of rod and cone cells that affects predominantly peripheral visual fields. Macular edema may cause additional central visual acuity decrease. Cystoid macular edema (CME) is one of the few treatable causes of visual loss in RP. The prevalence of CME in RP has been found to be between 10 and 20% on fluorescein angiography-based studies, and as high as 49% on reports based on optical coherence tomography. Macular edema can manifest at any stage of the disease and may be unilateral or bilateral. It can be found in any genetic form, but is more often associated with RP caused by CRB1 mutations. The origin of macular edema in RP patients still remains poorly understood. Some mechanisms have been suggested, including antiretinal antibodies (retinal, carbonic anhydrase, and enolase antibodies), vitreous traction, retinal pigment epithelium dysfunction, and Müller cell edema. There is no gold standard therapeutic strategy. Drug therapy is the primary treatment. Systemic carbonic anhydrase inhibitors, such as oral acetazolamide or topical dorzolamide, are still the mainstays of initial therapy. If CME is refractory to acetazolamide, intravitreal corticosteroid injections may be a therapeutic option. However, antivascular endothelium growth factor injections have limited effect and should be avoided. Vitrectomy has also been evaluated, but its exact role remains to be determined. The benefits of these therapies are variable among patients. The establishment of therapeutic approaches is limited by our poor understanding of the pathophysiology of CME in patients with RP. Autoimmune retinopathies (AIRs) are a group of rare diseases characterized by acute or subacute progressive vision loss and are thought to be mediated by autoantibodies specific to retinal antigens. The AIRs encompass paraneoplastic syndromes, such as cancer-associated retinopathy and melanoma-associated retinopathy, and a larger group of AIRs that have similar clinical and immunological findings but without underlying malignancy. These diseases may also be complicated by macular edema. RP is one of the most common forms of inherited retinal degeneration. It displays extensive clinical and genetic variations and leads to progressive blindness with variable onset.

Factors of Visual Acuity Decrease and Retinitis Pigmentosa

Retinitis pigmentosa (RP) is the most common group of inherited retinal disorders. It is a heterogeneous group of inherited retinal degenerations that primarily affect the rod photoreceptors and the retinal pigment epithelium (RPE) with mutations in over 100 genes identified underlying the disease.

The typical clinical features of RP include bone spicule retinal pigment, progressive atrophy of the RPE, 'waxy pallor' of the optic disc, and diffuse attenuation of the retinal arteries. Although rod photoreceptors are thought to be the main target of the disease, there is histological and functional evidence for cone photoreceptor damage that seems to develop secondarily to rod degeneration (Sahel et al., 2001)[1]. Most forms of RP are caused by mutations in genes coding for proteins restricted to rod photoreceptors (Travis, 1998)[2]. Cone survival, however, appears to depend on the presence of rod photoreceptors, even if they are not functional (Leveillard et al., 2004; Mohand-Said S, 2000)[3, 4].

Accordingly, the survival of cone receptors can be a promising target for development of future therapeutic options in useful visual acuity (VA) gain.

As RP progresses, symptoms worsen. One of the earliest symptoms of RP is difficulty in seeing at night (nyctalopia or night blindness), which is due to rod degeneration. Later in the disease course, a reduction in the peripheral visual field also develops, resulting in loss of central vision in some cases. The rate of central VA loss depends on the mutated gene, the type of mutation, and modifying factors (i.e., genetic and environmental interactions). Depending on the transmission mode, central vision loss appears at the age of 20–30 years in X-linked forms, at the age of 20–40 years in autosomal recessive forms, and at the age of 60 years in autosomal dominant forms. In particular cases, such as sector RP, VA can remain intact.

It is extremely important to note that in addition to the underlying degenerative pathology, other causes for decrease of the central VA in patients with RP can potentially exist (e.g., macular edema, epiretinal membrane, and posterior subcapsular cataract). While the gene therapies and other strategies to suspend or reverse photoreceptor degeneration in RP are not available yet, the treatment of macular edema, epiretinal membrane, and cataract are so far the only ways to improve vision in some patients.

Among the possible complications that may decrease the central VA in RP patients, we will focus our attention on the occurrence of cystoid macular edema (CME). CME may cause fast VA decline in patients with good central vision despite an abnormal visual field.

Retinitis Pigmentosa and Macular Edema

Epidemiology and Natural Course
Fluorescein angiography detects the presence of CME in 10–20% of RP patients (Fishman et al., 1977; Heckenlively, 1987; Pruett, 1983)[5-7]. Advances in in vivo optical imaging technologies, such as optical coherence tomography (OCT), have permitted more sensitive detection of CME (in about 20–50% of patients with RP), even in cases with no diffusion on angiography (Adackapara et al., 2008; Hajali et al., 2008; Hirakawa, 1999)[8-10].

The most common cause of autosomal dominant RP [mutations in rhodopsin (*RHO*)] accounts for approximately one third of the cases and may be associated with earlier and more severe CME (Kim et al., 2012)[11]. Mutations in CRB1 are more usually associated with CME (Bujakowska et al., 2012)[12]. CME can manifest at any stage of the disease and may be unilateral or bilateral. Interestingly, in the late stages of the degenerative pathology, CME seems less likely to appear. There are no differences in the prevalence of CME that are associated with the inheritance pattern (autosomal dominant, recessive, and sporadic forms) (Hajali and Fishman, 2009)[13]. Nevertheless, in X-linked forms, CME is very rare.

The high rate of macular edema that can be detected by OCT shows the importance of this type of investigation in case of VA decline. The indications for treatment of macular edema will be discussed later. Another point which must be kept in mind during OCT analysis is the imperfect correlation between retinal thickness and VA. The preservation of the ellipsoid zone may be a better correlation.

Physiopathology
Numerous hypotheses have been proposed to explain the origin of CME in various pathologies, including mechanical traction on the vitreoretinal interface (as in epiretinal membrane or vitreoretinal traction syndrome), retinal toxicity, and release of proinflammatory factors [e.g., cytokines (as in uveitis) or proangiogenic factors (as in patients with diabetes or venous occlusion)].

These mechanisms are implicated in a blood-retinal barrier breakdown and accumulation of liquid localized in the outer plexiform layer that may lead to the development of CME. Other factors, such as vascular endothelial growth factor or interleukin-6, also seem to play an important role in CME formation. At present, no correlation between the mechanisms underlying the formation of CME and its chronicity has been established.

In RP, the origin of CME still remains poorly understood. The possible pathophysiological role of some antibodies has been proposed (retinal, carbonic anhydrase, and enolase antibodies) (Heckenlively et al., 1996)[14]. We suggest that loss of retinoschisin levels secondary to photoreceptor loss should be considered as a mechanism. Other authors proposed that anomaly in the polarity of the pigment epithelium cells may result in a defective absorption of liquid in the outer neuroretina (Cox et al., 1988)[15]. It has also been hypothesized that Müller cell dysfunction is involved (Bringmann and Wiedemann, 2012; Iandiev et al., 2008; Wurm et al., 2009)[16–18]. Further studies are needed to understand CME physiopathology in patients with RP. Moreover, many cystic changes in RP do not show evidence of CME and a better term could therefore be 'intraretinal cysts'.

Clinical Diagnosis
When facing a patient with RP who presents a VA decrease that is neither explained by formation of a cataract nor by the progression of the retinal degeneration, the ophthalmologist must consider the presence of CME. For the diagnosis of CME, a macular contact lens should be used. This will reveal thickening of the macular profile and cystoid cavities of variable sizes. Detection of diffuse macular edema is more difficult. When performing fundus examination, posterior hyaloid and retinal vessels must be carefully examined in order to establish the differential diagnosis. Diagnosis and follow-up of macular edema have become easier with the introduction of OCT. This tool is critical to make the distinction between the evolution of RP as a degenerative pathology and the occurrence of macular edema. OCT allows accurate analysis of the vitreoretinal interface and quantitative measurement of retinal thickness. Currently, the assessment of macular edema progression can be precisely monitored with OCT. Fluorescein angiography should be reserved for cases of questionable etiology.

Treatments
Some treatments have been reported to improve vision and retinal thickness in CME secondary to RP. There is no gold standard therapeutic strategy and treatment should be individualized. The data evaluating these therapies are mainly from interventional case series. Topical and oral carbonic anhydrase inhibitors, intravitreal triamcinolone, intravitreal dexamethasone implants, and intravitreal anti-vascular endothelial growth factor (VEGF) agents may be of some benefit in treating CME in RP. However, there is only one prospective masked crossover study showing that oral acetazolamide improved macular edema and vision in 12 patients (Fishman et al., 1989)[19].

At present, drug therapy is the primary treatment modality for CME in patients with RP. Systemic carbonic anhydrase inhibitors, such as oral acetazolamide (Diamox[®]) or topical dorzolamide 2%, are still the mainstays of initial therapy. If CME is refractory to acetazolamide, intravitreal corticosteroid injections could be administered. Intravitreal antivascular endothelial growth factor therapy has also been used in cases of CME persistence after oral acetazolamide therapy (Melo et al., 2007; Yuzbasioglu et al., 2009)[20, 21], though with uncertain results. In cases of chronic and/or refractory CME despite oral and intravitreal therapies, vitrectomy can also be proposed, but its role is not yet clear. The most effective current therapies are described below.

Carbonic Anhydrase Inhibitors
Oral acetazolamide is considered the drug of first choice for treatment of CME in RP (Fishman et al., 1989; Apushkin et al., 2007; Chen et al., 1990; Orzalesi et al., 1993)[19, 22–24]. Different dosing regimens have been suggested, with the usual recommended dosage ranging from 250 to 500 mg per day. Daily oral acetazolamide decreases the central macular thickness and allows CME regression that can be seen on OCT imaging 7–15 days after the introduction of the treatment. VA improvement and disappearance of metamorphopsias, together with a normal foveal profile, can be noted in patients who respond to oral acetazolamide. There is no correlation between functional improvement and angiographic or OCT modifications. A rebound of CME has often been described, despite the continuity in the treatment with oral acetazolamide (Apushkin et al., 2007)[22]. The mechanisms by which acetazolamide reduce CME remain uncertain (Cox et al., 1988)[15]. There may be an effect on the RPE pumping function with subsequent fluid egress from the retina into the choroid. There may be an effect at the level of the perifoveal capillaries, suggesting a direct effect on retinal vasculature and the internal blood-retinal barrier. Topical carbonic anhydrase inhibitors have also been used in patients with RP, with a lower rate of systemic side effects than oral acetazolamide. One study has shown a functional improvement in 20% of the patients treated with topical acetazolamide and a rebound effect in 30% of the patients during the treatment (Grover et al., 1997)[25]. The largest cohort to date included 81 patients from the Moorfields Eye Hospital: 64 patients (125 eyes) were treated with topical dorzolamide 2% and 17 patients (32 eyes) with oral acetazolamide 250 mg twice a day. In this study, a higher proportion of eyes responded to topical dorzolamide (40%) on spectral domain OCT than to oral acetazolamide (28%) after a mean duration of treatment of 3 months (Liew et al., 2015)[26]. In this analysis, patients with autosomal recessive RP and greater initial central retinal thickness on spectral domain OCT were more likely to respond to treatment (Liew et al., 2015)[26]. Grover et al. (1997)[25] reported results from a prospective double-masked crossover study of 5 patients that all (100%) showed improvement of leakage on FA compared to 40% with topical dorzolamide. Genead and Fishman (2010)[27] evaluated 32 patients (64 eyes) treated with topical dorzolamide 3 times a day for a long time (6–58 months) and found that 67% showed a reduction of central retinal thickness on OCT and one third were nonresponders. Among the responders, one third of the patients showed sustained improvement over a mean period of 39.5 months. The changes in VA did not correlate with the changes of cystic macular lesions on OCT (Genead and Fishman, 2010)[27]. There is no way to predict which patients will respond to therapy. There appears to be less of a rebound rate with the use of topical dorzolamide over an extended period of time (Genead and Fishman, 2010)[27].

When comparing the efficacy of oral acetazolamide with topical dorzolamide, the rate of responders to oral therapy varies from 50% [12 patients FA based (Fishman et al., 1989)[19]] to 100% [5 patients FA based (Grover et al., 1997)[25] and 6 patients OCT based (Apushkin et al., 2007)[22]].

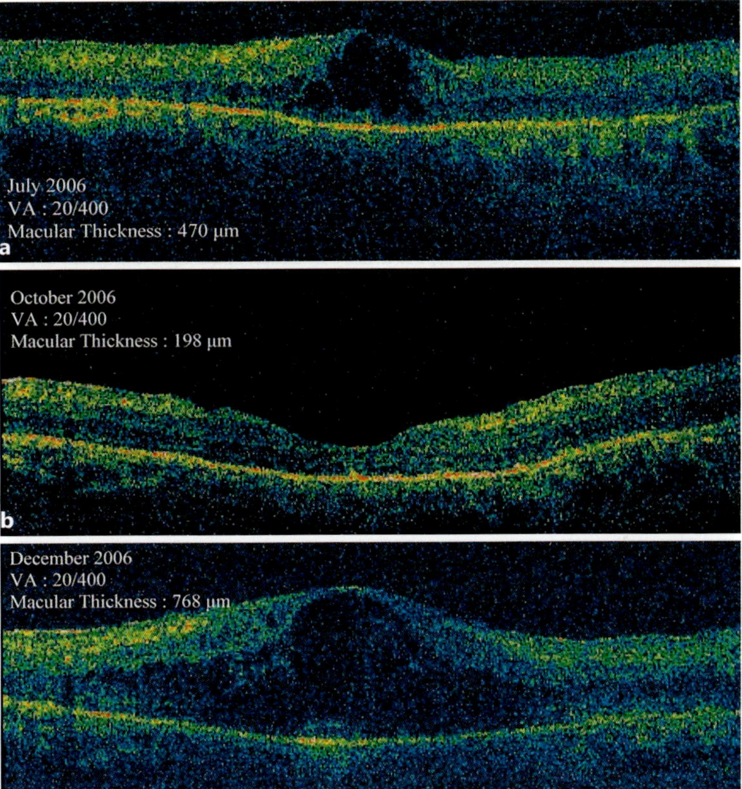

Fig. 1. OCT examination. Patient with macular edema secondary to RP. Before (**a**) and after (**b**) intravitreal triamcinolone acetonide. Five months after the injection a rebound effect was observed (**c**).

The rate of responders to topical dorzolamide varies from 40% (5 patients, FA-based (Grover et al., 1997)[25]] to 100% [8 patients, OCT-based (Fishman and Apushkin, 2007)[28]].

Differences in age, severity, and duration of CME, and methods of evaluating and monitoring CME may at least partially explain the variable results of these studies. However, all studies have consistently shown a poor correlation between change in VA and decrease in retinal thickness on OCT.

Intravitreal Triamcinolone Acetonide Injection
Intravitreal triamcinolone injection is another therapeutic option for the management of CME in RP patients. The therapeutic effect is fast and manifests with improvement in VA and normalization of the macular thickness profile (Ozdemir et al., 2005; Sallum et al., 2003; Saraiva et al., 2003; Scorolli et al., 2007)[29–32]. This therapeutic modality could be proposed in patients who do not or only partially respond to oral acetazolamide, and in cases of rebound.

The effect of intravitreal triamcinolone is often transient and may result in rebounds that sometimes lead to VA levels lower than those before treatment (fig. 1). Other disadvantages include possible reiterative injections (when necessary), cataract progression or development, and elevated intraocular pressure.

More recently, a sustained-release dexamethasone implant has become available and approved for ophthalmology (Ozurdex; Allergan Inc., Irvine, Calif., USA). Ozurdex is approved for ophthalmology in CME secondary to vein occlusion and diabetes, while intravitreal triamcinolone is an off-label corticosteroid for ophthalmology. A

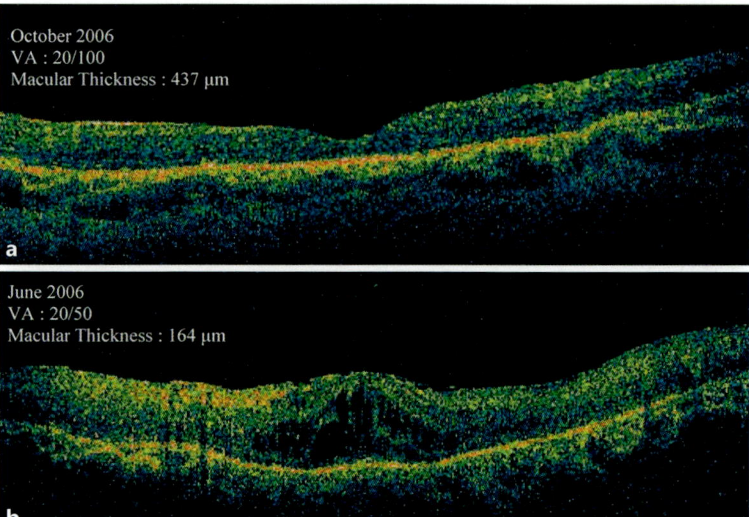

Fig. 2. OCT examination. A patient with macular edema secondary to RP before (**a**) and after (**b**) vitreoretinal surgery with limiting membrane peeling. Administration of oral acetazolamide and intravitreal triamcinolone was associated with rebound effects. Improvement in VA and reduction in macular thickness were observed for 2 years after surgery without additional treatment.

dexamethasone implant is less likely to give ocular side-effects such as cataract and increase in intraocular pressure than triamcinolone acetonide. It has been evaluated with anatomical and visual benefits in 3 patients with refractory CME due to RP (Srour et al., 2013)[33]. Recurrent CME occurred in 2/3 patients at 3 months and retreatment with Ozurdex was performed with good anatomical results and limited evidence for VA recovery. Ozurdex may represent a valuable treatment option in patients with CME refractory to carbonic anhydrase inhibitors, but its efficacy seems to be limited over time.

We are cautious about intravitreal injections of anti-VEGF for two main reasons: it does not target the main mechanisms involved in CME secondary to RP, and there is at least one theoretical risk of accelerating RPE atrophy by suppressing VEGF since VEGF maintains the choriocapillaris (Saint-Geniez et al., 2009)[34].

Vitreoretinal Surgery

One study has described vitreoretinal surgery with internal limiting membrane peeling in RP-associated CME not responding to acetazolamide. Twelve eyes with RP were operated using indocyanine green staining for internal limiting membrane peeling. The results after a 6-month follow-up showed a VA improvement (mean preoperative best-corrected VA: 20/115; mean postoperative best-corrected VA: 20/45) and a macular thickness decrease (mean preoperative foveal thickness: 477 μm; mean postoperative foveal thickness: 260 μm). Mechanisms of therapeutic action have not been discussed (Garcia-Arumi et al., 2003)[35]. More recently, Ikeda et al. (2015)[36] reported their experience with the long-term surgical outcomes of epiretinal membrane (ERM) peeling in 10 patients with RP. They found anatomical improvement without visual deterioration at 68 months.

Our personal experience with vitreoretinal surgery performing internal limiting membrane peeling without staining in patients who no longer responded to the therapies described above suggests that improvement in VA and reduction in macular thickness can be obtained in all patients (fig. 2). Significant adherence of the internal limiting membrane to the neuroretinal tissue was noted during surgery in all cases. Surprisingly, although some patients presented a macular edema recurrence, the fovea was spared. Such experience cannot be considered as evidence for efficiency until comparative studies are conducted on larger series.

How to Treat and When
The management of CME in RP patients may differ depending on the clinical presentation. For instance, CME without clinical manifestations (but OCT detectable) may need only follow-up but no treatment. It is important to keep in mind that there is not always a correlation between retinal thickness and VA.

The existence of a macular syndrome associated with VA decrease is a good indication for proposing a therapeutic approach. However, it is not known whether cysts themselves modify retinal ionic or trophic exchanges in the long term; therefore, we tend to treat cystic changes when the foveal region is involved regardless of decreased VA.

In our department, adults with bilateral CME are first treated with oral acetazolamide 250 mg. In children and adults with unilateral CME, we start with topical dorzolamide 2% three times a day. When oral acetazolamide is contraindicated, topical administration of dorzolamide can be considered. We evaluate the response to treatment at 3 months: if patients respond, the treatment is continued until the OCT has been stabilized for 6 months, and then decreased progressively. If the patients do not respond, the dosage can be increased to 250 mg twice a day, or even 3 times a day. After the first control at 3 months, patients are reevaluated every 6 months. Patients are considered refractory when they do not respond after 6 months of treatment with carbonic anhydrase inhibitors.

As a second option, only when the VA is significantly decreased, sub-Tenon triamcinolone acetonide injection can be proposed. The results can be satisfactory in some cases, but if not, an intravitreal injection can be proposed.

Intravitreal triamcinolone injection has a faster effect and restores ad integrum the foveal profile in most cases. The possibility of a rebound effect, which frequently takes place approximately 3 months after the injection, needs special attention. In addition, intraocular pressure follow-up has to be performed in those patients who usually respond after repeated injections of steroids. Furthermore, more frequent injections may be required as the efficacy and duration of the steroid therapy effect tend to decrease. More recently, intravitreal injection of an intravitreal dexamethasone implant approved for ophthalmology showed good anatomical results in small case series, with a similar rebound effect at 3 months, and possibly a lower rate of cataracts and elevated intraocular pressure. The risk of inducing a cataract with iterative steroid intravitreal injections in young phakic patients should be considered and discussed with the patient.

As a third line of therapy in patients with a significant functional deterioration, vitreoretinal surgery with internal limiting membrane peeling might be proposed. Surgery might be difficult to perform as the internal limiting membrane is very adherent. It should be kept as short as possible in order to avoid phototraumatism. Long-term efficacy of this surgical approach remains unknown.

Cataract Surgery and Macular Edema in RP
Posterior subcapsular cataract is typically associated with RP (Eshaghian et al., 1980)[37], and surgery improves the VA in patients with preserved central visual field. The capsular opacification rate is higher than in normal patients and anterior capsular contraction can occur.

The rate of occurrence or aggravation of CME after cataract surgery (comparing the preoperative and postoperative macular profile) has not yet been studied (Jackson et al., 2001)[38].

Optical Coherence Tomography and Macular Edema in RP: Anatomy and Function Correlation
All studies are consistent in showing a poor correlation between the change in VA and decrease

in retinal thickness on OCT. Battaglia Parodi et al. (2016)[39] evaluated the correlation between retinal changes on spectral domain OCT and visual function in patients with RP. They evaluated 22 patients (44 eyes), and 7 eyes had CME. Multivariate analysis revealed that the absence of outer segment/RPE and external limiting membrane layers were the only variables independently associated with a decrease in VA (Battaglia Parodi, 2016)[39].

These results suggest that the qualitative analysis of the preservation or disruption of the outer retinal layers on spectral domain OCT may be more predictive of the visual outcome than the quantitative measurement of CME.

Makiyama et al. (2014)[40] evaluated the topography and spatial distribution of cystoid spaces in RP in 275 patients (529 eyes) using spectral domain OCT. Cystoid spaces were present in 27% of patients. The layer most frequently involved with cysts was the inner nuclear layer (99%) followed by the outer nuclear layer (28%) and the ganglion cell layer (7%). Cystoid spaces were distributed in the relatively preserved retina, in the areas where the external limiting membrane was preserved (79%). The presence of epiretinal membrane or posterior vitreous adhesion was significantly associated with the presence of cysts (Makiyama et al., 2014)[40].

Melanoma and Cancer-Associated Retinopathy

The autoimmune retinopathies (AIRs) are a group of diseases characterized by acute or subacute progressive vision loss, and are thought to be mediated by autoantibodies specific to retinal antigens (Adamus, 2000; Heckenlively et al., 2000)[41, 42]. The prevalence of AIRs is unknown, although it is believed to be relatively uncommon. They are characterized by abnormal findings on electroretinogram (ERG) (either rod-cone or cone-rod patterns). The AIRs encompass the bet-ter-studied paraneoplastic syndromes, such as cancer-associated retinopathy and melanoma-associated retinopathy, and a larger group of AIRs that have similar clinical and immunological findings but without underlying malignancy.

This latter group is called *nonparaneoplastic autoimmune retinopathy* (npAIR). It has previously been called recoverin-associated retinopathy (Whitcup et al., 1998)[43] or autoimmune retinopathy in the absence of cancer (Mizener et al., 1997)[44]. Some npAIRs have CME as a prominent feature that appears to be a distinguishing factor (npAIR/CME).

Cancer-associated retinopathy, melanoma-associated retinopathy, npAIR, and npAIR/CME tend to have common clinical features despite the fact that no uniform set of antiretinal antibodies has been found in these patients (Chan, 2003; Hooks et al., 2001)[45, 46]. Patients may have a variety of antibody activity, sometimes multiple.

RP and AIRs share similar clinical features and many AIR patients may be referred with a diagnosis of RP. The figure is complicated by the fact that some cases of RP may develop secondary AIR with rapid visual field loss and severe CME (Hajali and Fishman, 2009; Heckenlively et al., 1999; Heckenlively et al., 1985)[13, 47, 48]. Ninety percent of patients with RP and cysts have circulating antiretinal antibodies by means of Western blot analysis, compared with 13% of patients with RP without macular cysts, and 6% of controls (Chant et al., 1985)[49]. However, it remains to be determined whether the presence of antiretinal antibodies is a direct cause of worsening of RP.

Common features of the presentation of patients with AIR include a rapidly progressive bilateral painless visual deterioration. The visual symptoms include rapid onset of photopsia, followed by night blindness, scotomata, and visual field loss. Some patients also develop diminished central vision. Frequently, npAIR patients have CME as a prominent feature. The presentation may be asymmetrical between eyes. Patients often reveal they have autoimmune family histories. On clinical examination, the fundus may appear normal or there can be changes suggesting retinal degeneration such as attenuated retinal vessels, optic disk pallor, or pigment mottling. A standardized ERG will show abnormal responses. Some cases have negative waveforms, consisting of a preserved a-wave with severely reduced b-wave amplitude with a b:a ratio inferior to 1 on dark-adapted bright-flash ERG response. Kinetic visual fields are better at measuring peripheral losses or scotomata, blind spot enlargement, or pericentral losses.

Although OCT can demonstrate intraretinal cystic spaces or schisis-like spaces, many of these cases do not show leakage on fluorescence angiography, and the AIR macular changes may be a form of degenerative schisis.

The diagnosis of AIRs involves clinical and electrophysiological evidence of retinal degeneration with concurrent detection of antiretinal antibodies. There is often a strong personal and family history or medical history of autoimmune disease. The detection of antiretinal antibodies can be performed using different techniques: Western blot, immunohistochemistry, and enzyme-linked immunosorbent assay (Grewal et al., 2014)[50]. Antibodies against recoverin, α-enolase, the inner plexiform layer, the inner retinal layer and rod-transducing α have been found in npAIR (Grewal et al., 2014)[50]. While most authors agree that the presence of antiretinal antibodies is required for the diagnosis of npAIRs, there is a strong need for standardization and validation of these antibody tests. To date, there has been no data in the literature validating the sensibility, specificity, positive predictive, and negative value of antiretinal antigen testing (Forooghian, 2016)[51]. Moreover, there is no proof of these antibodies' pathogenicity except for anti-recoverin (Forooghian, 2016)[51]. In fact, the detection of antiretinal antibodies in a patient can represent either the primary cause of the retinal disorder, a normal unrelated finding, or a secondary process

that may worsen a retinal disease (Grewal et al., 2014)[50].

Recently, a panel of experts met to reach a consensus on the definition and diagnostic criteria of npAIRs (Fox et al., 2016)[52]. This appears as a first step to evaluate and validate the diagnostic value of ARA testing and therapeutic strategy. The experts agreed on criteria considered essential for the diagnosis: (1) no apparent cause responsible for visual deterioration such as malignancy, inflammation, infection, surgery, trauma, toxicity, or hereditary retinal degeneration; (2) ERG abnormality with or without visual field abnormality; (3) presence of serum antiretinal antibodies; (4) absence of fundus lesions and retinal degeneration or dystrophy that may explain vision loss; and (5) absence of overt intraocular inflammation (Fox et al., 2016)[52].

The rarity of AIRs, and the difficulty in firmly establishing the diagnosis, has limited therapeutic investigations. No specific treatment regimens for autoimmune retinopathies have emerged during the past decade. Immunosuppression with oral or intravenous corticosteroids has shown mixed results. Generally, short courses of steroids are ineffective. In a series of 30 patients, Ferreyra et al. (2009)[53] reported their experience using immunosuppression to treat AIR. Long-term treatment with immunosuppression resulted in clinical improvement in all subgroups of AIR. The most responsive group was cancer-associated retinopathy, the last was npAIR. Sub-Tenon periocular injections of methylprednisolone have also been proposed (Ferreyra et al., 2009)[53].

The panel of experts agreed that corticosteroids or immunosuppressive agents should be used as the first or second line of treatment (Fox et al., 2016)[52]. Efforts will be made to develop a standardized way to test antiretinal antibodies and validate their diagnostic sensibility, specificity, and pathogenicity in npAIRs. This will be the first step towards evaluating a homogeneous cohort of patients and evaluate their response to therapy.

References

1 Sahel JA, Mohand-Said S, Leveillard T, et al: Rod-cone interdependence: implications for therapy of photoreceptor cell diseases. Prog Brain Res 2001;131:649–661.

2 Travis GH: Mechanisms of cell death in the inherited retinal degenerations. Am J Hum Genet 1998;62:503–508.

3 Leveillard T, Mohand-Said S, Lorentz O, et al: Identification and characterization of rod-derived cone viability factor. Nat Genet 2004;36:755–759.

4 Mohand-Said S, Hicks D, Dreyfus H, Sahel JA: Selective transplantation of rods delays cone loss in a retinitis pigmentosa model. Arch Ophthalmol 2000;118:807–811.

5 Fishman GA, Fishman M, Maggiano J: Macular lesions associated with retinitis pigmentosa. Arch Ophthalmol 1977;95:798–803.

6 Heckenlively JR: RP cone-rod degeneration. Trans Am Ophthalmol Soc 1987;85:438–470.

7 Pruett RC: Retinitis pigmentosa: clinical observations and correlations. Trans Am Ophthalmol Soc 1983;81:693–735.

8 Adackapara CA, Sunness JS, Dibernardo CW, et al: Prevalence of cystoid macular edema and stability in oct retinal thickness in eyes with retinitis pigmentosa during a 48-week lutein trial. Retina 2008;28:103–110.

9 Hajali M, Fishman GA, Anderson RJ: The prevalence of cystoid macular oedema in retinitis pigmentosa patients determined by optical coherence tomography. Br J Ophthalmol 2008;92:1065–1068.

10 Hirakawa H, Iijima H, Gohdo T, Tsukahara S: Optical coherence tomography of cystoid macular edema associated with retinitis pigmentosa. Am J Ophthalmol 1999;128:185–191.

11 Kim C, Chung H, Yu HG: Association of p.P347L in the rhodopsin gene with early-onset cystoid macular edema in patients with retinitis pigmentosa. Ophthalmic Genet 2012;33:96–99.

12 Bujakowska K, Audo I, Mohand-Saïd S, et al: CRB1 mutations in inherited retinal dystrophies. Hum Mutat 2012;33:306–315.

13 Hajali M, Fishman GA: The prevalence of cystoid macular oedema on optical coherence tomography in retinitis pigmentosa patients without cystic changes on fundus examination. Eye (Lond) 2009;23:915–919.

14 Heckenlively JR, Aptsiauri N, Nusinowitz S, et al: Investigations of antiretinal antibodies in pigmentary retinopathy and other retinal degenerations. Trans Am Ophthalmol Soc 1996;94:179–200; discussion 200–176.

15 Cox SN, Hay E, Bird AC: Treatment of chronic macular edema with acetazolamide. Arch Ophthalmol 1988;106:1190–1195.

16 Bringmann A, Wiedemann P: Müller glial cells in retinal disease. Ophthalmologica 2012;227:1–19.

17 Iandiev I, Wurm A, Hollborn M, et al: Müller cell response to blue light injury of the rat retina. Invest Ophthalmol Vis Sci 2008;49:3559–3567.

18 Wurm A, Lipp S, Pannicke T, et al: Involvement of A(1) adenosine receptors in osmotic volume regulation of retinal glial cells in mice. Mol Vis 2009;15:1858–1867.

19 Fishman GA, Gilbert LD, Fiscella RG, et al: Acetazolamide for treatment of chronic macular edema in retinitis pigmentosa. Arch Ophthalmol 1989;107:1445–1452.

20 Melo GB, Farah ME, Aggio FB: Intravitreal injection of bevacizumab for cystoid macular edema in retinitis pigmentosa. Acta Ophthalmol Scand 2007;85:461–463.

21 Yuzbasioglu E, Artunay O, Rasier R, et al: Intravitreal bevacizumab (Avastin) injection in retinitis pigmentosa. Curr Eye Res 2009;34:231–237.

22 Apushkin MA, Fishman GA, Grover S, Janowicz MJ: Rebound of cystoid macular edema with continued use of acetazolamide in patients with retinitis pigmentosa. Retina 2007;27:1112–1118.

23 Chen JC, Fitzke FW, Bird AC: Long-term effect of acetazolamide in a patient with retinitis pigmentosa. Invest Ophthalmol Vis Sci 1990;31:1914–1918.

24 Orzalesi N, Pierrottet C, Porta A, Aschero M: Long-term treatment of retinitis pigmentosa with acetazolamide. A pilot study. Graefes Arch Clin Exp Ophthalmol 1993;231:254–256.

25 Grover S, Fishman GA, Fiscella RG, Adelman AE: Efficacy of dorzolamide hydrochloride in the management of chronic cystoid macular edema in patients with retinitis pigmentosa. Retina 1997;17:222–231.

26 Liew G, Moore AT, Webster AR, Michaelides M: Efficacy and prognostic factors of response to carbonic anhydrase inhibitors in management of cystoid macular edema in retinitis pigmentosa. Invest Ophthalmol Vis Sci 2015;56:1531–1536.

27 Genead MA, Fishman GA: Efficacy of sustained topical dorzolamide therapy for cystic macular lesions in patients with retinitis pigmentosa and usher syndrome. Arch Ophthalmol 2010;128:1146–1150.

28 Fishman GA, Apushkin MA: Continued use of dorzolamide for the treatment of cystoid macular oedema in patients with retinitis pigmentosa. Br J Ophthalmol 2007;91:743–745.

29 Ozdemir H, Karacorlu M, Karacorlu S: Intravitreal triamcinolone acetonide for treatment of cystoid macular oedema in patients with retinitis pigmentosa. Acta Ophthalmol Scand 2005;83:248–251.

30 Sallum JM, Farah ME, Saraiva VS: Treatment of cystoid macular edema related to retinitis pigmentosa with intravitreal triamcinolone acetonide: case report. Adv Exp Med Biol 2003;533:79–81.

31 Saraiva VS, Sallum JM, Farah ME: Treatment of cystoid macular edema related to retinitis pigmentosa with intravitreal triamcinolone acetonide. Ophthalmic Surg Lasers Imaging 2003;34:398–400.

32 Scorolli L, Morara M, Meduri A, et al: Treatment of cystoid macular edema in retinitis pigmentosa with intravitreal triamcinolone. Arch Ophthalmol 2007;125:759–764.

33 Srour M, Querques G, Leveziel N, et al: Intravitreal dexamethasone implant (Ozurdex) for macular edema secondary to retinitis pigmentosa. Graefes Arch Clin Exp Ophthalmol 2013;251:1501–1506.

34 Saint-Geniez M, Kurihara T, Sekiyama E, et al: An essential role for RPE-derived soluble VEGF in the maintenance of the choriocapillaris. Proc Natl Acad Sci USA 2009;106:18751–18756.

35 Garcia-Arumi J, Martinez V, Sararols L, Corcostegui B: Vitreoretinal surgery for cystoid macular edema associated with retinitis pigmentosa. Ophthalmology 2003;110:1164–1169.

36 Ikeda Y, Yoshida N, Murakami Y, et al: Long-term surgical outcomes of epiretinal membrane in patients with retinitis pigmentosa. Sci Rep 2015;5:13078.

37 Eshaghian J, Rafferty NS, Goossens W: Ultrastructure of human cataract in retinitis pigmentosa. Arch Ophthalmol 1980;98:2227–2230.

38 Jackson H, Garway-Heath D, Rosen P, et al: Outcome of cataract surgery in patients with retinitis pigmentosa. Br J Ophthalmol 2001;85:936–938.

39 Battaglia Parodi M, La Spina C, Triolo G, et al: Correlation of SD-OCT findings and visual function in patients with retinitis pigmentosa. Graefes Arch Clin Exp Ophthalmol 2016;254:1275–1279.

40 Makiyama Y, Oishi A, Otani A, et al: Prevalence and spatial distribution of cystoid spaces in retinitis pigmentosa: investigation with spectral domain optical coherence tomography. Retina 2014; 34:981–988.

41 Adamus G: Antirecoverin antibodies and autoimmune retinopathy. Arch Ophthalmol 2000;118:1577–1578.

42 Heckenlively JR, Fawzi AA, Oversier J, et al: Autoimmune retinopathy: patients with antirecoverin immunoreactivity and panretinal degeneration. Arch Ophthalmol 2000;118:1525–1533.

43 Whitcup SM, Vistica BP, Milam AH, et al: Recoverin-associated retinopathy: a clinically and immunologically distinctive disease. Am J Ophthalmol 1998;126: 230–237.

44 Mizener JB, Kimura AE, Adamus G, et al: Autoimmune retinopathy in the absence of cancer. Am J Ophthalmol 1997; 123:607–618.

45 Chan JW: Paraneoplastic retinopathies and optic neuropathies. Surv Ophthalmol 2003;48:12–38.

46 Hooks JJ, Tso MO, Detrick B: Retinopathies associated with antiretinal antibodies. Clin Diagn Lab Immunol 2001;8: 853–858.

47 Heckenlively JR, Jordan BL, Aptsiauri N: Association of antiretinal antibodies and cystoid macular edema in patients with retinitis pigmentosa. Am J Ophthalmol 1999;127:565–573.

48 Heckenlively JR, Solish AM, Chant SM, Meyers-Elliott RH: Autoimmunity in hereditary retinal degenerations. II. Clinical studies: antiretinal antibodies and fluorescein angiogram findings. Br J Ophthalmol 1985;69:758–764.

49 Chant SM, Heckenlively J, Meyers-Elliott RH: Autoimmunity in hereditary retinal degeneration. I. Basic studies. Br J Ophthalmol 1985;69:19–24.

50 Grewal DS, Fishman GA, Jampol LM: Autoimmune retinopathy and antiretinal antibodies: a review. Retina 2014;34: 827–845.

51 Forooghian F: Consensus on the diagnosis and management of nonparaneoplastic autoimmune retinopathy using a modified Delphi approach. Am J Ophthalmol 2016;170:241–242.

52 Fox AR, Gordon LK, Heckenlively JR, et al: Consensus on the diagnosis and management of nonparaneoplastic autoimmune retinopathy using a modified Delphi approach. Am J Ophthalmol 2016;168:183–190.

53 Ferreyra HA, Jayasundera T, Khan NW, et al: Management of autoimmune retinopathies with immunosuppression. Arch Ophthalmol 2009;127:390–397.

Prof. José-Alain Sahel
Institut de la Vision
17, Rue Moreau
FR–75012 Paris (France)
E-Mail j.sahel@gmail.com

Coscas G (ed): Macular Edema. 2nd, revised and extended edition.
Dev Ophthalmol. Basel, Karger, 2017, vol 58, pp 202–219 (DOI: 10.1159/000455282)

Macular Edema of Choroidal Origin

Gisèle Soubrane

Hotel Dieu de Paris, Université Paris V Centre, Paris, France

Abstract

Macular edema is most often clinically defined as an accumulation of serous fluid within the neurosensory retina with increased thickness of the central retina. In exudative age-related macular degeneration the leakage of fluid from the choroidal new vessels may be the origin of macular edema. Their abnormal permeability and the inflammatory reaction are mechanisms involved in this accumulation of fluid, which occurs in all layers. Cystoid macular edema is more often associated with subepithelial occult choroidal neovascularization (CNV) than it is with pre-epithelial classic CNV. The simultaneous presence of choroidal new vessels and ME implies a number of cellular dysfunctions especially of Müller cells and subsequently metabolic alterations. The leakage from the choroidal new vessels, predominantly vascular endothelial growth factor (VEGF)-induced, may produce a large accumulation of fluid under the neurosensory retina. It is also likely that the key signaling steps occur prior to the upregulation of VEGF either initiated by, or facilitated by, cytokines, which act under normal basic conditions to counterbalance the integral VEGF effects and, in pathologic circumstances, may either counteract or serve to amplify the process.

Age-related macular degeneration (AMD) is the result of an involvement of the choriocapillaris, retinal pigment epithelium (RPE), and photoreceptor layer triad. The neural retina is only partially involved, and additional pathways are required for the development of edema within the retina.

Age-related maculopathy is the initial clinical manifestation affecting the RPE and begins with drusen of various types and RPE mottling, clumping, or patches of atrophy. Age-related maculopathy can progress to the degenerative stage, which is referred to as AMD. The atrophic or dry form of macular degeneration does not generally present with macular edema, but sometimes with small pseudocysts located in the inner nuclear layer of the retina that might correspond to Müller cell degeneration (Cohen et al., 2010)[1]. The exudative form is due to choroidal neovascularization (CNV) that causes a serous detachment of the RPE and neurosensory retina.

Macular edema is most often clinically defined as an accumulation of serous fluid within the neurosensory retina with increased thickness of the central retina. In exudative AMD, the leakage of fluid from the choroidal new vessels may be the origin of macular edema. Their abnormal permeability and the associated inflammatory reaction are mechanisms involved in this accumulation of fluid.

The presence of cystoid macular edema is more likely if the retinal serous detachment is long-standing and if the choroidal neovascular membrane has involved most of the subfoveal region. In addition, after prolonged detachment, the retinal capillaries may become damaged and contribute to the leakage of dye into the extra cellular compartment of the retina.

Pathophysiology: Theories of Macular Edema in Age-Related Macular Degeneration

CNV being of choroidal origin presents the same histological structure as the choriocapillaris and thus, in pathological conditions, leads to an exudation within the subretinal space. The consequent damage of the outer retinal layers determines alterations of the overlying (and underlying) tissues. In addition, several inflammatory mediators and inflammatory cells, which secrete numerous cytokines such as vascular permeability factor, referred to as vascular endothelial growth factor (VEGF), are present at the site of the angiogenic stimulus and interact in a complex chain reaction, which is not yet completely understood.

Cellular Components
Choriocapillaris
The choriocapillaris is a key player in choroidal new vessel development and is implicated to a lesser degree in retinal vascular disease. Due to the presence of the fenestrations facing Bruch's membrane (Burns et al., 1986)[2], the capillaries leak more plasma components, even large proteins (Connolly et al., 1989)[3]. In addition, the high choroidal flow rate aids metabolic exchanges and maintains a high concentration gradient across the vessel walls.

With increasing age, there is a loss of choroidal vascular elements and a progressive decrease in the thickness of the choroid (from 200 µm at birth to 80 µm by the age of 90) (Ramrattan et al., 1994)[4]. Numerous publications have demonstrated an age-related decrease in the density and lumen diameter of the vessels of the choriocapillaris (Sarks, 1976; Bird et al., 1990; Olver et al., 1990)[5–7].

The decrease in the density and dimension of the choroidal capillary bed, and thus the blood flow, is likely to globally reduce the amount of fluid – as well as the potential for metabolic support – to the photoreceptors. Related to age, however, no change of the diffusion capability of the choriocapillaris has ever been described.

Bruch's Membrane
The overlying Bruch's membrane has a hydraulic conductivity that decreases with age (Fisher, 1987)[8]. In the elderly, Bruch's membrane and choriocapillaris prominent fibrillar structures represent choroidal structure and permeability alteration (Han et al., 2007)[9]. Deposition of material under the basal surface of the RPE resulting from the metabolic turnover of the polyunsaturated fatty acids from the photoreceptor outer segment membranes contributes to thickening of Bruch's membrane. With age, the amount of deposited lipids increases exponentially. All these changes are more marked in the macula than in the periphery (Moore et al., 1995; Holtz et al., 1994)[10, 11].

Although Bruch's membrane has been found to contain neutral fats (Sheraidah et al., 1993)[12], the predominant classes of lipids are phospholipids (Pauleikoff et al., 1992)[13]. The lipid deposition in Bruch's membrane limits the diffusion of oxygen and metabolites.

The reduction of the hydraulic conductivity of Bruch's membrane may be implicated in fluid accumulation to form a RPE detachment. RPE cells normally pump fluid out toward the choroid through Bruch's membrane. In AMD, Bruch's membrane is made hydrophobic by the accumulation of lipids (Curcio et al., 2001)[14]. The trapped fluid spreads within the neurosensory retina and collects in cystic spaces. Impedance of metabolic exchange between the choroid and RPE across Bruch's membrane (Löffler and Lee, 1986)[15] may also compromise photoreceptor function and eventually lead to cell death.

Photoreceptors
Photoreceptors are dependent on the RPE for renewal of spent outer segments and on the choriocapillaris for nutrients and elimination of waste products. An age-related decrease in delivery or diffusion of oxygen or metabolites to the photoreceptors of the macula region has been theorized as the key event in the initiation of a compensatory mechanism, which ultimately leads to the formation of new vessels in AMD.

Among retinal cells, photoreceptors are most exposed to light stress and are the most fragile cells in the face of environmental or genetic stress. Conversely, photoreceptors have developed strong mechanisms of protection. Rods are more vulnerable than cones to senescence.

The external limiting membrane (ELM) is composed of junctional complexes linking Müller cells to the photoreceptor inner segments. This barrier can partially limit the movement of large molecules and retain the proteins in the extracellular space. Intracellular accumulation of fluid in these cells may result in cell death.

Outer Retinal Barrier; Retinal Pigment
Epithelium
The physiological roles of the RPE are numerous. Only those most relevant to the genesis of macular edema with CNV will be considered.

Fluid Movement
RPE cells are joined near the apical side by tight junctions (formed by transmembrane molecules). This outer part of the retinal barrier blocks the free passage of water, ions, and proteins in normal conditions and regulates the environment of the retinal cells. The ability of the RPE to transport water by active mechanisms is very powerful.

Healthy RPE transports proteins and resorbs fluid. Passive mechanisms such as hydrostatic and osmotic pressure also work to drive water out of the subretinal space into the choroid. In AMD, a large amount of protein extravagates through the immature new vessels. This increases the oncotic pressure in the tissues, impedes the resorption of fluid from the tissue to the plasmatic compartment, and results in water accumulation in the surrounding extracellular space, which causes extracellular edema. The proteins that have diffused into the retinal tissue will remain there and only diffuse in a limited amount into the vitreous cavity or subretinal space. Nevertheless, this amount of protein will be replaced by the constant leakage coming from the choroidal new vessels, resulting in possible development of macular edema. In addition, the protein retained in the retina will also be retained by osmosis. This mechanism then aggravates the macular edema due to the breakdown of the outer retinal barrier.

Extracellular matrix changes affect the formation of macular edema. Matrix metalloproteinases cause a degradation and modulation of the extracellular matrix. The breakdown and the dysfunction of the blood-retinal barrier cause changes in endothelial cell resistance. The fluid movement is thus profoundly disturbed in neovascular AMD.

Metabolism of the Retinal Pigment Epithelium Cells
The enzymatic machinery of the RPE assumes a large number of functions including membrane transport, waste product digestion, and elaboration of growth factors. The RPE is involved in photoreceptor outer segment renewal. This phagocytosis process is involved in residual bodies within the cell and deposition of lipids in Bruch's membrane.

The RPE constitutively expresses VEGF to maintain the choriocapillaris. VEGF is also the major mediator of AMD related to CNV (Lopez et al., 1996)[16]. The RPE also produces neuronal traffic, neuronal protective and antiangiogenic factor (pigment epithelium-derived factor) (Imai et al., 2005)[17]. The presence of macrophages in Bruch's membrane has also been implicated in the synthesis of VEGF since activated macrophages have long been recognized as stimulating blood vessel growth (Killingsworth et al., 1990)[18].

Müller Cells

Müller glial cells span the thickness of the retina from the vitreous to the outer limiting membrane (OLM) and ensheath all retinal neurons. The morphological relationship between neurons and Müller cells is reflected by a multitude of functional interactions. The maintenance of the homeostasis of the retinal extracellular milieu (ions, water, neurotransmitter molecules, and pH) is regulated by different ionic channels, inevitably coupled to water fluxes. The cells express a complex microtopographically optimized pattern of transporters and channels for osmolytes and water in their plasma membrane. The major are water channel aquaporin (AQP4) and potassium channels (Kir4.1). The glial cell-mediated transport of extracellular K^+ away from excited neurons is dependent on the cooperation of different Kir channel subtypes absorbing extracellular K^+ into the cell body, and subsequently eliminating the K to retinal blood vessels and the vitreous at the endfoot membranes facing the vitreous and the retinal vessels (Kofuji et al., 2002)[19]. The apical processes of Müller cells are attached to each other and to the inner segments of the photoreceptor cells by continuous heterotypic adherens junctions type that collectively form the OLM. Adherens junctions in the OLM provide a semipermeable barrier, preventing the diffusion of some proteins out of the extracellular space that surrounds the photoreceptors. Occludin with ZO-1 and claudin are the main plasma-membrane proteins located at the tight junctions. During diabetic retinopathy, glial Müller cells are not only swollen, but they also lose their occludin content at the OLM level, which leads to cyst formation (Omri et al., 2010)[20].

The relation of Müller cells and retinal vessels suggests their role in the maintenance of angiogenesis control and regulation of retinal blood flow.

The removal and metabolism of neurotransmitters in the neural retina contributes to the protection of neurons by the uptake of glutamate, N-acetylaspartyl glutamate, γ-aminobutyric acid, glycine, and the secretion of the antioxidant, glutathione. Müller cells regulate the excitability of neurons through release of d-serine and glutamate. The production and release of lactate by Müller cells serves to maintain the photoreceptors glycolysis elevated and to fuel mitochondrial oxidative metabolism and glutamate resynthesis in photoreceptors (Bringmann et al., 2009)[21].

Müller cells may display a dysregulation of the neuron-supportive functions. Disturbance of glutamate metabolism and ion homeostasis causes the development of retinal edema and neuronal cell death (Bringmann, 2006)[22]. Serum leakage from intraretinal vessels causes cysts mainly in the inner nuclear layer while leakage from choroid/pigment epithelium generates (in addition to subretinal fluid accumulation) cyst formation in the Henle fiber layer. Ischemic/hypoxic alterations of the retinal microvasculature result in gliotic responses which involve downregulation of K^+ channels in the perivascular Müller cell endfeet. This means a closure of the main pathway which normally generates the osmotic drive for the redistribution of water from the inner retina into the blood. The result is an intracellular K^+ accumulation which, then, osmotically drives water from the blood into the glial cells (i.e., in the opposite direction) and causes glial cell swelling, edema, and cyst formation (Bringmann et al., 2004)[23].

Vitreous

The development of macular edema may correlate with the presence of an attached posterior hyaloid as suggested in a number of publications about diabetic edema. Similarly, the traction of the posterior hyaloid has been implicated in the increase and possibly occurrence of CNV (Robison et al., 2009)[24] and subsequent macular edema. Vitreomacular traction resulting from an incomplete or anomalous posterior vitreous detachment is suspected to play a role in the pathogenesis of different forms of exudative AMD along with other mechanisms.

It is probable that the fundamental pathomechanisms of AMD formation have already begun by the time tractional forces lead to a change. Hyaloid adhesion to the macula is associated with AMD and frequently causes vitreomacular traction in eyes with CNV. As shown on optical coherence tomography (OCT), there is a clinically high co incidence of vitreomacular traction and CNV in a number of eyes. The area of hyaloid adhesion is claimed to be concentric to the area of CNV complex in such eyes (Mojana et al., 2008; Lee et al., 2009)[25, 26]. Vitreomacular traction seems to be associated with the severity of AMD.

The concept of the pathogenesis of AMD should be extended to include the influence of the vitreous (Schulze et al., 2008)[27]. Persistent attachment of the posterior vitreous cortex to the macula may be a risk factor for the development of exudative AMD (Lee et al., 2009)[26] via vitreoretinal traction inducing chronic low-grade inflammation, by maintaining macular exposure to cytokines or free radicals in the vitreous gel, or by interfering in transvitreous oxygenation and nutrition of the macula (Krebs et al., 2007)[28]. However, there is no evidence presently that vitreous traction is crucial in the genesis of CNV.

Vascular Endothelial Growth Factor

VEGF is an important mediator of CNV by a selective mitogenic activity, but it is also a survival factor for endothelial cells and vessel maintenance. VEGF is involved in ocular pathologic processes such as new vessel formation and is also implicated in the development of macular edema.

VEGF is primarily expressed in endothelial cells as well as in pericytes, monocytes, and neural cells. Its effects are launched when VEGF binds to its receptors on vessel endothelial cells. Basic and clinical studies have shown expression of VEGF on choroidal endothelial cells of new vessels and synthesis of VEGF in RPE cells (Lopez et al., 1996)[16].

Furthermore, eyes with AMD also showed VEGF expression in photoreceptors overlying CNV. In experimentally induced CNV, increased expression was found in macrophages, in RPE cells, and in Müller cells (Kliffen et al., 1997)[29]. In vitro, RPE expressing VEGF promotes experimental choroidal angiogenesis.

Vascular ischemia is one of the major mechanisms inducing VEGF synthesis and release. Increased expression of VEGF in CNV supports the controversial hypothesis that tissue hypoxia may be involved since hypoxia stimulates VEGF expression in the RPE.

It has been theorized that age-related changes in Bruch's membrane may also limit the diffusion of oxygen and therefore create an ischemic environment. The RPE cells on top of drusen were thought to be particularly ischemic (Pauleikhoff et al., 1999)[30]. The ordinary daily exposure of the lipids in the photoreceptor outer segments helps to maintain the constitutive secretion of VEGF by the RPE cells.

This raises the possibility that excessive exposure to oxidative damage may lead the RPE cells to secrete excessive VEGF. The reactive oxygen species and peroxidized lipids increase the production of VEGF (Monte et al., 1997; Kuroki et al., 1996)[31, 32], which is involved in supporting vascular endothelial cells.

VEGF causes vascular hyperpermeability that is leukocyte-mediated. This results in an opening of interendothelial junctions. Elevated oxidative stress levels induce tissue inflammation.

Inflammation induces breakdown of the VEGF-mediated inner blood-retinal barrier via leukocyte binding and by inducing their recruitment to the site of inflammation. The cells involved in the pathogenesis of AMD and macular edema are macrophages and leukocytes that present VEGF receptors. These inflammatory cells also produce and release cytokines (Penfold et al., 1986)[33].

Clinical Findings

The accumulation of serous fluid within the retina occurs in all layers: under the RPE as a pigment epithelial detachment (PED) under the neurosensory retina as subretinal fluid or a serous retinal detachment, within the retina, between the inner limiting membrane and the RPE band, either as diffuse fluid leakage or organized as cysts of various locations, importance, and size. The location is easily identifiable and quantifiable on OCT.

Cystoid macular edema is more often associated with subepithelial occult CNV than it is with pre-epithelial classic CNV. The occurrence of macular edema is probably related to the slow growth rate of these new vessels, the constant leakage through their fenestrations, and their usual subfoveal location. The serous fluid originating from the choriocapillaris, the choroidal new vessels, and in some cases from the deep plexus of the retinal capillaries spreads posteriorly and laterally where it accumulates within the inner nuclear and outer plexiform layers. The extension of the large cellular space available in the outer plexiform layer of Henle causes the typical biomicroscopic and angiographic picture of cystoid macular edema (Gass, 1997)[34].

The functional consequences of macular edema associated with CNV have never been precisely evaluated. It is quite challenging to attempt to do so, as the location, the extent, and the activity of the foveal CNV are predominantly responsible for the visual degradation. Controversy still exists regarding the timing of the occurrence of this cystoid macular edema: early (Soubrane et al., 1988)[35] or late (Bressler et al., 1991)[36].

Biomicroscopy
Biomicroscopic examination with a contact lens is the only way to clinically identify the optically empty clear spaces located within the shallow neurosensory retina elevation overlying a deep gray-green mound. The use of a slit lamp with a 10° angle best provides visualization. Subepithelial occult CNV is usually associated with an RPE detachment and in some instances may be surrounded by hard exudates.

Fluorescein Angiography
Fluorescein angiography was the method previously used to identify macular edema despite the fact that it does not always clearly contrast the hyperfluorescence of the leaking neovascularization (fig. 1).

The pre-injection fluorescein frames are helpful, especially in blue light, as they enable visualization of the cysts encroaching upon the xanthophyll pigment. The central cysts compress the foveal center, especially the Henle fibers, which contain a high concentration of yellow xanthophyll enhanced by the complementary wavelength.

Fluorescein angiography has been instrumental in identifying the 2 major types of CNV.

Pre-epithelial classic CNV manifests as a discrete, well-demarcated focal area of hyperfluorescence (Fine et al. 1986; Coscas, 1991; Soubrane, 2007)[37–39] with late leakage beyond the boundaries of the early hyperfluorescence (Bressler et al., 2006)[40]. Fluorescein may pool in the subsensory retinal fluid overlying the new vessels, which is best seen on stereoscopic images.

Subepithelial occult CNV (formerly named 'late leakage of undetermined source') refers to late choroidal-based leakage without identifiable vessels and poorly demarcated boundaries. This ill-defined area of hyperfluorescence at the level

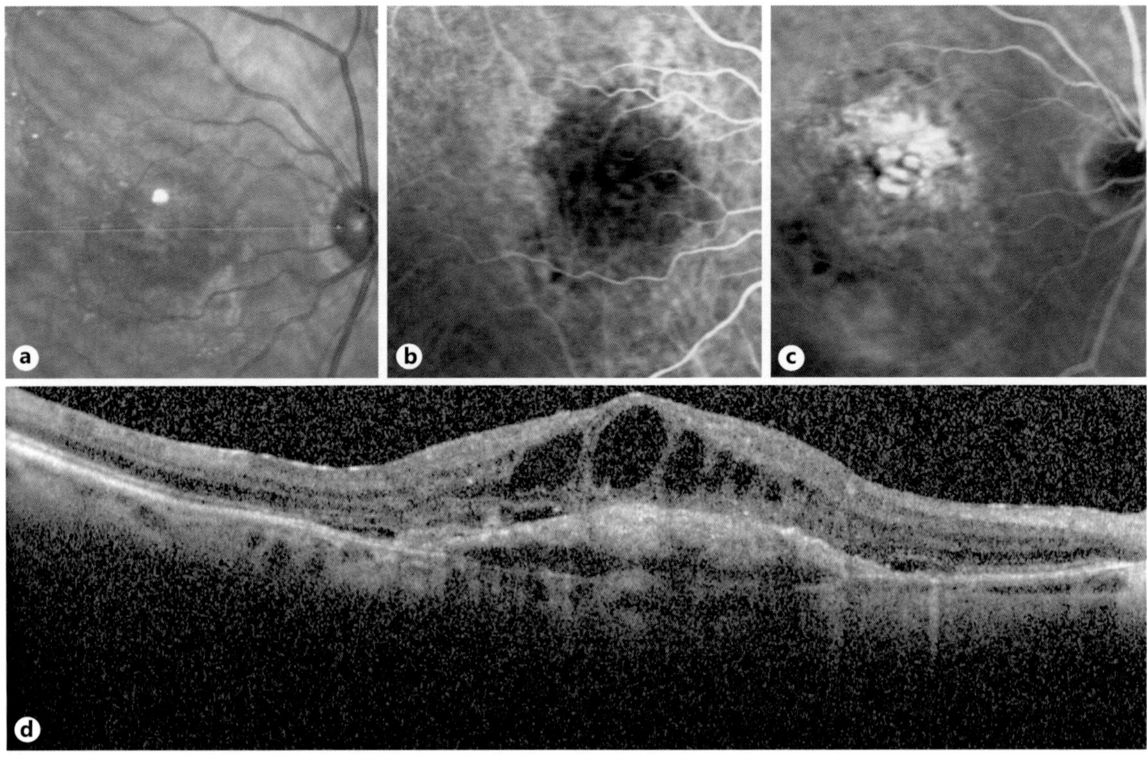

Fig. 1. Cystoid macular edema in a case of advanced subepithelial occult CNV. **a** Monochromatic green light. **b** Fluorescein angiography, early phase: 3 DD central area is dark. **c** Fluorescein angiography, late phase: the central area became heavily hyperfluorescent with at least 4 large macular cysts, distinctly visible. **d** SD-OCT (Spectralis): extensive multiple cysts occupying the complete thickness of the neurosensory retina. Some remaining Müller cell pillars. The retinal outer layers are modified by a hyperreflective dense spindle corresponding to a fibrovascular membrane. The ELM and the IS/OS interface are unrecognizable. Note the fibrovascular PED partially organized.

of the RPE is later followed by pinpoints of leakage (ooze). Progressively faint leakage will take place (Soubrane et al., 1990; Bressler et al., 1992)[41, 42]. The angiographic appearance of the subepithelial CNV depends on the location, the density, and the maturity of the new vessels as well as the associated vascularized PED (Coscas, 2009)[43].

A second pattern of subepithelial occult CNV previously separated is fibrovascular PED (Macular Photocoagulation Study Group, 1991)[44]. Due to the progress of imaging it has been identified as a stage in the natural history of subepithelial occult CNV (Soubrane, 2007)[39].

In the late phase, the hyperfluorescence of the cystoid spaces superimposes on the deep uneven fluorescence of the CNV. A careful analysis of mid and late phase is necessary in order to delineate each component. The cysts are usually encroaching upon the central avascular zone, but may be difficult to identify in most instances. A large central cyst may be the cause of a hypofluorescent area seen on angiography if the RPE is not altered. In addition, a PED can be clinically evident in the cleavage site created by the subepithelial occult CNV (Gass, 1997)[34].

The intraretinal collection of fluid caused by macular edema alters the structure of the macula and affects its function. The breakdown of the outer blood-retinal barrier gives rise to fluorescein leakage from the choroidal circulation and the choroidal new vessels. But the retinal vasculature may also be involved in exudative AMD and contribute to macular edema. The retinal capillaries may become damaged, develop microaneurysms, and contribute to the leakage of dye into the extracellular compartment of the retina after a prolonged retinal detachment.

Extension of a choroidal neovascular membrane in the capillary-free zone, as is the rule in subepithelial occult CNV, may destroy the ELM and facilitate the collection of fluid in cystic spaces. The predisposition for the spaces to be located in the capillary-free zone may be related to structural weaknesses of the ELM where Müller cell processes are reduced in number as well as to the paucity of retinal capillaries which drain the extracellular fluid in the intravascular compartment.

Indocyanine Green Angiography
Indocyanine green (ICG) angiography designed to reveal choroidal abnormalities is able to confirm the fluorescein angiography appearance of pre-epithelial classic CNV (Hayashi and De Laey, 1985)[45]. With the improvement of the instruments, especially the scanning laser ophthalmoscope (SLO), ICG angiography was shown to be very useful in the conversion of subepithelial CNV into a well-delimited network (Yannuzzi et al., 1992)[46]. Further studies have demonstrated a variety of patterns of subepithelial occult CNV in ICG angiography (Soubrane, 1995)[47].

Areas of CNV that appear poorly defined on fluorescein angiography can be revealed as a clearly delineated network at the early phase of ICG angiography, contrasting with a larger hypofluorescent macular area. At the late phase, some subepithelial occult CNV may present as relatively large, well-defined staining plaques whereas others, active lesions, present an early washout. This difference is possibly related to the development stage of the lesion or to the speed of the blood flow as assessed by OCT angiography. In rare cases, mainly at the inversion (late) phase,

cystoid spaces may fill with ICG dye. Furthermore, ICG angiography is useful in identifying CNV with and without PED (Scheider and Schroedel, 1989)[48]. SLO-ICG angiography is particularly helpful in chorioretinal anastomosis, demonstrating anastomosis in the area of a uniformly dark PED and late intraretinal leakage (fig. 2).

ICG angiography has been essential for imaging subepithelial occult CNV and the associated PED (Coscas, 2005)[49]. Thus, the best imaging strategy was to perform both fluorescein angiography and ICG angiography to detect CNV (Bressler et al., 2006)[40].

Optical Coherence Tomography
Optical coherence tomography (OCT) generates axial cross-sectional images of the retina. It allows a visualization of the CNV beneath and in front of the RPE as well as the cystoid macular edema overlying the choroidal new vessels. Following OCT variations and correlations with angiographic techniques is of primary interest in the study of the natural history or the result of treatment and may provide additional prognostic clues (fig. 1d) (Coscas, 2009)[43].

Neurosensory Retina
Serous fluid in the neurosensory retina becomes manifest either within the retinal tissue (as diffuse infiltration) or is collected in intraretinal cysts. The association of both patterns induces an increase in the retinal thickness and an attenuation of the foveal depression.

Fluid
The diffuse fluid can infiltrate all the retinal layers associated or not associated with cystoid spaces. The fluid accumulation probably induces a swelling of Müller cells, which consequently may distort the photoreceptor segments and alter the ELM. This accumulation of fluid is usually associated with an inflammatory reaction that might account for the intraretinal hyperreflective dots (Coscas, 2009)[43]. The increase in fluid and in-

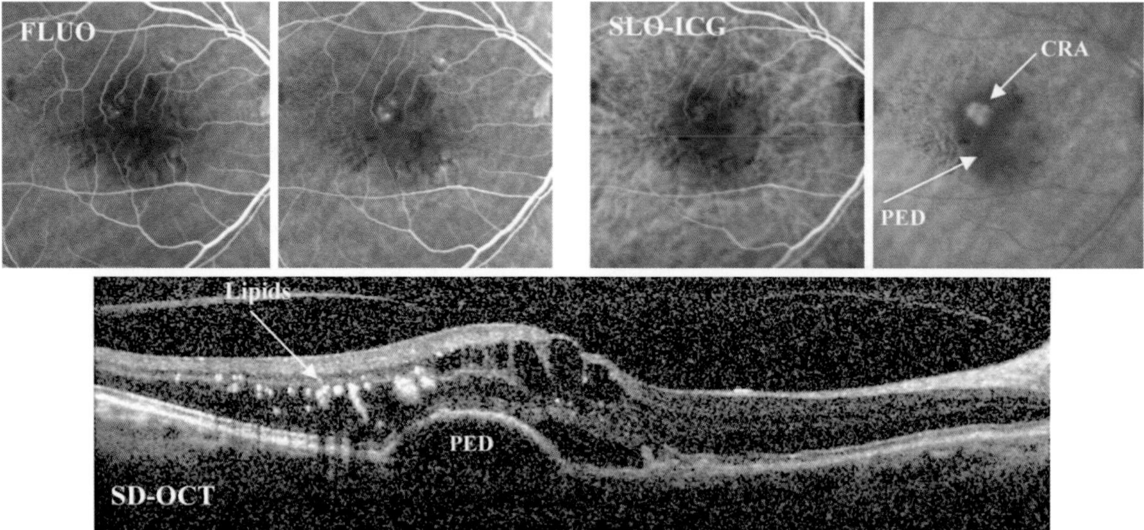

Fig. 2. Chorioretinal anastomoses. SD-OCT horizontal section (Spectralis), associated with fluorescein angiography (early and late stage) and SLO-ICG (early and late stage). Note the hyperfluorescent leakage on the late stage of the ICG angiography contrasting in the dark area of the PED. Also note the extensive and marked intraretinal accumulation of fluid within large cystic spaces.

flammatory reaction may subsequently be revealed as a dense, uneven hyperreflectivity in the disorganized photoreceptor layer.

Cysts

The cysts are spaces that are optically empty, homogenous, and thus dark in the neurosensory retina. The size of the cysts is variable according to the stage of the disease. They are mostly small (70%) or tightly packed and confluent (30%). They are more or less extensive in the advanced stage. Their distribution in one layer (42%) or in two (58%) is of similar frequency. The swelling of the retina induces the loss of the foveal depression that is occupied early by 3–4 large cysts or by a single huge cyst, which is sometimes prolonged by a row of smaller cysts (fig. 3, 4).

A study of 150 consecutive cases of exudative AMD showed the presence of the cystoid spaces in nearly half of the eyes (41%), often multiple (97%), rarely isolated and centrally located (3%). These cysts are present in recent or active lesions with hyperreflective dots and areas of intraretinal densification. During treatment, improvement or degradation is parallel to the importance of the cysts. After 3 intravitreous injections of anti-VEGF, the cysts were noted in 35% of the treated eyes. They vanish relatively slowly when compared with the functional improvement. The recurrence of the leakage results in the reemergence of the cysts (Coscas, 2009)[43].

On the other hand, in the advanced form, cysts are associated with various amounts of fibrosis. The persistence of the cysts in 30% of the eyes without fluorescein leakage means an irreversible degeneration of the neural tissue with severe vision loss (Coscas, 2009)[43].

Central Thickness

Central retinal thickness is often used in clinical studies. The normal thickness of the central retina is between 180 and 360 μm according to the OCT instrument used. Central retinal thickness helps to determine the indication for treatment or re-

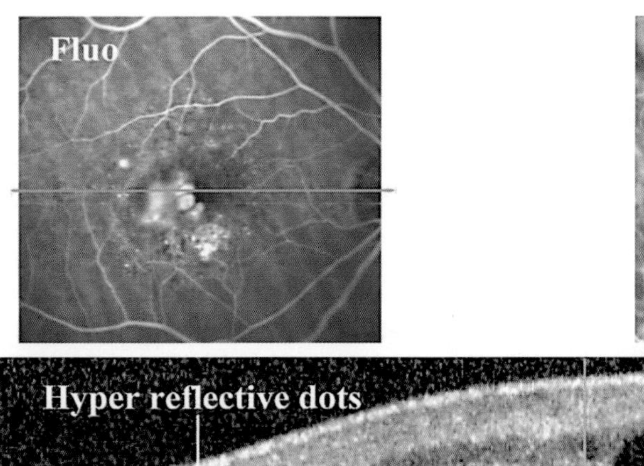

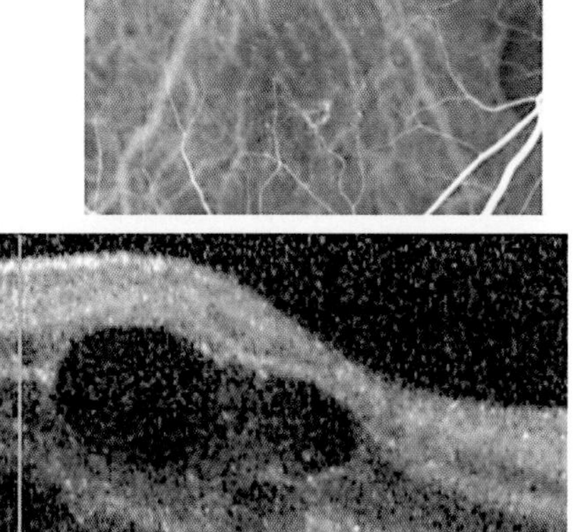

Fig. 3. Active CNV in AMD: SD-OCT horizontal section (Spectralis), associated with fluorescein and SLO-ICG angiography. Increased retinal thickness, intraretinal large cysts, hyperreflective dots, intraretinal dense area. Disorganization of the outer retinal layers [courtesy of Coscas (2009)[36]].

treatment as well as the prognosis and the follow-up of exudative AMD. This criterion of central thickness is quite easy to use but is obviously insufficient for a precise justification for retreatment due to the polymorphism of the disease.

Retinal Pigment Epithelium
CNV proliferation is manifested either as a pre-RPE zone of hyperreflectivity (pre-epithelial classic CNV) or as an irregular thickening of the RPE (subepithelial occult CNV). It is then associated with the RPE elevation, which is ascertained by the visibility of Bruch's membrane. A large, prominent bullous PED with numerous packed cystic spaces in elevated retina is almost pathognomonic of anastomoses between retinal and choroidal vessels (Coscas et al., 2007)[50].

The accumulation of intraretinal and subretinal fluid and the intraretinal cysts parallels with the progression of the underlying disease but, un-til now, at an unpredictable speed, sometimes delayed or sometimes rapid. The most difficult problem is to predict which residual lesion is likely to vanish and which cyst confirms an irreversible alteration of the retinal tissue. Review of the different OCT sections and correlations with the angiographic examinations are therefore of major value.

OCT Angiography
OCT angiography (OCTA) is a recent high-resolution imaging method for visualizing the retinal and choroidal circulation. The comparison between sequential OCT-B scans at the exact same location shows the modifications from one to another slab, thus the moving red cells.

Structural OCT-B scans cannot reliably discriminate CNV tissue from the surrounding tissues that has similar reflectivity as drusenoid material, hemorrhage, RPE, and choroid. OCTA

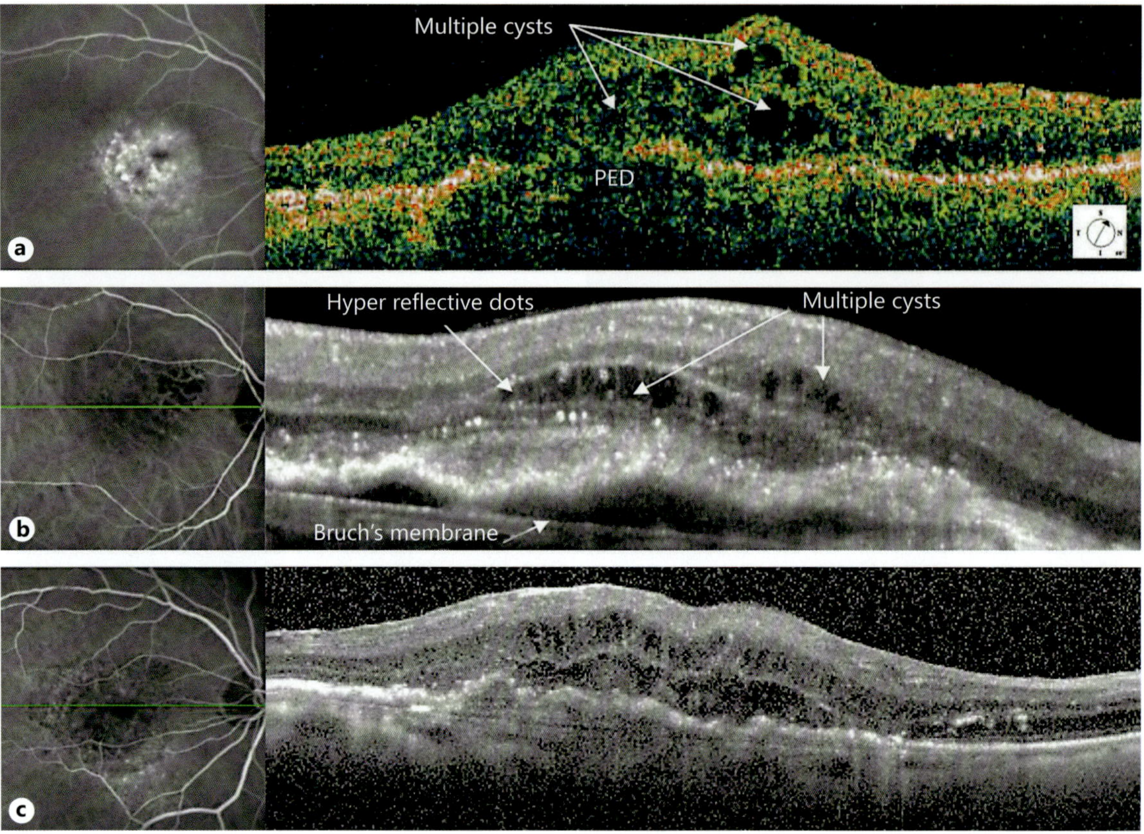

Fig. 4. Multiple intraretinal cysts and increased retinal thickness: OCT horizontal section, associated with fluorescein angiograph. **a** Advanced multiple chorioretinal anastomosis: multiple confluent cysts. **b** Persistent vascularized PED: presence of many hyperreflective dots and intraretinal dense area. Disorganization of the outer retinal layers. **c** Late advanced lesion not responding to treatment. Visual acuity: 20/800. Large number of cysts in the inner nuclear layer and between the outer plexiform layer and the outer nuclear layer [courtesy of Coscas (2009)[43]].

provides noninvasive 3D in-depth location of the CNV, information on the architecture of new vessels, and quantification of the blood flow within CNV. The pattern and the position of the CNV relative to the RPE and Bruch's membrane is easily determined: underneath the RPE and above Bruch's membrane, (subepithelial so-called type I or occult) or in front of the RPE (pre-epithelial so-called classic or type II) (Hong et al., 2013)[51]. Hemorrhages do not obscure the CNV. The network is surrounded by focal regions adjacent to CNV where there was total absence of choriocapillaris with loss of both inner and deeper choroidal vessels. These focal areas of choroidal hypoperfusion suggest a possible outer retinal ischemia that may have a role in CNV pathogenesis. (Jia et al., 2014)[52].

Cysts in the deep capillary plexus manifest as dark spaces surrounded by capillary dilations and sometimes microaneurysms. The superficial plexus is pushed aside by the large foveal cysts.

The determinant mechanism of intraretinal macular edema is still debatable. One of the hypotheses implies the breakdown of the outer retinal barrier, which would allow the influx of exudation towards the central avascular zone (Gass,

1997)[34]. An alternative hypothesis suggests the possibility of an intracellular edema of the Müller cells (Yannoff et al., 1984)[53]. The role of vitreous traction in AMD is still questionable: is it an initiating mechanism or, on the contrary, an aggravation for the development of CNV and of the macular edema? The leakage from choroidal new vessels is the determinant factor in the occurrence of macular edema; the initiating mechanism of which, however, remains to be clarified.

Treatment Approaches

The exudative form of AMD accounts for a large number of cases of legal blindness in the elderly, and efforts have been made to develop drugs to address this problem (Ambati et al., 2003)[54]. Visual loss results from the proliferation of new capillaries accompanied by exudation, bleeding, and secondary fibrosis with disorganization of the RPE and outer retina. Further, secondary alterations in both the subretinal and retinal capillaries and the pigment epithelial permeability lead to the accumulation of fluid and induce more visual dysfunction. The treatment should achieve a common goal by reducing the accumulation of intraretinal fluid.

Laser Treatment
Destruction and occlusion of the CNV resolves leakage from the abnormal new capillaries and thus induces reduction of the macular edema. However, it also destroys the neurosensory retina and the pigment epithelium in the area of laser burns.

Photocoagulation
If precisely applied, the heat produced by this direct laser treatment technique will occlude and destroy the new vessels causing the new vessel leakage to disappear. As a result, the cystoid macular edema will resolve. A side effect of the treatment, however, includes the occurrence of a definitive localized scotoma due to the destruction of the complete thickness of the neurosensory retina.

Photodynamic Therapy
Another means of neovascular occlusion is using a pharmacologic photosynthesizer verteporfin). The product injected into the veins has to be activated by the adapted laser wavelength. The healing process involves the formation of a glial scar. Clinical trial results were very encouraging regarding stabilization of visual acuity. Unfortunately the generation of free radicals necessary for the photothrombotic effect may also serve as a proangiogenic stimulus, possibly accounting for the apparent benefit associated with concomitant administration of steroids (Rudolf et al., 2004)[55].

Pharmacotherapy
Anti-VEGF
VEGF produces an important increase in hydrolytic conductivity and is the central player of leakage both in choroidal new vessels and in macular edema. A variety of methods are available to directly block the VEGF165 molecule and its various other isoforms. Bevacizumab (Avastin®), ranibizumab (Lucentis®; recombinant humanized Fab fragment of a murine monoclonal anti-VEGF antibody), and aflibercept (Eylea®; a recombinant fusion protein with binding domains from human VEGF receptors) block this protein which results in a decrease in leakage clearly visible on fluorescein angiography and OCT.

The randomized clinical trials, which included pre-epithelial CNV or subepithelial occult CNV, clearly demonstrated that visual acuity is stabilized and sometimes increased. However, the decrease of leakage of the choroidal new vessels requires multiple injections for a period of 12–24 months and regular follow-up later on. The effectiveness of aflibercept is comparable to ranibizumab for visual acuity and morphological outcomes in eyes with neovascular AMD (Sarwar et al., 2016)[56].

A number of attempts have been made to decrease the frequency of injections. Most were able to stabilize visual acuity, but no attempt resulted in a functional improvement as was obtained by the regular injections. This suggests that a decrease in leakage from the choroidal vessels and also from the altered blood-retinal barrier is necessary in order to obtain a positive result. In the eyes in which the treatment failed, one of the most prominent features is the persistence of cystic spaces. In addition, chronic degenerative cysts may be disseminated in the inner retina, which will not resorb despite treatment.

Retrospective analyses of medical records from patients with neovascular AMD receiving bevacizumab for 9–12 months demonstrated that the presence of cystoid macular edema at baseline was significantly associated with a worse visual outcome (Byun et al., 2010)[57]. Subanalysis of the EX-CITE study demonstrated that lower mean best corrected visual acuity at month 12 in patients receiving ranibizumab was significantly correlated with intraretinal cysts (IRC) at baseline compared with patients without (Simader et al., 2014)[58]. In a post hoc analysis of randomized multicenter clinical trials of 1,240 patients treated in 189 sites, only intraretinal cysts at baseline and persistent OCT through week 12 had a negative impact on best corrected visual acuity. With either regimen, fixed or flexible, or substance, ranibizumab or aflibercept, intraretinal cysts consistently showed the lowest visual gains. PED appears to be the primary indicator for progressive disease activity, whereas secondary cystoid degeneration is the most relevant imaging marker for visual function (Schmidt-Erfurth et al., 2015)[59].

Direct and Indirect Vascular Endothelial Growth

Factor Modulators
Cytokines may be divided into two classes: those that upregulate VEGF or VEGF-associated effects and those that act in an inhibitory capacity. Naturally occurring inhibitory factors include interferon-α, thrombospondin, angiostatin, endostatin, and metalloproteinases. Intracellular adhesion molecules (ICAM-1) mediate leukocyte adhesion and transmigration. They are expressed on the RPE and choroidal vascular endothelial cell surfaces and mediate extravasation from retinal and choroidal capillaries in response to inflammation. Naturally occurring downregulators include pigment epithelial-derived growth factor (PEGF) secreted by the RPE. Because VEGF is thought to initiate a cascade of intracellular signals followed by subsequent extracellular events, it is possible to inhibit VEGF effects either through prevention of secretion of the molecule, direct inhibition of the molecule in the extracellular space, blockade of the receptors, or through interruption in the downstream intracellular signaling pathway leading to both an intracellular and extracellular event (Campochiaro, 2004)[60].

A large body of evidence exists to support the critical and probably rate-limiting role of VEGF in the neovascular form of AMD (Ambati et al., 2003; Grossniklaus et al., 2002)[54, 61]. Additionally, there are strong indicators that elevated levels of VEGF are the proximal causes for the hyperpermeability seen in eyes with subsensory and intraretinal fluid associated with CNV. These alterations are able to be either reversed by direct blockade of VEGF receptors or prevented as in a NOS knockout model (Senger et al., 1983; Fukumura et al., 2001; Sennlaub et al., 2002)[62–64]. Inactivation of soluble VEGF by monoclonal antibodies directed against it or inhibition of ICAM also appears to be effective.

Other methods of direct inhibition of VEGF include inhibition of its tyrosine kinase receptors (VEGF-R1/FLT-1 and VEGF-R2/KDR-1) either by systemic administration or gene transfer. The VEGF inhibitors share an attempt to mitigate the proliferative and permeability effect of VEGF on normal and neovascular tissue. It remains unclear and the point of some debate as to the relative desirability and safety of a complete blockade of all major VEGF isoforms compared to selective VEGF165 blockade. Similarly, it is undetermined if the global blockade would stop all leakage from the retinal capillaries and restore the blood-retinal barrier in its integrity.

Steroids and Other Immunomodulators
Steroids have been associated with neovascularization reduction by mechanisms that are complex. It is known that corticosteroids reduce expression of VEGF and other permeability factors and suppress influx of leukocytes into the retina. Clinical studies using conventional steroids alone have shown relatively unimpressive effects on the progression of AMD (Ranson et al., 2002)[65].

A double-masked, placebo-controlled, randomized, clinical trial of intravitreal TA (4 mg) injection was performed in 151 patients with classic CNV and 1-year follow-up. The results showed no effect on the risk of vision loss with a single dose of intravitreal TA. Moreover, there were no differences in the size of CNV membranes between the TA and control groups after 1 year, even though CNV membranes were smaller after 3 months in the TA group (Gillies et al., 2003)[66]. The change in size of the neovascular membrane was significantly less in the treated eyes, but there were no significant differences in the visual acuity outcomes between the two groups.

The use of conventional steroids with glucocorticoid and mineralocorticoid activity, including triamcinolone, has an inhibitory effect on ICAM and thus they inhibit VEGF.

Recently, a number of steroids have come on the market for the treatment of macular edema due to retinal vein occlusion (RVO) and diabetic retinopathy. For RVO, the SCORE study using 4 mg of triamcinolone steroids without preservative, and the GENEVA study using an implant with dexamethasone steroids demonstrated a best corrected visual acuity improvement of ≥15 letters from baseline at month 12. In the SCORE study the repeated intravitreal injections resulted in an improvement in about a quarter of patients versus laser or observation. In the GENEVA study an increase in visual acuity was experienced in 29.3% of RVO patients in a 2-month period and in 21.8% of patients in a 3-month period over the 12-month follow-up.

The adverse event rate, however, was quite important: 36% of patients with BRVO and 15.7% of patients with CRVO had an intraocular pressure (IOP) increase >10 mm Hg above baseline and 10 and 9% in both treated groups, or 3.7% in the control group, had an IOP >35 mm Hg at 2 or 12 months. Over 12 months, fewer patients treated with dexamethasone (23%) required IOP-lowering medication versus 35–41% of patients treated with triamcinolone. The major advantage of the implant versus repeated injections was a prolonged effect over 4–6 months. A nonbiodegradable implant containing fluocinolone was announced to be efficient in diabetic retinopathy.

In these studies, the results can be attributed, at least in part, to the effect on macular edema of retinal vascular origin. None of the eyes presented with choroidal new vessels.

The suggestion to use intravitreal triamcinolone for CNV has been generally greeted with enthusiasm, but the association with conventional photodynamic therapy has been disappointing. However, the effect of steroids on the inflammatory component of retinal vascular permeability may suggest that a similar effect can be expected on the inflammatory component of choroidal new vessels in AMD either alone or in association with ranibizumab.

In order to target multiple components of CNV in AMD, a dexamethasone intravitreal implant was added to ranibizumab. In a 6-month, singlemasked, multicenter study, the dexamethasone implant and ranibizumab (123 patients) provided the same efficacy and allowed a modest statistically significant reduction in the frequency of ranibizumab injections compared with ranibizumab used alone (120 patients). Increased IOP in this study (IOP ≥25 mm Hg) occurred in 18.2% of patients treated with the dexamethasone implant (Kuppermann et al., 2015)[67]. A sustained drug intravitreal delivery system with fluocinolone acetonide had the same goal in diabetic macular edema. Despite the common drug-related serious adverse events (cataract and more importantly IOP increase with a 3.7% risk of incisional glaucoma surgery over a 2-year period), significant improved visual acuity was demonstrated in 375 patients with DME over 2 years compared to 185 sham-injected patients (Campochiaro et al., 2011)[68]. However, no study has been initiated to evaluate this long-lasting implant in AMD that requires long-term treatment.

Vitrectomy

In cystoid macular edema, there are 3 ways in which the vitreous contributes to macular edema. First, vitreoretinal traction via the internal limiting membrane leads directly to vessel distortion and damage, causing them to leak (Schepens et al., 1984)[69]. The second role of the vitreous is to sequester cytokines and alter the pathways of their removal (Sebag and Balazs, 1984)[70]. Finally, it is thought that traction may contribute to the release of the cytokines via direct action on neuroretinal cells (Lewis, 2001)[71]. Thus, this traction can lead to vascular leakage both directly and through the release of cytokines that might be relieved by surgical vitrectomy (Aylward, 1999)[72]. There is a rationale for surgery that aims to relieve vitreomacular traction and remove the cytokine-laden vitreous.

Pharmacologic vitreolysis may improve vitreoretinal surgery and, ultimately, prevent disease by mitigating the contribution of the vitreous to retinopathy. Enzymatic-assisted posterior vitreous detachment with microplasmin increases vitreal O_2 levels and increases the rate of O_2 exchange within the porcine vitreous cavity (Quiram et al., 2007)[73]. Despite the fact that AMD formation has already begun before the persistent attachment of the posterior vitreous to the macula, it may be a risk factor for the development of exudative AMD (Lee et al., 2009)[26]. In addition to vitrectomy, vitreolysis is presently being evaluated in a phase II study in order to determine if the injection of microplasmin, inducing a vitreous detachment, would decrease the CNV proliferation and possibly the persistence of CME.

Conclusion

The simultaneous presence of choroidal new vessels and macular edema implies a number of cellular dysfunctions and metabolic alterations. The implication of both circulations, retinal associated with choroidal, is not mandatory. The leakage from the choroidal new vessels, predominantly VEGF-induced, may produce a large accumulation of fluid under the neurosensory retina.

Without the participation of the retinal circulation, a major disturbance of 3 barriers must have taken place: the outer retinal barrier and the blood-retinal barrier both presented tight junctions that failed and the OLM loosened. The shift of the RPE pump and the oncotic pressure are additional forces providing an opportunity for fluid invasion of the whole retina.

Also, the contribution of the retinal circulation as observed in chorioretinal anastomosis results in the maximum influx of fluid further depending upon VEGF-induced inflammation.

Finally, the mechanic traction of the vitreous delimiting the premacular pocket described by Worst may constitute a cytokine reservoir. VEGF is, in all likelihood, the rate-limiting step rather than the initiating step in AMD.

It is also likely that the key signaling steps occur prior to the upregulation of VEGF either initiated by, or facilitated by, cytokines, which act under normal basic conditions to counterbalance the integral VEGF effects and, in pathologic circumstances, may either counteract or serve to amplify the process. The major factors implied in this complex construction are the cytokines under the control of inflammation that upregulate or downregulate a large number of mechanisms. The initiating mechanisms still remain to be identified.

References

1 Cohen SY, Dubois L, Nghiem-Buffet S, Ayrault S, Fajnkuchen F, Guiberteau B, Delahaye-Mazza C, Quentel G, Tadayoni R: Retinal pseudocysts in age-related geographic atrophy. Am J Ophthalmol 2010;150:211–217.

2 Burns MS, Bellhorn RW, Korte GE, Heriot WJ: Plasticity of the retinal vasculature; in Osborne N, Chader G (eds): Progress in Retinal Research. Oxford, Pergamon Press, 1986, pp 253–308.

3 Connolly DT, Heuvelman DM, Nelson R, Olander JV, Eppley BL, Delfino JJ, Siegel NR, Leimgruber RM, Feder J: Tumor vascular permeability factor stimulates endothelial cell growth and angiogenesis. J Clin Invest 1989;84:1470–1478.

4 Ramrattan RS, van der Schaft TL, Mooy CM, de Bruijn WC, Mulder PG, de Jong PT: Morphometric analysis of Bruch's membrane, the choriocapillaris, and the choroid in aging. Invest Ophthalmol Vis Sci 1994;35:2857–2864.

5 Sarks SH: Ageing and degeneration in the macular region: a clinico-pathological study. Br J Ophthalmol 1976;60:324–341.

6 Bird AC, Pauleikhoff D, Olver J, Maguire J, Sheraidah G, Marshall J: The correlation of choriocapillaris and Bruch membrane changes in ageing. Invest Ophthalmol Vis Sci 1990;31:228.

7 Olver J, Pauleikhoff D, Bird AC: Morphometric analysis of age changes in the choriocapillaris. Invest Ophthalmol Vis Sci 1990;31:229.

8 Fisher RF: The influence of age on some ocular basement membranes. Eye 1987;1:184–189.

9 Han M, Giese G, Schmitz-Valckenberg S, Bindewald-Wittich A, Holz FG, Yu J, Bille JF, Niemz MH: Age-related structural abnormalities in the human retina-choroid complex revealed by two-photon excited autofluorescence imaging. J Biomed Opt 2007;12:024012.

10 Moore DJ, Hussain AA, Marshall J: Age-related variation in the hydraulic conductivity of Bruch's membrane. Invest Ophthalmol Vis Sci 1995;36:1290–1297.

11 Holz FG, Sheraidah G, Pauleikhoff D, Bird AC: Analysis of lipid deposits extracted from human macular and peripheral Bruch's membrane. Arch Ophthalmol 1994;112:402–406.

12 Sheraidah G, Steinmetz R, Maguire J, Pauleikhoff D, Marshall J, Bird AC: Correlation between lipids extracted from Bruch's membrane and age. Ophthalmology 1993;100:47–51.

13 Pauleikhoff D, Zuels S, Sheraidah GS, Marshall J, Wessing A, Bird AC: Correlation between biochemical composition and fluorescein binding of deposits in Bruch's membrane. Ophthalmology 1992;99:1548–1553.

14 Curcio CA, Millican CL, Bailey T, Kruth HS: Accumulation of cholesterol with age in human Bruch's membrane. Invest Ophthalmol Vis Sci 2001;42:265–274.

15 Löffler KU, Lee WR: Basal linear deposit in the human macula. Graefes Arch Clin Exp Ophthalmol 1986;224:493–501.

16 Lopez PF, Sippy BD, Lambert HM, Thach AB, Hinton DR: Transdifferentiated retinal pigment epithelial cells are immunoreactive for vascular endothelial growth factor in surgically excised age-related macular degeneration-related choroidal neovascular membranes. Invest Ophthalmol Vis Sci 1996;37:855–868.

17 Imai D, Yoneya S, Gehlbach PL, Wei LL, Mori K: Intraocular gene transfer of pigment epithelium-derived factor rescues photoreceptors from light-induced cell death. J Cell Physiol 2005;202:570–578.

18 Killingsworth MC, Sarks JP, Sarks SH: Macrophages related to Bruch's membrane in age-elated macular degeneration. Eye 1990;4:613–621.

19 Kofuji P, Biedermann B, Siddharthan V, Raap M, Iandiev I, Milenkovic I, Thomzig A, Veh RW, Bringmann A, Reichenbach A: Kir potassium channel subunit expression in retinal glial cells: implications for spatial potassium buffering. Glia 2002;39:292–303.

20 Omri S, Omri B, Savoldelli M, et al: The outer limiting membrane (OLM) revisited: clinical implications. Clin Ophthalmol 2010;4:183–195.

21 Bringmann A, Pannicke T, Biedermann B, Francke M, Iandiev I, Grosche J, Wiedemann P, Albrecht J, Reichenbach A: Role of retinal glial cells in neurotransmitter uptake and metabolism. Neurochem Int 2009;54:143–160.

22 Bringmann A, Pannicke T, Grosche J, et al: Müller cells in the healthy and diseased retina. Prog Retin Eye Res 2006;25:397–424.

23 Bringmann A, Reichenbach A, Wiedemann P: Pathomechanisms of cystoid macular edema. Ophthalmic Res 2004;36:241–249.

24 Robison CD, Krebs I, Binder S, Barbazetto IA, Kotsolis AI, Yannuzzi LA, Sadun AA, Sebag J: Vitreomacular adhesion in active and end-stage age-related macular degeneration. Am J Ophthalmol 2009;148:79–82.

25 Mojana F, Cheng L, Bartsch DU, Silva GA, Kozak I, Nigam N, Freeman WR: The role of abnormal vitreomacular adhesion in age-related macular degeneration: spectral optical coherence tomography and surgical results. Am J Ophthalmol 2008;146:218–227.

26 Lee SJ, Lee CS, Koh HJ: Posterior vitreomacular adhesion and risk of exudative age-related macular degeneration: paired eye study. Am J Ophthalmol 2009;147:621–626.

27 Schulze S, Hoerle S, Mennel S, Kroll P: Vitreomacular traction and exudative age-related macular degeneration. Acta Ophthalmol 2008;86:470–481.

28 Krebs I, Brannath W, Glittenberg C, Zeiler F, Sebag J, Binder S: Posterior vitreomacular adhesion: a potential risk factor for exudative age-related macular degeneration? Am J Ophthalmol 2007;144:741–746.

29 Kliffen M, Sharma HS, Mooy CM, Kerkvliet S, de Jong PT: Increased expression of angiogenic growth factors in age-related maculopathy. Br J Ophthalmol 1997;8:154–162.

30 Pauleikhoff D, Spital G, Radermacher M, Brumm GA, Lommatzsch A, Bird AC: A fluorescein and indocyanine green angiographic study of choriocapillaris in age-related macular disease. Arch Ophthalmol 1999;117:1353–1358.

31 Monte M, Davel LE, Sacerdote de Lustig E: Hydrogen peroxide is involved in lymphocyte activation mechanisms to induce angiogenesis. Eur J Cancer 1997;33:676–682.

32 Kuroki M, Voest EE, Amano S, Beerepoot LV, Takashima S, Tolentino M, Kim RY, Rohan RM, Colby KA, Yeo KT, Adamis AP: Reactive oxygen intermediates increase vascular endothelial growth factor expression in vitro and in vivo. J Clin Invest 1996;98:1667–1675.

33 Penfold PL, Killingsworth MC, Sarks SH: Senile macular degeneration. The involvement of giant cells in atrophy of the retinal pigment epithelium. Invest Ophthalmol Vis Sci 1986;27:364–371.

34 Gass JDM: Stereoscopic Atlas of Macular Diseases. Diagnosis and Treatment, ed 4. Saint Louis, Mosby, 1997.

35 Soubrane G, Coscas G, Larcheveque F: Macular degeneration related to age and cystoid macular edema. Apropos of 95 cases (100 eyes) (in French). J Fr Ophtalmol 1988;11:711–720.

36 Bressler NM, Bressler SB, Alexander J, Javornik N, Fine SL, Murphy RP: Loculated fluid. A previously undescribed fluorescein angiographic finding in choroidal neovascularization associated with macular degeneration. Macular Photocoagulation Study Reading Center. Arch Ophthalmol 1991;109:211–215.

37 Fine AM, Elman MJ, Ebert JE, Prestia PA, Starr JS, Fine SL: Earliest symptoms caused by neovascular membranes in the macula. Arch Ophthalmol 1986;104:513–514.

38 Coscas G: Dégénérescences maculaires acquises liées à l'âge et néovaisseaux sous-rétiniens. Paris, Masson, 1991, pp 213–258.

39 Soubrane G: Les DMLA(s). Paris, Masson, 2007, pp 253–266.

40 Bressler N, Bressler S, Fine SL: Neovascular (exudative) age-related macular degeneration; in Ryan SJ (ed): Retina. Philadelphia, Mosby, 2006, pp 1075–1113.

41 Soubrane G, Coscas G, François C, Koenig F: Occult subretinal new vessels in age-related macular degeneration. Natural history and early laser treatment. Ophthalmology 1990;97:649–657.

42 Bressler SB, Silva JC, Bressler NM, Alexander J, Green WR: Clinicopathologic correlation of occult choroidal neovascularization in age-related macular degeneration. Arch Ophthalmol 1992;110:827–832.

43 Coscas G: Optical Coherence Tomography in Age-Related Macular Degeneration (OCT in AMD). Heidelberg, Springer, 2009, pp 1–389.

44 Macular Photocoagulation Study Group: Subfoveal neovascular lesions in age-related macular degeneration. Guidelines for evaluation and treatment in the macular photocoagulation study. Arch Ophthalmol 1991;109:1109–1114.

45 Hayashi K, De Laey JJ: Indocyanine green angiography of neovascular membranes. Ophthalmologica 1985;190:30–39.

46 Yannuzzi LA, Slakter JS, Sorenson JA, Guyer DR, Orlock DA: Digital indocyanine green videoangiography and choroidal neovascularization. Retina 1992;12:191–223.

47 Soubrane G: Affections acquises de la rétine et de l'épithélium pigmentaire rétinien. Bull Soc Ophtalmol Fr 1995;324–327.

48 Scheider A, Schroedel C: High resolution indocyanine green angiography with a scanning laser ophthalmoscope. Am J Ophthalmol 1989;108:458–459.

49 Coscas G: Atlas of Indocyanine Green Angiography. Paris, Elsevier, 2005, pp 1–383.

50 Coscas F, Coscas G, Souied E, Ticks S, Soubrane G: Optical coherence tomography identification of occult choroidal neovascularization in age-related macular degeneration. Am J Ophthalmol 2007;144:592–599.

51 Hong YJ, Miura M, Makita S, et al: Noninvasive investigation of deep vascular pathologies of exudative macular diseases by high-penetration optical coherence angiography. Invest Ophthalmol Vis Sci 2013;54:3621–3631.

52 Jia Y, Bailey ST, Wilson DJ, Tan O, Klein ML, Flaxel CJ, Potsaid B, Liu JJ, Lu CD, Kraus MF, Fujimoto JG, Huang D: Quantitative optical coherence tomography angiography of choroidal neovascularization in age-related macular degeneration. Ophthalmology 2014;121:1435–1444.

53 Yanoff M, Fine BS, Brucker AJ, Eagle RC Jr: Pathology of human cystoid macular edema. Surv Ophthalmol 1984;28(suppl):505–511.

54 Ambati J, Ambati BK, Yoo SH, Ianchulev S, Adamis AP: Age-related macular degeneration: etiology, pathogenesis, and therapeutic strategies. Surv Ophthalmol 2003;48:257–293.

55 Rudolf M, Michels S, Schlötzer-Schrehardt U, Schmidt-Erfurth U: Expression of angiogenic factors by photodynamic therapy (in German). Klin Monbl Augenheilkd 2004;221:1026–1032.

56 Sarwar S, Clearfield E, Soliman MK, Sadiq MA, Baldwin AJ, Hanout M, Agarwal A, Sepah YJ, Do DV, Nguyen QD: Aflibercept for neovascular age-related macular degeneration. Cochrane Database Syst Rev 2016;2:CD011346.

57 Byun YJ, Lee SJ, Koh HJ: Predictors of response after intravitreal bevacizumab injection for neovascular age-related macular degeneration. Jpn J Ophthalmol 2010;54:571–577.

58 Simader C, Ritter M, Bolz M, et al: Morphologic parameters relevant for visual outcome during anti-angiogenic therapy of neovascular age-related macular degeneration. Ophthalmology 2014;121:1237–1245.

59 Schmidt-Erfurth U, Waldstein SM, Deak GG, Kundi M, Simader C: Pigment epithelial detachment followed by retinal cystoid degeneration leads to vision loss in treatment of neovascular age-related macular degeneration. Ophthalmology 2015;122:822–832.

60 Campochiaro PA: Ocular neovascularisation and excessive vascular permeability. Expert Opin Biol Ther 2004;4:1395–1402.

61 Grossniklaus HE, Ling JX, Wallace TM, Dithmar S, Lawson DH, Cohen C, Elner VM, Elner SG, Sternberg P Jr: Macrophage and retinal pigment epithelium expression of angiogenic cytokines in choroidal neovascularization. Mol Vis 2002;8:119–126.

62 Senger DR, Galli SJ, Dvorak AM, Perruzzi CA, Harvey VS, Dvorak HF: Tumor cells secrete a vascular permeability factor that promotes accumulation of ascites fluid. Science 1983;219:983–985.

63 Fukumura D, Gohongi T, Kadambi A, Izumi Y, Ang J, Yun CO, Buerk DG, Huang PL, Jain RK: Predominant role of endothelial nitric oxide synthase in vascular endothelial growth factor-induced angiogenesis and vascular permeability. Proc Natl Acad Sci USA 2001;98:2604–2609.

64 Sennlaub F, Courtois Y, Goureau O: Inducible nitric oxide synthase mediates retinal apoptosis in ischemic proliferative retinopathy. J Neurosci 2002;22:3987–3993.

65 Ranson NT, Danis RP, Ciulla TA, Pratt L: Intravitreal triamcinolone in subfoveal recurrence of choroidal neovascularisation after laser treatment in macular degeneration. Br J Ophthalmol 2002;86:527–529.

66 Gillies MC, Simpson JM, Luo W, Penfold P, Hunyor AB, Chua W, et al: A randomized clinical trial of a single dose of intravitreal triamcinolone acetonide for neovascular age-related macular degeneration: one-year results. Arch Ophthalmol 2003;121:667–673.

67 Kuppermann BD, Goldstein M, Maturi RK, Pollack A, Singer M, Tufail A, Weinberger D, Li X-Y, Liu C-C, Lou J, Whitcup SM; Ozurdex® ERIE Study Group: Dexamethasone intravitreal implant as adjunctive therapy to ranibizumab in neovascular age-related macular degeneration: a multicenter randomized controlled trial. Ophthalmologica 2015;234:40–54.

68 Campochiaro PA, Brown DM, Pearson A, Ciulla T, Boyer D, Holz FG, Tolentino M, Gupta A, Duarte L, Madreperla S, Gonder J, Kapik B, Billman K, Kane FE; FAME Study Group: Long-term benefit of sustained-delivery fluocinolone acetonide vitreous inserts for diabetic macular edema. Ophthalmology 2011;118: 626–663.

69 Schepens CL, Avila MP, Jalkh AE, Trempe CL: Role of the vitreous in cystoid macular edema. Surv Ophthalmol 1984; 28(suppl):499–504.

70 Sebag J, Balazs EA: Pathogenesis of cystoid macular edema: an anatomic consideration of vitreoretinal adhesions. Surv Ophthalmol 1984;28(suppl):493–498.

71 Lewis H: Macular translocation with chorioscleral outfolding: a pilot clinical study. Am J Ophthalmol 2001;132:156–163.

72 Aylward GW: The place of vitreoretinal surgery in the treatment of macular oedema. Doc Ophthalmol 1999;97:433–438.

73 Quiram PA, Leverenz VR, Baker RM, Dang L, Giblin FJ, Trese MT: Microplasmin-induced posterior vitreous detachment affects vitreous oxygen levels. Retina 2007;27:1090–1096.

74 Folkman J, Ingber DE: Angiostatic steroids. Method of discovery and mechanism of action. Ann Surg 1987;206:374–383.

75 Folkman J, Weisz PB, Joullié MM, Li WW, Ewing WR: Control of angiogenesis with synthetic heparin substitutes. Science 1989;243:1490–1493.

Prof. Gisèle Soubrane
Hotel Dieu, University Paris V Centre
1, place du Parvis Notre Dame
FR–75004 Paris (France)
E-Mail soubraneg@gmail.com

Coscas G (ed): Macular Edema. 2nd, revised and extended edition.
Dev Ophthalmol. Basel, Karger, 2017, vol 58, pp 220–237 (DOI: 10.1159/000455283)

Miscellaneous

Catherine Creuzot-Garcher

Service d'Ophtalmologie, CHU Dijon, Dijon, France

Abstract

This chapter provides the reader with practical information to be applied to the various remaining causes of macular edema. Some clinical cases of macular edema linked to ocular diseases like postradiotherapy for ocular melanomas remained of poor functional prognosis due to the primary disease. On the contrary, macular edema occurring after retinal detachment or after diverse systemic or local treatment use is often temporary. Macular edema associated with epiretinal membranes or vitreomacular traction is the main cause of poor functional recovery. In other cases, as in tractional myopic vitreoschisis, the delay to observe a significant improvement of the vision after surgery should be long. Finally, macular edema associated with hemangiomas or macroaneurysms should be treated, if symptomatic, using the same current treatment as in diabetic macular edema or exudative macular degeneration. The miscellaneous chapter is always a challenging one, laden with two serious caveats: being too exhaustive or forgetting common circumstances. The author has attempted to provide the reader with useful, practical information that can be applied to the various causes of macular edema.   © 2017 S. Karger AG, Basel

Radiation Therapy

Radiation retinopathy is a sight-threatening complication that mainly occurs after irradiation for tumors involving the choroid, retina, orbit, and paranasal sinuses (Finger, 1997)[1]. Theoretically, this complication can occur in industrial and military activities. Ionizing radiation leads to cell death related to cellular DNA damage and can take years to appear (Finger et al., 2009)[2].

Clinically, it is characterized by an aspect of ischemic vasculopathy with microaneurysms, vessel occlusion, and capillary dropout. It is generally associated with exudative signs with retinal hemorrhage, edema, and exudation, which fluorescein angiography visualizes as leakage (fig. 1).

Histopathology shows impaired vascular endothelial vessels and pericytes with progressive closure and thickening of tumor vessel walls (occurring as well in normal adjacent retina), but also thickening of normal retinal vessels in the targeted zone treated by the radioactive plaque.

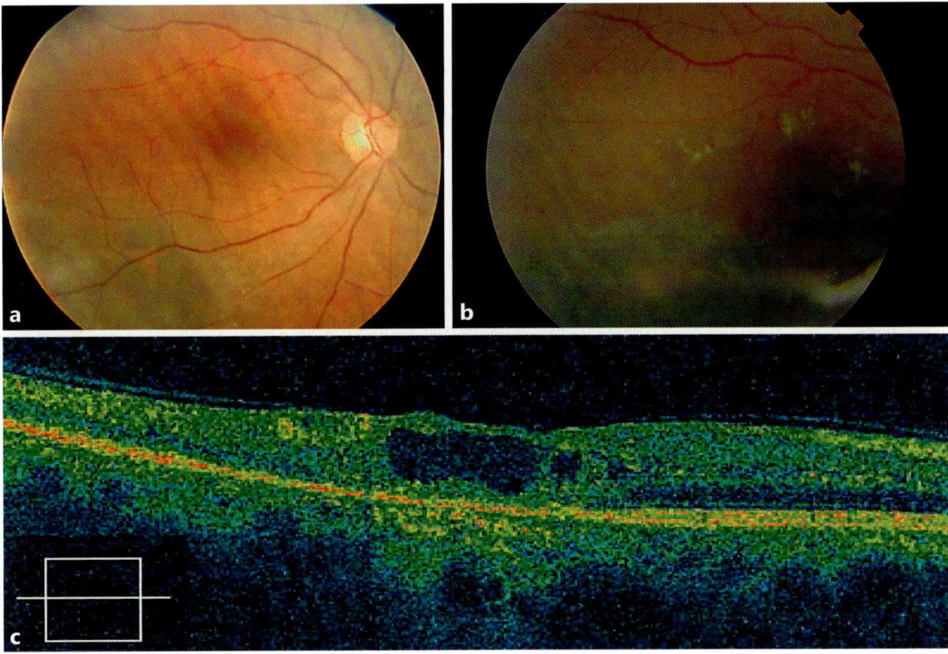

Fig. 1. a Temporoinferior melanoma with no visual loss, before treatment. **b** Same patient after treatment (1 year later), with macular edema. **c** OCT of the patient: increased macular thickness with visual loss.

Risk factors for radiation therapy are: the use of larger doses and more rapid dose rates delivering the effective dose, the potential radiation sensitizers used with the radiation treatment, and systemic risk factors such as diabetes, which potentiates the ischemic response (Finger, 2000)[3]. This progressive obliterative endarteritis can lead to progressive tissue ischemia with intraocular neovascularization.

In this disease, visual loss results from ischemic retinopathy with neovascularization and macular edema. Neovascular glaucoma is a frequent complication of neovascularization (Finger, 1997)[1].

To treat these severe complications, different treatments have been proposed:

- *Laser photocoagulation* was reported by some authors to obliterate the irradiated zone surrounding the plaque (Hykin et al., 1998)[4]. While neovascular glaucoma can be prevented with panretinal photocoagulation, the efficacy of grid or focal laser in treating macular edema has remained only somewhat successful regarding visual acuity recovery. Improvement in visual acuity has been reported in 70% of cases of radiation macular edema with a follow-up of 39 months (Kinyoun et al., 1995)[5]. The method for treating these edemas does not differ from the procedure used in macular edema found in diabetic retinopathy.

- *Intravitreal steroid* use was reported to treat refractory macular edema in a 64-year-old woman with a parotid carcinoma (Sutter and Gillies, 2003)[6]. This patient was treated with a triamcinolone injection (4 mg) after long-lasting macular edema refractory to macular grid laser treatment. The clinical outcome showed visual acuity improvement and a decrease in macular thickness on optical coherence tomography (OCT). However, a relapse of macular edema 9 months later led to another intravitreal injection with the same efficacy but no recurrence during a 1-year follow-up. The pathophysiology of the mechanism of action remains unclear but is probably based on restoration of a compromised inner blood-retinal barrier (Gillies, 1999)[7]. The effect of steroids seems to be transient with current relapse (Shields et al., 2005)[8]. Interesting results have been found with dexamethasone implants (Baillif et al., 2013)[9].

- *Intravitreal antiangiogenic injection* was reported in refractory macular edema caused by radiation therapy. The authors reported the results of intravitreal injections of bevacizumab in 6 patients suffering from macular edema stemming from ocular melanomas treated with plaque irradiation. They reported visual acuity improvement with reduced exudative signs documented on angiogram and OCT with no serious adverse events. The patients were treated with an average of 2.8 injections (range: 1–4) with a mean follow-up of 4.7 months (range: 2–8 months). Interestingly, the delay between the plaque insertion and the onset of the radiation therapy ranged from 9 to 150 months (Finger et al., 2008)[10]. However, while anatomical results seem interesting, functional recovery is usually poor. In very severe forms, combined anti-VEGF (vascular endothelial growth factor) and steroids can be proposed (Shah et al., 2013)[11].

The best way to prevent radiation damage is to decrease as much as possible the dosage and the area to be treated with irradiation.

Macular Edema Resulting from Systemic or Topical Treatment

Prostaglandin Analogs
There have been a number of contradictory results suggesting an association between the development of anterior uveitis and cystoid macular edema (CME) and prostaglandin (PG) use. However, these cases were anecdotal without good evidence from controlled clinical trials. Indeed, in most cases a nonindependent risk factor for the development of uveitis such as previous ocular surgery, pseudophakia or aphakia, posterior capsule rupture, or past history of uveitis were associated (Hoyng et al., 1997; Schumer et al. 2000; Wand and Gaudio, 2002)[12–14]. The pathophysiology of this effect may be the proinflammatory action of PGs. However, PG analogs have a high affinity for the FP prostanoid receptor but a very low effect on vasoactive prostanoid receptors. Furthermore, experimental studies have failed to demonstrate a prochemotactic effect of PGs (Schumer et al., 2002)[15]. Additionally, no blood barrier breakdown should be observed in eyes treated for increased ocular pressure caused by PGs (Linden, 2001)[16].

A retrospective study demonstrated that PG analogs are not associated with increased risk of CME or anterior uveitis, although they can lead to substantially decreased intraocular pressure (Chang et al., 2008)[17]. In 163 eyes of 84 consecutive patients with uveitis, the author compared the rate of uveitis and CME in eyes treated with PG and control eyes treated by non-PG-lowering treatment. No statistically significant difference between the two groups was found: neither patients with previous history of anterior uveitis or CME, nor patients with no CME history expressed significantly increased CME or uveitis once treated with PG in comparison with non-PG use.

Anticancer Drugs
In most cases, macular edema will resolve when the treatment can be stopped. If not, some definitive lesions involving photoreceptors can persist.

Certain agents used in cancer can induce some toxicity. While most of them are reversible, with or without treatment and with or without stopping cancer treatment, some can induce definitive lesions. Early detection of these side effects

Table 1. Macular edema related to anticancer drugs

Treatment	Incidence, %	Signs	Outcome
Tamoxifen	1.5	Macular edema associated with white refractile opacities involving internal plexiform layer and nerve fiber layer	Reversible when treatment stopped Macular atrophy if photoreceptors damages
Taxane	–	Bilateral ME with external plexiform layer involvement on the OCT No leakage on angiography	Usually reversible if stopped NSAIA or acetazolamide proposed
Fingolimob	1.3–2.2	Bilateral ME with fluid accumulation in outer and inner plexiform layer on OCT	Usually reversible Steroids or NSAIA proposed
Nicotinic acid	0.67	Bilateral ME with inner nuclear layer involvement on OCT	Reversible if stopped
Interferon	15–86 (cotton wool spot)	Cotton wool spots, CME with inner nuclear and external plexiform layer involvement on the OCT	Reversible in most cases Rare cases of macular atrophy
MEK inhibitors	1–4	Retinal vein occlusion, serous retinal detachment, central serous retinopathy	Reversible Usually no discontinuation
Tyrosine kinase inhibitor	–	CME, retinal hemorrhages	Reversible
BRAF kinase inhibitor	–	Uveitis and central macular edema	Reversible, treatment with topical corticosteroid

NSAIA = Nonsteroid anti-inflammatory agent.

can prevent these complications (Liu et al., 2014)[18]. Some authors have proposed steroidal and nonsteroidal anti-inflammatory agents or acetazolamide to treat the macular edema occurring in these situations (table 1).

Fingolimob

Fingolimob is a systemic treatment used to treat multiple sclerosis. Macular edema has been reported in 0–1.6% of the cases, 3–4 months after the treatment was initiated. Macular edema disappears after fingolimob is discontinued (Afshar et al., 2013)[19].

Glitazone Use

Glitazones belong to a class of drugs used to reduce insulin resistance in diabetic patients. These peroxisome proliferator-activated receptor-γ activators were implicated in a potential induction of diabetic macular edema (DME) by a few reports in limited series (Colucciello, 2005; Ryan et al., 2006; Sivagnanam, 2006)[20–22].

Until now, there have been controversial results concerning this secondary macular edema. Indeed, a large cohort study involving 17,000 glitazone users was performed to evaluate the 1-year incidence of DME (Fong and Contreras, 2009)[23].

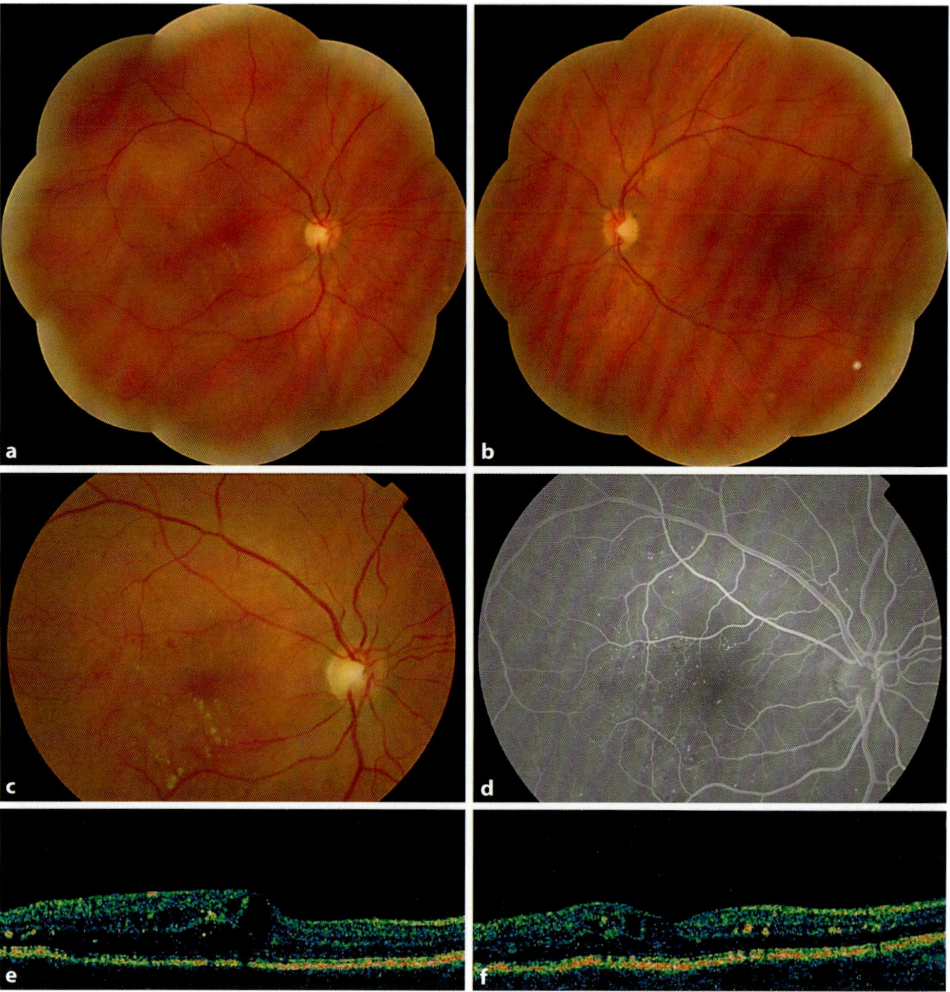

Fig. 2. a Patient treated with glitazone with focal macular edema (right eye). **b** Patient treated with glitazone with focal macular edema (left eye). **c** Patient with worsened focal macular edema in spite of grid treatment (right eye) – color retinophotography but good systemic diabetic control. **d** Patient with worsened focal macular edema in spite of grid treatment (right eye) – fluorescein angiogram. **e** Same patient, macula OCT, 3 months later with diffuse macular edema. **f** Same patient, 3 months later after glitazone was stopped.

The authors found that glitazone users were more likely to develop DME [odds ratio = 2.5 (2.4–3)], with an increased risk still present when adjusting for confounding factors [odds ratio = 1.6 (1.4–1.8)]. However, some confounding factors such as high blood pressure, renal status, and hyperlipidemia were not available in this electronically collected database study, and the diagnosis of macular edema was made upon computer data only, without assessed clinical data (fig. 2). These controversial results clearly emphasize the need for large-scale studies to assess the risk-benefit ratio of these drugs. In all cases, the macular edema disappeared when the glitazone was stopped as long as no confounding factors such as poor diabetic balance or increased high blood pressure were associated (Colucciello, 2005)[20]. This treatment has been recently stopped in some countries.

Epiretinal Membrane and Traction Syndrome

Epiretinal membrane (ERM) can be either idiopathic or associated with various conditions such as retinal breaks, diabetic retinopathy, branch retinal vein occlusion, inflammation, and exudative vitreoretinopathy. It also frequently appears after intraocular surgery, especially retinal detachment surgery (Margherio et al., 1985; Gaudric et al.,1993)[24, 25].

In vitreomacular traction syndrome (VMTS), the presence of a persistent attachment of the vitreous to the macula with incomplete posterior vitreous detachment (PVD) is responsible for the thickening of the macular area (Smiddy et al., 1989)[26]. Many studies have found a clear visual improvement after vitreomacular traction removal (Smiddy et al., 1989; Smiddy et al., 1990; Rouhette and Gastaud, 2001)[26–28] (fig. 3).

The additional benefit of internal limiting membrane (ILM) peeling for VMTS remains unknown (Gandorfer et al., 2002)[29]. VMTS leads to a persistent traction of the macula, producing macular edema and visual loss. Idiopathic VMTS occurs without ERM or macular hole, but most cases are secondary to ERM (Puliafito et al., 1995)[30].

The Role Played by OCT in the Surgical Decision: A Histologic-Like Assessment
OCT plays a major role in decision making in ERM and VMTS management (Do et al., 2007)[31]. Do et al. found that the diagnosis of macular edema was made in 67.9% of the cases by clinical examination in comparison with 83.3% with OCT. In contrast, OCT leads to fewer surgical decisions than clinical examination (42.4 vs. 57.6%). In patients recommended for surgery, macular edema was more pronounced. Macular edema was thought to be associated with lower visual acuity (Gaudric and Cohen, 1992)[32].

OCT has shown that it can take a long time to obtain complete resolution of macular changes. Subretinal fluid can persist as long as 1 year after surgery, the delay required for almost normal retinal tissue organization (Uchino et al., 2001)[33].

Recent OCT techniques have provided a better understanding of the relation between the vitreous and retina in ERM and VMTS.

The problem linked to the precise phenotyping of vitreomacular traction was greatly improved with the classification of the International Vitreomacular Traction Study Group that associates signs observed on OCT and clinical features (Duker et al., 2013)[34]. Indeed, this classification has defined precisely different types of vitreomacular interface with: vitreomacular adhesion (i.e., vitreous separation with remaining vitreomacular attachment but with normal macular morphologic features), vitreomacular traction (where abnormal posterior vitreous detachment is accompanied by an anatomic distortion of the macula), and finally macular hole. This classification strengthened the role of evolving vitreous detachment to induce macular changes. The preoperative aspect revealed by OCT is important in VMTS, as demonstrated by Yamada and Kishi (2005)[35]. These authors reported two different aspects of PVD. One was an incomplete-shaped detachment, while the other one was only partial with remaining attached vitreous on the nasal part of the fovea. The former aspect was associated with a good visual outcome with a tomographic recovery within 4 months in almost all cases. In contrast, the latter was associated with greater preoperative macular thickness with a prominent CME in 3 out of 4 patients as well as an increased rate of postoperative complications (macular hole and macular atrophy). This complicated outcome resulted in decreased visual acuity (fig. 3).

Several authors have underlined poor visual outcome in VMTS (Smiddy et al., 1989; McDonald et al., 1994; Melberg et al., 1995)[26, 36, 37], but their observations of PVD status were mainly intraoperative. One of the main advantages of OCT is to detail PVD status as a histologic-like aspect.

Is ILM Peeling Necessary to Avoid CME after ERM or VMTS?

The influence of ILM peeling on CME remains unclear. The ILM is the structural boundary between the retina and the vitreous. This 2.5-μm-thick membrane is closely associated with the plasma membrane of the Müller cells, suggesting that it derives from glial cells (Abdelkader et al., 2008)[38]. There is no general agreement on whether or not the ILM should be peeled during ERM removal. To ease ILM peeling, several dyes have been successively used with different histologic consequences (Haritoglou et al., 2003; Haritoglou et al., 2004)[39, 40]. There is currently no reason for not using dye to peel the ILM safely. Up to now, there is no proof that ILM peeling decreases the risk of ME after ERM peeling. The histologic studies on ILM specimens have shown Müller cell plasma membranes and retinal elements on the retinal side of the indocyanine green-peeled ILM, suggesting that this dye alters the cleavage plane during ILM peeling (Haritoglou et al., 2004)[41] (fig. 4). Pathology studies have found cellular elements such as glial cells, fibroblasts, macrophages, and collagen fibers, suggesting a multifactorial aspect combining inflammation, proliferation, and fibrosis (Kampik et al., 1980)[42]. ILM associated with ERM probably acts as a scaffold for cell proliferation and the authors suggested removing the ILM during epiretinal peeling to decrease the recurrence rate (Park et al., 2003; Sakamoto et al., 2003)[43, 44]. The presence of a thin layer of collagen between the ILM and ERM found by Haritoglou et al. (2004)[41] strongly suggests that ILM removal should decrease the risk of recurrence by this means. Several case-control studies or case series showed that combined ILM and epiretinal peeling does not seem to alter the outcome after surgery.

However, as ILM peeling is a delicate technical procedure, the need for ILM peeling has to be confirmed. This remains unclear given the controversial results: some authors found the ILM remnants on epiretinal specimens were associated with better visual outcomes (Bovey et al., 2004)[45], whereas others have found the opposite (Sivalingam et al., 1990)[46]. Some authors have reported that preexisting CME and increased preoperative central foveal thickness should increase the risk of postoperative CME (Frisina et al., 2015)[47]. This is even more crucial as some authors have hypothesized that ILM peeling can induce some macular sensitivity loss (Tadayoni et al., 2012)[48].

The value of ILM peeling in CME combined with ERM was studied by Geerts et al. (2004)[49]. They showed that when they compared the outcome of CME in patients, the relief was better in patients with ILM removal than in patients without. However, these were diabetic patients, which could bias the results. Indeed, there have been many studies suggesting a potential role of vitrectomy and ILM peeling in the outcome of CME during diabetes, but to date no studies have clearly demonstrated the benefit of a surgical approach to CME during diabetes except for tractional macular edema (see chapter on diabetic retinopathy by Bandello et al. (this vol., pp. 102–138). Although a lower recurrence of ERM was found after ILM peeling (Gan-

Fig. 3. a Tractional macular edema gives the typical aspect of honeycomb macular edema. It remains the only validated indication of ERM peeling in diabetic macular edema. **b** Vitreomacular traction in the nasal part of the fovea. Posterior hyaloid remains strongly attached. **c** VMTS with severe macular edema (preoperative aspect). **d** VMTS after ERM and ILM peeling. Macular thickness is strongly decreased with a partial recovery of normal macular profile on the OCT. **e** Macular edema secondary to a thick macular ERM (preoperative aspect). **f** Same patient, postoperative aspect (after 6 months): the macula remained thickened without normal macular profile. **g** ERM with macular edema (preoperative). Triamcinolone was injected during surgery. **h** Same patient, 1 month postoperatively: complete recovery of normal macular thickness with a partial recovery of visual acuity (20/80). **i** Same patient, macular edema recurrence: 1 year later without recovery of visual acuity (20/80). *(For figure see next page.)*

Creuzot-Garcher

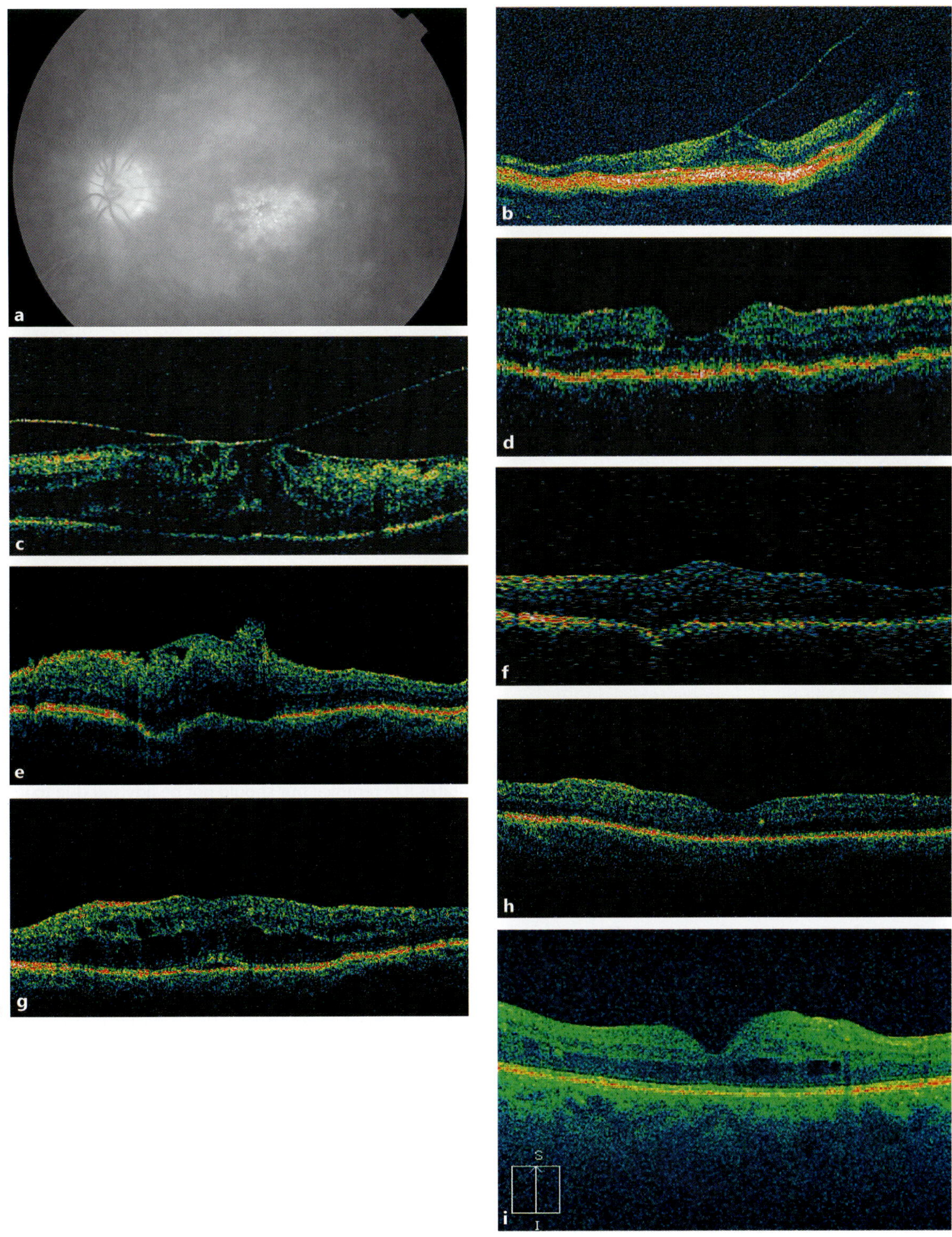

a
b
c
d
e
f
g
h
i
S
I
3

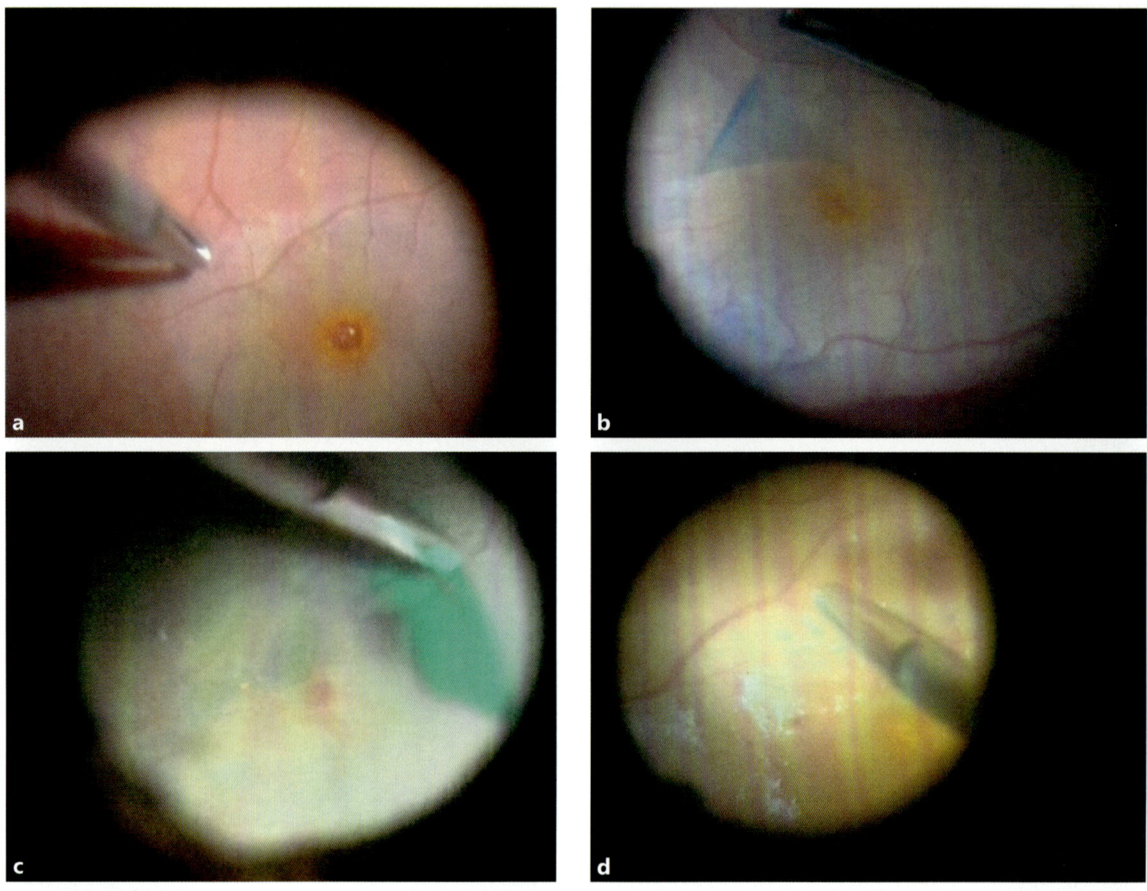

Fig. 4. a ILM peeling without any dye: the whitening of the retina clearly shows the limits where ILM was removed. **b** ILM peeling with indocyanine green: the dye strongly facilitates ILM removal but should not be advised due to its potential toxicity. **c** ILM peeling with brilliant blue peel: the dye seems to stain exclusively ILM without any retinal toxicity. **d** Vitreous removal can be facilitated by triamcinolone use: the crystals are trapped in the vitreous gel and improve vitreous visualization.

dorfer et al., 2000; Kuhn et al., 2004; Kimura et al., 2005)[50–52], some studies have reported controversial results regarding the outcome of CME with positive results (Tachi and Ogino,1996; Stolba et al., 2005)[53, 54] and negative ones (Thomas et al., 2005)[55].

Retinal Detachment

Many studies have focused on the postoperative analysis of the macula by OCT after retinal detachment. A study by Kiss et al. (2007)[56] investigated the aspect of the macula after complicated retinal detachment with proliferative vitreoretinopathy. They found that the macula remained normal in only 12.8% of cases and 17.1% of patients presented with macular edema (fig. 5). This rate was lower than that reported by Bonnet (1994)[57] who found a 51.7% rate in 1994, but the surgical technique was probably different. Macular edema can be present alone or combined with subretinal fluid (Benson et al., 2006)[58]. In about one third of patients, macular disease is eligible for treatment, namely in the cases of macular pucker or macular edema.

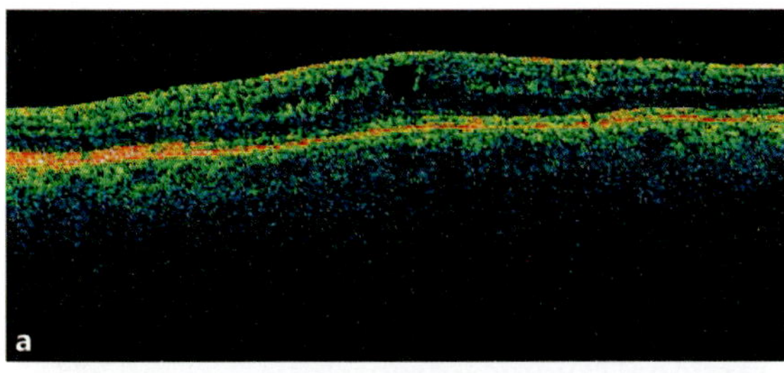

Fig. 5. Macular edema after a retinal detachment. **a** Six months after retinal detachment. **b** Same patient, 4 years later. **c–e** Subretinal fluid after retinal detachment: 1 month after the operation (**c**), 6 months after the operation (**d**), and 12 months after the operation (**e**).

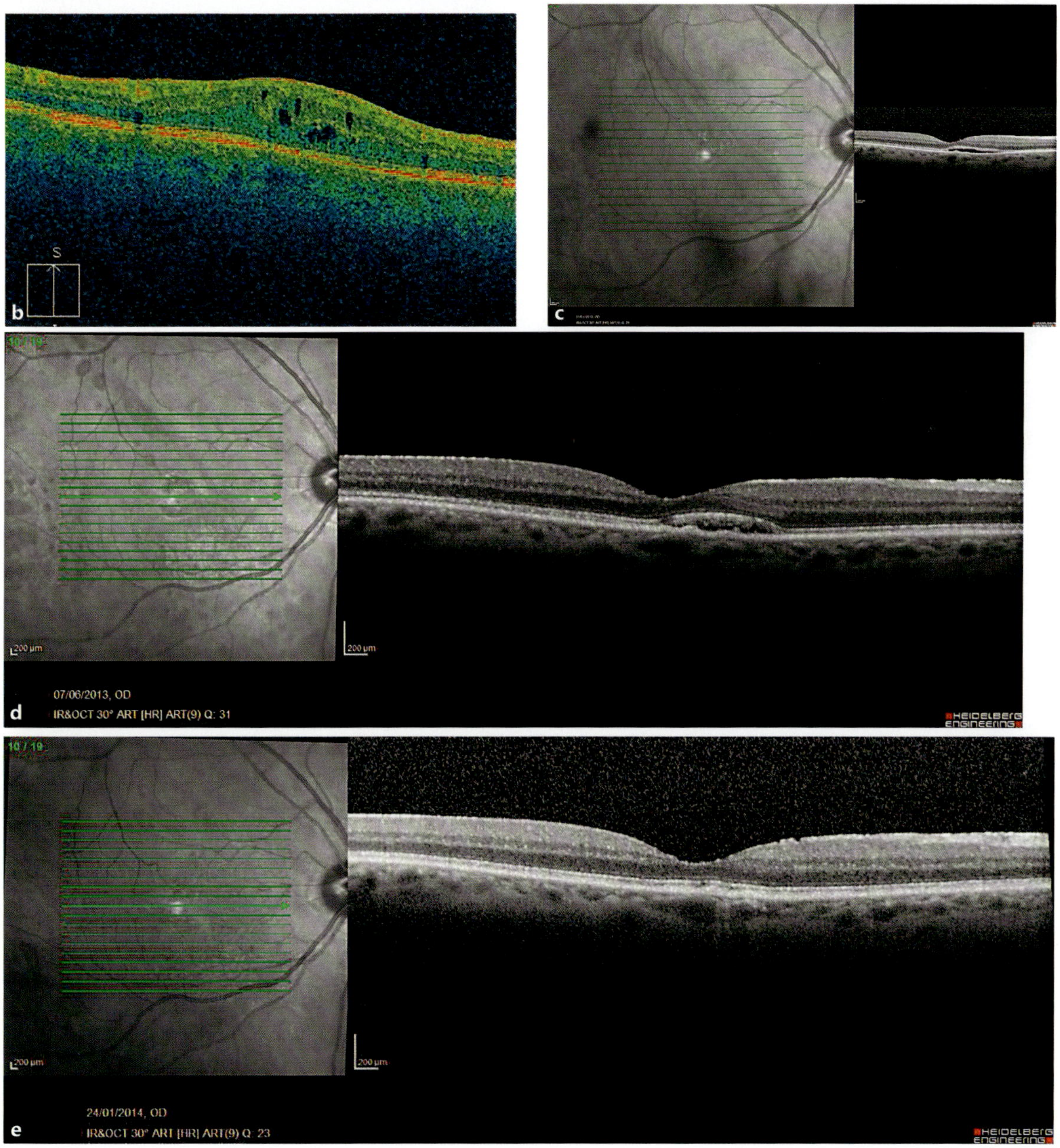

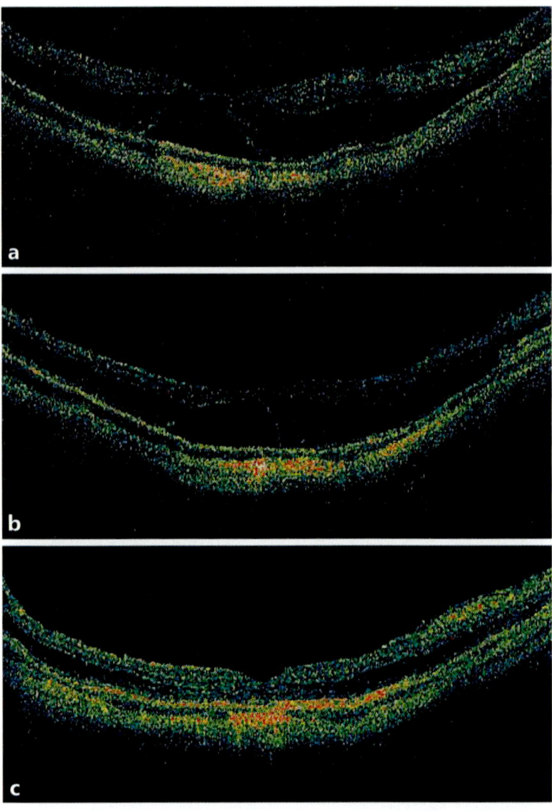

Fig. 6. Vitreofoveal schisis in a myopic patient with visual loss. The delay to recover a normal aspect is very long (sometimes 1 year): preoperative (**a**), **1** month later (**b**), and **6** months later (**c**).

Ultrahigh-resolution OCT provides a very precise assessment of the vitreoretinal interface. Schocket et al. (2006)[59] studied the microstructural changes in the retina in patients suffering from poor recovery after retinal detachment surgery. They found an isolated macular edema in 12% of their patients and an ERM in 59% of the cases. In a prospective study involving more than 100 retinal detachments with a 12-month follow-up, we have found a steady CME rate of 8% without pre- or perioperative identified risk factors. This macular edema should be differentiated from subretinal fluid found in almost 18% of cases after 1 month. This later seems to be more frequent after scleral buckling procedures (fig. 5c, d). Macu-

lar edema is one of the features known to influence visual outcome after retinal detachment. The rule is to consider macular edema occurring after retinal detachment as a postoperative inflammatory macular edema and to treat it with steroids.

Tractional Myopic Vitreoschisis

Macular schisis is a vitreoretinal disease caused by splitting of the macular area. This condition is not really macular edema but corresponds to a thickening of the macular area and can be difficult to distinguish from macular edema in myopic patients.

OCT provides a very precise comprehensive mechanism. The usual presentation is an outer schisis where the retina is split into the outer retinal layers with a thick inner layer. In contrast, inner schisis involves the inner layers leading to a thick outer layer. This condition can be stable: Gaucher et al. (2007)[60] reported a progression in 20 eyes of 29 patients with a follow-up of 31 months. Premacular structure (44.8%), foveal detachment (34.5%), and lamellar macular hole (20.7%) were the most common OCT findings. Visual acuity can be preserved even with severe macular thickening (fig. 6). The authors found that a hyperreflective premacular structure and foveal detachment were associated with a worse outcome. Vitrectomy with cortex removal, with or without ILM peeling, and internal tamponade can be useful to treat the cases with impaired visual acuity (Ikuno et al., 2004; Kwok et al., 2005)[61, 62], with some risk of postoperative macular hole.

Choroidal Hemangioma

Choroidal hemangioma is a rare benign vascular tumor that occurs in two circumstances: either in its diffuse form associated with Sturge-Weber syndrome or in its circumscribed form [circumscribed choroidal hemangioma (CCH)], and is usually sporadic without any systemic manifestations.

These orange-red, smooth lesions can be discovered incidentally, but can lead to severe loss of vision especially in cases of exudative detachment and CME. The diagnosis is made by angiography. Fluorescein angiography only shows an early and then persisting hyperfluorescence but indocyanine green angiography shows the typical 'washout' phenomenon, characteristic for CCH (with an early hyperfluorescence in the early frame followed by a relative hypofluorescence in the 15 min late frame) (fig. 7).

A long-term report of CCH concluded that about 50% of patients will suffer from a visual loss <20/200 due to a chronic macular edema (Shields et al., 2001)[63].

Asymptomatic CCHs not causing visual loss are usually not treated and only need periodical observation. By contrast, symptomatic CCHs require treatment (Gunduz, 2004)[64]. Treatment options have varied during the last decade: initial treatments were based mainly on laser photocoagulation but led to nerve fiber layer consequences and did not lead to regression of the tumor. Radiation therapy and transpupillary thermotherapy were also used and led to a good control of the tumor, but all these techniques have limited efficacy with common recurrences. Recent studies underlined the interest in photodynamic therapy (PDT). PDT allows a selective photochemical injury to the vascular endothelial cells, but the protocols (mean radiation exposure between 50 and 100 J/cm^2) and exposure time (between 83 and 186 s) used in the literature remain a matter of debate. Authors reported on treatments with a number of sessions ranging between 1 and 5 with intervals from 6 to 12 weeks. The aim of the treatment remained the elimination of subretinal fluid and not the tumor regression, although PDT can lead to a decrease in CCH thickness. CME regressed in almost all the cases after PDT and subretinal fluid disappeared with a single treatment only in most cases (Boixadera et al., 2009)[65].

However, this treatment does not seem efficient in hemangioma with thickness >4 mm with frequent relapses.

More recently, proton beam irradiation has been proposed with both good anatomical and functional results with a mean of 4 sequences to deliver 20 Gy (Zeisberg et al., 2014)[66].

Ocular Melanoma

Ocular melanoma can be associated with macular edema with different mechanisms: retinal degeneration sometimes associated with subretinal fluid, secondary retinal detachment, inflammatory reaction, or VEGF secretion linked to the tumor. Macular edema can also be a complication of the treatment with irradiation. Risk factors for macular edema are female gender, tumor thickness, the distance between the tumor and the macula, and a preexisting macular thickening on the treated eye (Shields et al., 2005)[67].

Retinal Macroaneurysm

Retinal arterial macroaneurysm (MA) is an acquired dilation of a retinal artery occurring usually in the elderly. It is marked by a strong female predominance in a context of systemic hypertension and arteriosclerosis with a lesion present in one eye only in the majority of cases.

Although the most common presenting symptom remains the loss of vision, MAs should remain asymptomatic with a diagnosis found incidentally during a routine exam. MA usually involves the temporal arcade arteries. Vision loss depends on the involvement of the macula and should be progressive in case of exudation and edema or more sudden and severe in case of hemorrhage.

Hemorrhages can reach all retinal layers from the subretinal space to the subhyaloidal layer, and can be associated with a vitreous hemorrhage in

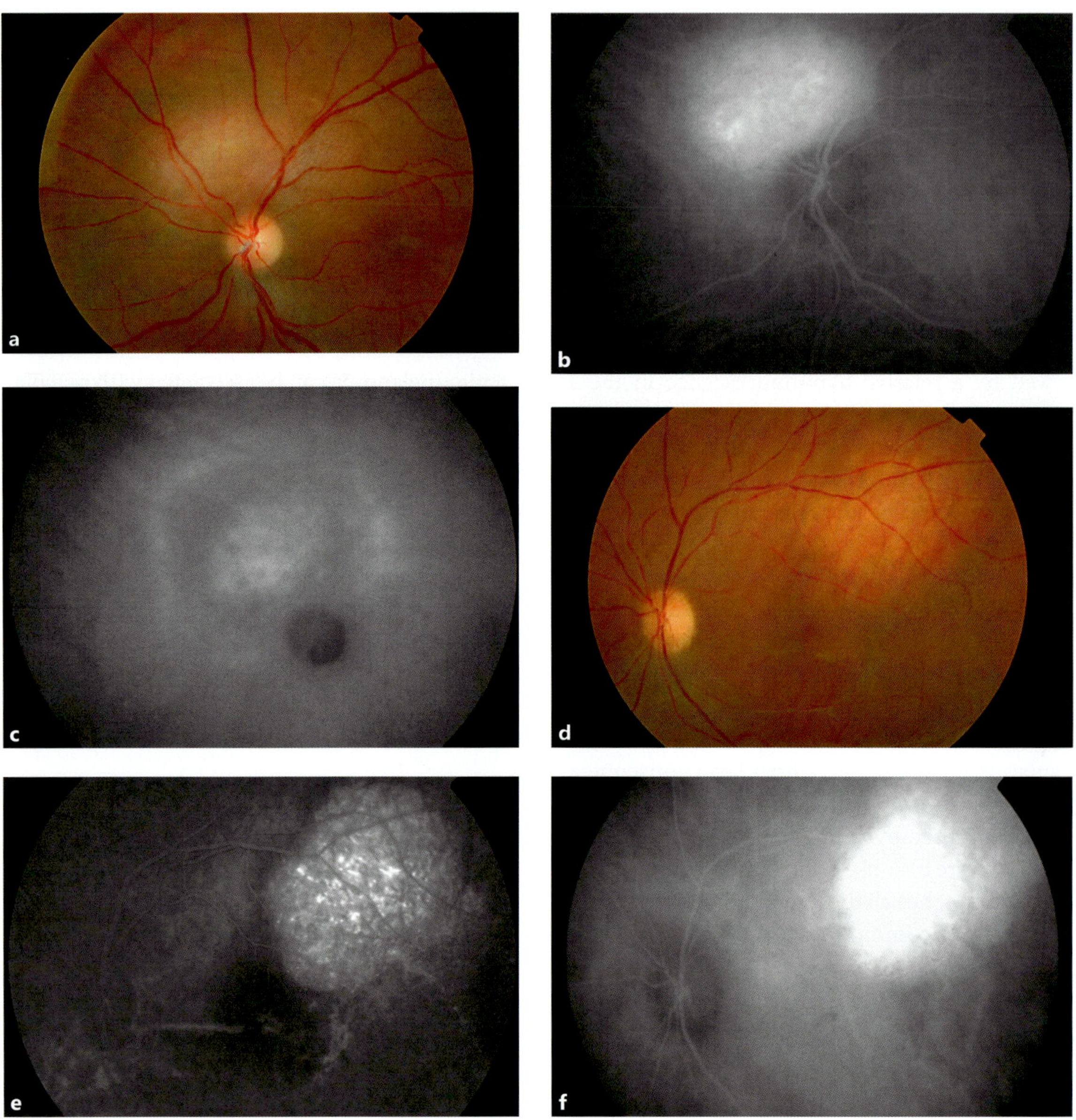

Fig. 7. Choroidal hemangioma. **a–c** Color images, fluorescein, and indocyanine green angiogram with a washout of the indocyanine green in the late frame. **a** Hemangioma located in the superior part of the optic nerve head. **b** Hemangioma early frame. **c** Hemangioma late frame. **d–g** Patients operated for retinal detachment with subretinal folds. During the follow-up, the remaining subretinal fluid was in fact due to a temporal choroidal hemangioma. **d** Hemangioma, color image. **e** Hemangioma fluorescein angiogram. **f** Hemangioma, indocyanine green, early frame.

Creuzot-Garcher

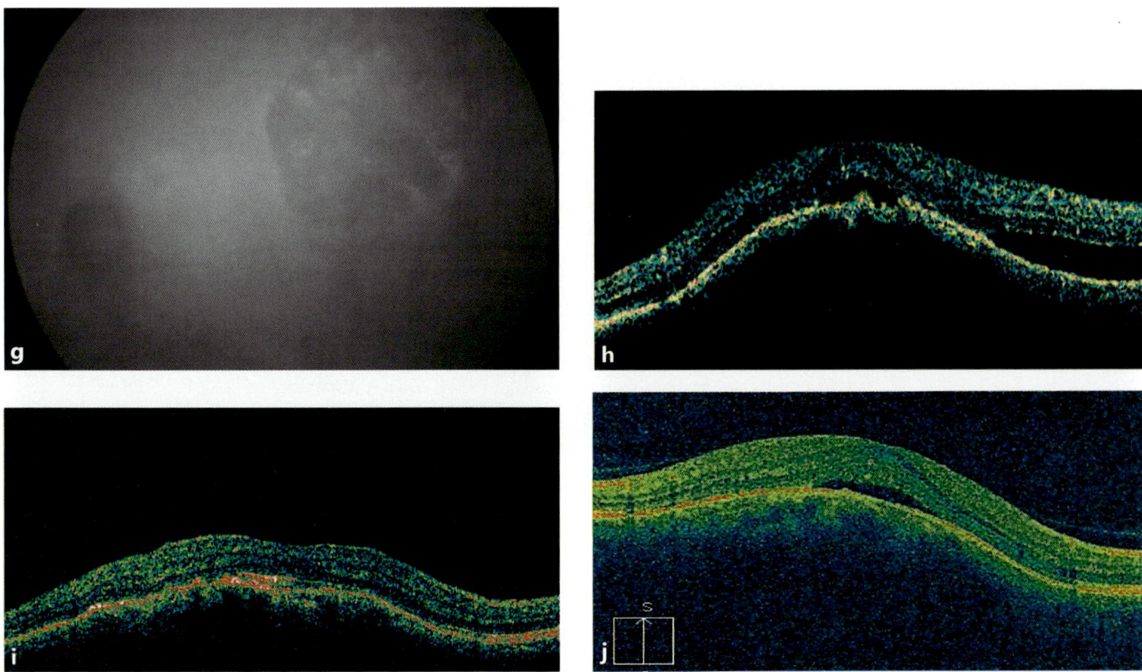

Fig. 7. Choroidal hemangioma. **g** Hemangioma, indocyanine green, late frame. **h** Subretinal fluid before treatment. **i** Three months after PDT. **j** Recurrence of subretinal fluid, 9 months after initial treatment.

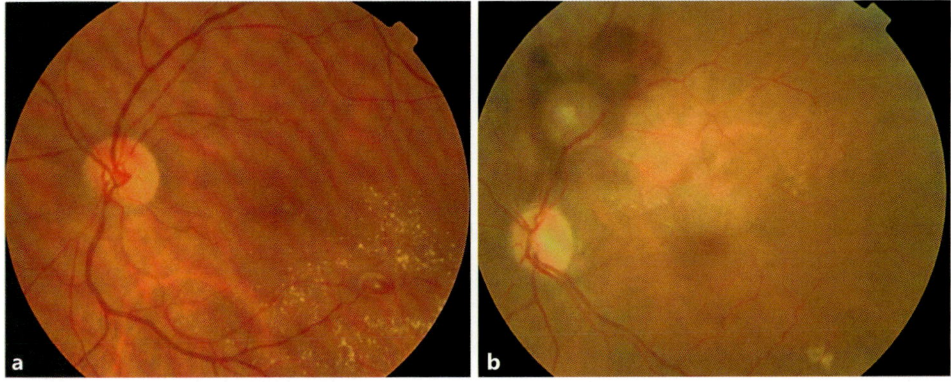

Fig. 8. a Temporal MA with exudative deposits in the temporal part of the fovea. **b** Superior MA with hemorrhage and macular edema.

10% of the cases. Exudative retinopathy looks like a circinate pattern around the MA, and neurosensory retinal detachment can be associated with edema, hemorrhage, or exudate. However, some MAs exhibit severe exudative changes.

The usual outcome of MA follows a course from thrombosis, fibrosis to spontaneous involution. This is the reason why, in most cases, it does not exhibit any macular leakage after hemorrhage disappearance (Rabb et al., 1988)[68]. Indeed, once

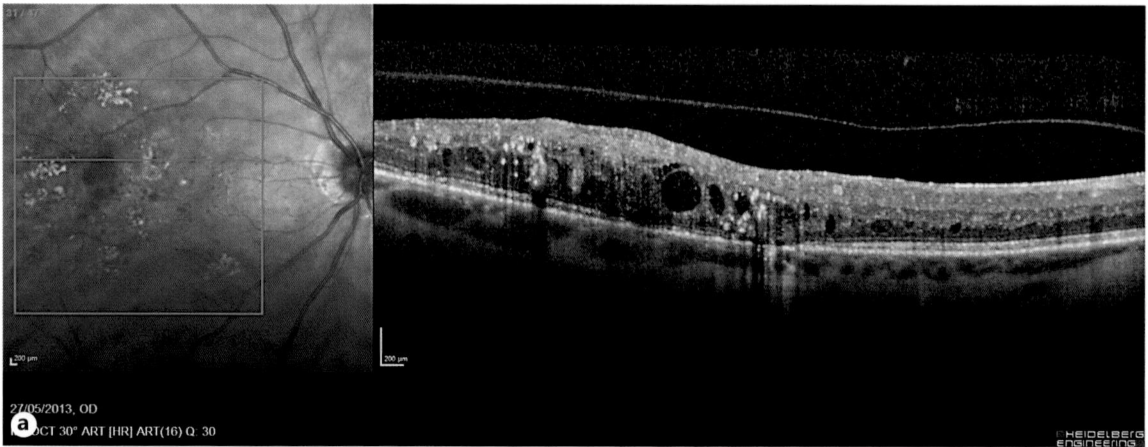

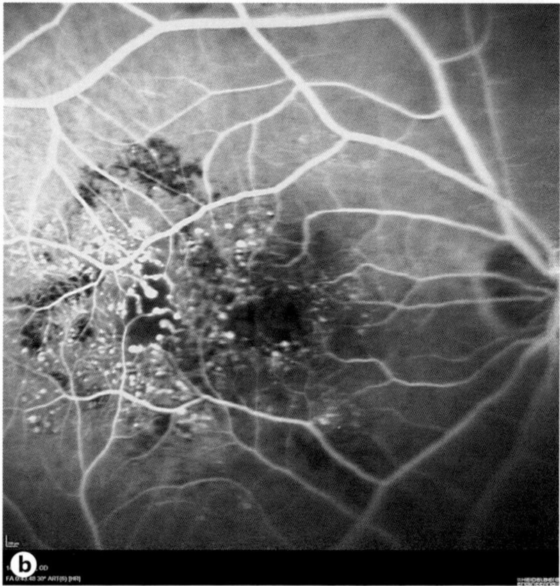

Fig. 9. Type 1 telangiectasia: OCT (**a**) and angiography (**b**)

the aneurysm ruptures, it usually spontaneously regresses (fig. 8).

Initially, if present, macular edema usually involves the outer layer. Most MAs exhibit vascular leakage leading to macular edema with secondary lipid deposits. Macular edema and its consequences are considered as the main cause of vision loss as it occurs in about 1/3 of patients. Chronic macular edema will cause destruction of the foveal outer photoreceptor layer responsible for a poor vision (Tsujikawa et al., 2009)[69].

As the majority of MAs resolve spontaneously with good vision, the indications of laser photocoagulation are recommended only in case of severe macular edema with exudates lasting for more than 3 months or in case of recurrent bleeding with vitreous hemorrhage. This situation is rare as bleeding leads most often to a spontaneous thrombosis with secondary involution. In few cases, a photocoagulation therapy should be used with either direct treatment of the MA (with low dosage but long-lasting im-

Creuzot-Garcher

pacts) or an indirect treatment of the surrounding retina.

In eyes with exudative change, laser photocoagulation usually leads to a flattening of the fovea. However, after hemorrhage resolution, retinal structure and outer layers are usually impaired even if minimal hemorrhagic complications were found initially. The prognosis after laser photocoagulation of the MA depends on the amount of lipid deposits in the macular area and of the (irreversible) changes of the outer layers which could prevent from a good visual acuity recovery.

Recently, there have been reports of using intravitreal injection of bevacizumab to treat the exudative changes and the hemorrhage (Cho et al., 2013)[70]. In some cases with subretinal hemorrhage, vitrectomy can be proposed with intravitreal or subretinal injection of recombinant tissue plasminogen activator (Inoue et al., 2015)[71].

Idiopathic Juxtafoveolar Retinal Telangiectasia

Type 1 Idiopathic juxtafoveolar retinal telangiectasia belongs to the spectrum of Coats' disease. It is characterized by exudative dilations of perifoveal retinal capillaries occurring typically in a single eye of a male patient. Vision loss is linked to macular edema with diffusing telangiectasia (fig. 9a, b). OCT can show thickening of the mac-

ula, and fluorescein angiography can show the diffusion, but not as precisely as obtained recently with OCT angiography, which showed a global and capillary depletion (Matet et al., 2016)[72]. The treatment remains poor with laser or photodynamic therapy with frequent recurrences. Some authors have reported controversial results with anti-VEGF treatments (Takayama et al., 2010)[73] (fig. 9).

Conclusions

Macular edema remains a common clinical situation. Diabetes and vein occlusion still remain the main causes of macular edema. However, some circumstances should be associated with these diseases like ERM. Moreover, macular edema linked to topical or systemic treatment should be found in some diabetic or in uveitic patients. The learning from clinical trials for DME will provide us with very interesting results to be used in other circumstances like hemangioma or MA as these situations are not supposed to benefit from large-scale studies.

Finally, the more precise analysis of the foveal region and especially of the consequences of macular edema with new-generation OCT will probably enable us to better define the surgical indication and outcome of ERM and VMTS.

References

1 Finger PT: Radiation therapy for choroidal melanoma. Surv Ophthalmol 1997; 42:215–232.
2 Finger PT, Chin KJ, et al: Palladium-103 ophthalmic plaque radiation therapy for choroidal melanoma: 400 treated patients. Ophthalmology 2009;116:790–796, 796e1.
3 Finger PT: Tumour location affects the incidence of cataract and retinopathy after ophthalmic plaque radiation therapy. Br J Ophthalmol 2000;84:1068–1070.
4 Hykin PG, Shields CL, et al: The efficacy of focal laser therapy in radiation-induced macular edema. Ophthalmology 1998;105:1425–1429.
5 Kinyoun JL, Zamber RW, et al: Photocoagulation treatment for clinically significant radiation macular oedema. Br J Ophthalmol 1995;79:144–149.
6 Sutter FK, Gillies MC: Intravitreal triamcinolone for radiation-induced macular edema. Arch Ophthalmol 2003;121: 1491–1493.
7 Gillies MC: Regulators of vascular permeability: potential sites for intervention in the treatment of macular edema. Doc Ophthalmol 1999;97:251–260.
8 Shields CL, et al: Intravitreal triamcinolone acetonide for radiation maculopathy after plaque radiotherapy for choroidal melanoma. Retina 2005;25:868–874.

9   Baillif S, et al: Intravitreal dexamethasone 0.7-mg implant for radiation macular edema after proton beam therapy for choroidal melanoma. Retina 2013; 33:1784–1790.

10 Finger RP, Charbel Issa P, et al: Intravitreal bevacizumab for choroidal neovascularisation associated with pseudoxanthoma elasticum. Br J Ophthalmol 2008; 92:483–487.

11 Shah NV, et al: Combination therapy with triamcinolone acetonide and bevacizumab for the treatment of severe radiation maculopathy in patients with posterior uveal melanoma. Clin Ophthalmol 2013;7:1877–1882.

12 Hoyng PF, Rulo AH, et al: Fluorescein angiographic evaluation of the effect of latanoprost treatment on blood-retinal barrier integrity: a review of studies conducted on pseudophakic glaucoma patients and on phakic and aphakic monkeys. Surv Ophthalmol 1997;41(suppl 2):S83–S88.

13 Schumer RA, Camras CB, et al: Latanoprost and cystoid macular edema: is there a causal relation? Curr Opin Ophthalmol 2000;11:94–100.

14 Wand M, Gaudio AR: Cystoid macular edema associated with ocular hypotensive lipids. Am J Ophthalmol 2002;133: 403–405.

15 Schumer RA, Camras CB, et al: Putative side effects of prostaglandin analogs. Surv Ophthalmol 2002;47(suppl 1):S219.

16 Linden C: Therapeutic potential of prostaglandin analogues in glaucoma. Expert Opin Investig Drugs 2001;10:679–694.

17 Chang JH, McCluskey P, et al: Use of ocular hypotensive prostaglandin analogues in patients with uveitis: does their use increase anterior uveitis and cystoid macular oedema? Br J Ophthalmol 2008;92:916–921.

18 Liu C, et al: Retinal toxicities of cancer therapy drugs: biologics, small molecule inhibitors, and chemotherapies. Retina 2014;34:1261–1280.

19 Afshar AR, et al: Cystoid macular edema associated with fingolimod use for multiple sclerosis. JAMA Ophthalmol 2013; 131:103–107.

20 Colucciello M: Vision loss due to macular edema induced by rosiglitazone treatment of diabetes mellitus. Arch Ophthalmol 2005;123:1273–1275.

21 Ryan EH Jr, Han DP, et al: Diabetic macular edema associated with glitazone use. Retina 2006;26:562–570.

22 Sivagnanam G: Rosiglitazone and macular edema. CMAJ 2006;175:276.

23 Fong DS, Contreras R: Glitazone use associated with diabetic macular edema. Am J Ophthalmol 2009;147:583–586e1.

24 Margherio RR, Cox MS Jr, et al: Removal of epimacular membranes. Ophthalmology 1985;92:1075–1083.

25 Gaudric A, Fardeau C, et al: Ablation of the internal limiting membrane, macular unfolding and visual outcome in surgery of idiopathic epimacular membranes (in French). J Fr Ophtalmol 1993; 16:571–576.

26 Smiddy WE, Green WR, et al: Ultrastructural studies of vitreomacular traction syndrome. Am J Ophthalmol 1989; 107:177–185.

27 Smiddy WE, Michels RG, et al: Morphology, pathology, and surgery of idiopathic vitreoretinal macular disorders. A review. Retina 1990;10:288–296.

28 Rouhette H, Gastaud P: Idiopathic vitreomacular traction syndrome. Vitrectomy results (in French). J Fr Ophtalmol 2001;24:496–504.

29 Gandorfer A, Rohleder M, et al: Epiretinal pathology of vitreomacular traction syndrome. Br J Ophthalmol 2002;86: 902–909.

30 Puliafito CA, Hee MR, et al: Imaging of macular diseases with optical coherence tomography. Ophthalmology 1995;102: 217–229.

31 Do DV, Cho M, et al: Impact of optical coherence tomography on surgical decision making for epiretinal membranes and vitreomacular traction. Retina 2007; 27:552–556.

32 Gaudric A, Cohen D: Surgery of idiopathic epimacular membranes. Prognostic factors (in French). J Fr Ophtalmol 1992;15:657–668.

33 Uchino E, Uemura A, et al: Postsurgical evaluation of idiopathic vitreomacular traction syndrome by optical coherence tomography. Am J Ophthalmol 2001; 132:122–123.

34 Duker JS, et al: The International Vitreomacular Traction Study Group classification of vitreomacular adhesion, traction, and macular hole. Ophthalmology 2013;120:2611–2619.

35 Yamada N, Kishi S: Tomographic features and surgical outcomes of vitreomacular traction syndrome. Am J Ophthalmol 2005;139:112–117.

36 McDonald HR, Johnson RN, et al: Surgical results in the vitreomacular traction syndrome. Ophthalmology 1994;101: 1397–1402, discussion 1403.

37 Melberg NS, Williams DF, et al: Vitrectomy for vitreomacular traction syndrome with macular detachment. Retina 1995;15:192–197.

38 Abdelkader E, Lois N: Internal limiting membrane peeling in vitreo-retinal surgery. Surv Ophthalmol 2008;53:368–396.

39 Haritoglou C, Gandorfer A, et al: The effect of indocyanine-green on functional outcome of macular pucker surgery. Am J Ophthalmol 2003;135:328–337.

40 Haritoglou C, Eibl K, et al: Functional outcome after trypan blue-assisted vitrectomy for macular pucker: a prospective, randomized, comparative trial. Am J Ophthalmol 2004;138:1–5.

41 Haritoglou C, Gandorfer A, et al: Anatomic and visual outcomes after indocyanine green-assisted peeling of the retinal internal limiting membrane in idiopathic macular hole surgery. Am J Ophthalmol 2004;138:691–692, author reply 692.

42 Kampik A, Green WR, et al: Ultrastructural features of progressive idiopathic epiretinal membrane removed by vitreous surgery. Am J Ophthalmol 1980;90: 797–809.

43 Park DW, Dugel PU, et al: Macular pucker removal with and without internal limiting membrane peeling: pilot study. Ophthalmology 2003;110:62–64.

44 Sakamoto H, Yamanaka I, et al: Indocyanine green-assisted peeling of the epiretinal membrane in proliferative vitreoretinopathy. Graefes Arch Clin Exp Ophthalmol 2003;241:204–207.

45 Bovey EH, Uffer S, et al: Surgery for epimacular membrane: impact of retinal internal limiting membrane removal on functional outcome. Retina 2004;24: 728–735.

46 Sivalingam A, Eagle RC Jr, et al: Visual prognosis correlated with the presence of internal-limiting membrane in histopathologic specimens obtained from epiretinal membrane surgery. Ophthalmology 1990;97:1549–1552.

47 Frisina R, et al: Cystoid macular edema after pars plana vitrectomy for idiopathic epiretinal membrane. Graefes Arch Clin Exp Ophthalmol 2015;253:47–56.

                                                                    Creuzot-Garcher

48 Tadayoni R, et al: Decreased retinal sensitivity after internal limiting membrane peeling for macular hole surgery. Br J Ophthalmol 2012;96:1513–1516.

49 Geerts L, Pertile G, et al: Vitrectomy for epiretinal membranes: visual outcome and prognostic criteria. Bull Soc Belge Ophtalmol 2004;293:7–15.

50 Gandorfer A, Messmer EM, et al: Resolution of diabetic macular edema after surgical removal of the posterior hyaloid and the inner limiting membrane. Retina 2000;20:126–133.

51 Kuhn F, Kiss G, et al: Vitrectomy with internal limiting membrane removal for clinically significant macular oedema. Graefes Arch Clin Exp Ophthalmol 2004;242:402–408.

52 Kimura T, Kiryu J, et al: Efficacy of surgical removal of the internal limiting membrane in diabetic cystoid macular edema. Retina 2005;25:454–461.

53 Tachi N, Ogino N: Vitrectomy for diffuse macular edema in cases of diabetic retinopathy. Am J Ophthalmol 1996; 122:258–260.

54 Stolba U, Binder S, et al: Vitrectomy for persistent diffuse diabetic macular edema. Am J Ophthalmol 2005;140:295–301.

55 Thomas D, Bunce C, et al: A randomized controlled feasibility trial of vitrectomy versus laser for diabetic macular oedema. Br J Ophthalmol 2005;89:81–86.

56 Kiss CG, Richter-Muksch S, et al: Anatomy and function of the macula after surgery for retinal detachment complicated by proliferative vitreoretinopathy. Am J Ophthalmol 2007;144:872–877.

57 Bonnet M: Macular changes and fluorescein angiographic findings after repair of proliferative vitreoretinopathy. Retina 1994;14:404–410.

58 Benson SE, Schlottmann PG, et al: Optical coherence tomography analysis of the macula after vitrectomy surgery for retinal detachment. Ophthalmology 2006;113:1179–1183.

59 Schocket LS, Witkin AJ, et al: Ultrahigh resolution optical coherence tomography in patients with decreased visual acuity after retinal detachment repair. Ophthalmology 2006;113:666–672.

60 Gaucher D, Haouchine B, et al: Long term follow-up of high myopic foveo schisis: natural course and surgical outcome. Am J Ophthalmol 2007;143:455–462.

61 Ikuno Y, Sayanagi K, et al: Vitrectomy and internal limiting membrane peeling for myopic foveoschisis. Am J Ophthalmol 2004;137:719–724.

62 Kwok AK, Lai TY, et al: Vitrectomy and gas tamponade without internal limiting membrane peeling for myopic foveoschisis. Br J Ophthalmol 2005;89:1180–1183.

63 Shields CL, Honavar SG, et al: Circumscribed choroidal hemangioma: clinical manifestations and factors predictive of visual outcome in 200 consecutive cases. Ophthalmology 2001;108:2237–2248.

64 Gunduz K: Transpupillary thermotherapy in the management of circumscribed choroidal hemangioma. Surv Ophthalmol 2004;49:316–327.

65 Boixadera A, Arumi JG, et al: Prospective clinical trial evaluating the efficacy of photodynamic therapy for symptomatic circumscribed choroidal hemangioma. Ophthalmology 2009;116:100–105e1.

66 Zeisberg A, et al: Long-term (4 years) results of choroidal hemangioma treated with proton beam irradiation. Graefes Arch Clin Exp Ophthalmol 2014;252: 1165–1170.

67 Shields CL, et al: Intravitreal triamcinolone acetonide for radiation maculopathy after plaque radiotherapy for choroidal melanoma. Retina 2005;25:868–874.

68 Rabb MF, Gagliano DA, et al: Retinal arterial macroaneurysms. Surv Ophthalmol 1988;33:73–96.

69 Tsujikawa A, Sakamoto A, et al: Retinal structural changes associated with retinal arterial macroaneurysm examined with optical coherence tomography. Retina 2009;29:782–792.

70 Cho HJ, et al: Intravitreal bevacizumab for symptomatic retinal arterial macroaneurysm. Am J Ophthalmol 2013; 155:898–904.

71 Inoue M, et al: Subretinal injection of recombinant tissue plasminogen activator for submacular hemorrhage associated with ruptured retinal arterial macroaneurysm. Graefes Arch Clin Exp Ophthalmol 2015;253:1663–1669.

72 Matet A, et al: Macular telangiectasia type 1: capillary density and microvascular abnormalities assessed by optical coherence tomography angiography. Am J Ophthalmol 2016;167:18–30.

73 Takayama K, et al: Intravitreal bevacizumab for type 1 idiopathic macular telangiectasia. Eye (Lond) 2010;24: 1492–1497.

Prof. Catherine Creuzot-Garcher, MD, PhD
Service d'Ophtalmologie, CHU Dijon
Boulevard Gaffarel
FR–21000 Dijon (France)
E-Mail catherine.creuzot-garcher@chu-dijon.fr

Subject Index